医学影像学英语教程

English Tutorial of Medical Imaging

主编　曲晓峰　边　杰　郭冬梅

中国协和医科大学出版社

图书在版编目（CIP）数据

医学影像学英语教程 / 曲晓峰，边杰，郭冬梅主编. —北京：中国协和医科大学出版社，2014.10

ISBN 978-7-5679-0221-3

Ⅰ. ①医… Ⅱ. ①曲… ②边… ③郭… Ⅲ. ①医学摄影-英语-教材 Ⅳ. ①H31

中国版本图书馆 CIP 数据核字（2014）第 281559 号

医学影像学英语教程

主　　编：曲晓峰　边　杰　郭冬梅
责任编辑：顾良军　沈冰冰

出版发行：中国协和医科大学出版社
（北京市东城区东单三条 9 号　邮编 100730　电话 010-65260431）
网　　址：www. pumcp. com
经　　销：新华书店总店北京发行所
印　　刷：北京联兴盛业印刷股份有限公司

开　　本：710×1000　1/16
印　　张：30
字　　数：300 千字
版　　次：2014 年 10 月第 1 版
印　　次：2021 年 1 月第 3 次印刷
定　　价：60.00 元

ISBN 978-7-5679-0221-3

医学影像学英语教程

English Tutorial of Medical Imaging

主　编　曲晓峰　边　杰　郭冬梅

副主编　赵一平　董　洋　崔洪岩　岳　鑫

编　者（以姓氏首个拼音字母为序）

边　杰（大连医科大学附属二院）
崔洪岩（大连医科大学附属二院）
崔　倩（大连医科大学附属二院）
郭冬梅（大连医科大学附属二院）
刘　伟（大连医科大学附属二院）
李　响（大连医科大学附属二院）
曲晓峰（大连医科大学附属二院）
王戌娜（大连医科大学附属二院）
王林省（济宁医学院附属医院）
徐　楠（大连医科大学附属二院）
岳　鑫（厦门大学附属中山医院）
周　杨（大连医科大学附属一院）
薄华颖（大连医科大学附属二院）
曹　倩（大连医科大学附属二院）
董　洋（大连医科大学附属二院）
孔子璇（大连医科大学附属二院）
刘　棠（大连医科大学附属二院）
赖声远（大连医科大学附属二院）
秦冬雪（大连医科大学附属二院）
王魁阳（大连医科大学附属二院）
王皆欢（济宁医学院附属医院）
杨　超（大连医科大学附属二院）
赵一平（大连医科大学附属二院）
张喜友（大连医科大学附属二院）

前　言

随着我国临床医学水平的提高，对外科技交流机会的不断增多，有大量国际留学生到我国的医学院校学习医学影像诊断学。这些留学生和任课教师迫切需要一本系统讲述医学影像学的英文教材。同时，医学专业英语是阅读英文文献和发表 SCI 论文的语言基础。系统地学习医学影像学专业英语也可以提高广大临床医学专业本科生的英语水平，为今后的科研工作奠定良好的英语写作基础。

本书按照临床医学专业本科生医学影像学教学大纲编写，全部使用英文详细地讲解医学影像学的重点知识内容，包括普通 X 线、多层螺旋 CT、磁共振和超声成像的原理及临床应用。本书涵盖了临床医学各系统的常见病和多发病的影像诊断及鉴别诊断，内容丰富、讲解清楚、图文并茂，是一本供临床五年制、七年制、研究生和留学生使用的医学影像学英文教材，同时也是适合临床医生学习医学影像学专业英语的参考用书。

编　者

2015 年 5 月

English Tutorial of Medical Imaging

With the improvement of clinical medicine in China, chances of international scientific exchanges continuously increase. More and more international students enroll at Chinese medical schools to study medical imaging. These international students and their teachers urgently need an English textbook that explains medical imaging in a systematic way. At the same time, reading medical documents in English and publishing SCI papers require good knowledge in medical English. Finally, systematic study of medical imaging English can improve the English proficiency of the general medical students and help them to set solid foundation for English writing in their future careers.

This course follows the outline of medical imaging for undergraduates majored in clinical medicine, and uses English to illustrate the key knowledge of medical imaging, including ordinary X-ray, multi-slice spiral CT, magnetic resonance imaging, and ultrasound imaging. With clear narration and rich pictures, this book covers imaging diagnosis and differential diagnosis of common diseases in clinical settings. It can serve as an English textbook of medical imaging for students of five-or seven-year programs, graduates and international students, as well as a reference book for clinicians who are interested in medical imaging English.

目 录

Chapter 1

Brief Introduction to Medical Imaging

Lesson 1 X-ray Imaging

X-ray imaging has been applied in clinical settings to help physicians diagnose diseases for over one hundred years. Today it is still an important and irreplaceable imaging technique.

Section 1 The principles of X-ray imaging

X-ray can make the structures inside human body visible on fluorescent screens or films, which is attributed to both the properties of X-ray (namely, its penetrating, fluorescent, and sensitization effects) and the differences in density and thickness among different human tissues. When X-ray penetrates different tissues and structures with varying X-ray absorption degrees inside human body, there exist differences in the amount of X-ray photons that reach the fluorescent screens or films. Furthermore, because of the fluorescence effect and sensitization effect, the differences in X-ray absorption can produce shades of gray that contain information on radiography or fluoroscopy.

The human body is composed of different materials containing different elements that absorb X-ray in varying degrees. Based on the density, the tissues inside human body can be divided into three categories: a) high-density tissues such as bones and calcification; b) moderate-density tissues such as cartilages, muscles, nerves, parenchymal organs, connective tissues, and body fluid; and c) low-density tissues such as fatty tissues, respiratory tract, gastrointestinal tract, paranasal sinus, and mastoid sinus. High-density tissues such as bone absorb more X-ray and allow less X-ray to penetrate, thus presenting white on X-ray films. In contrast, low-density materials such as lung with air appear black. Moderate-density tissues such as solid organ appear gray between high density-tissues and low-density tissues (Fig 1-1-1). The relationship between X-ray absorption and thickness is intuitively obvious: a thick piece of any material absorbs more X-ray than a thin one; thus, the degree of black-white image on X-ray films is related with the density of organizational structures and affected by their thickness.

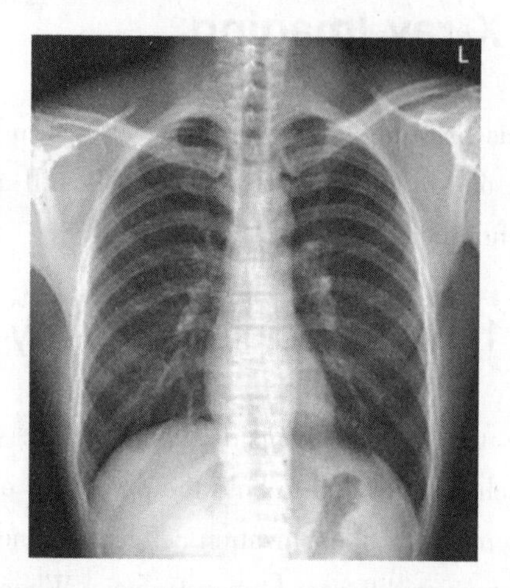

Fig 1-1-1 Normal chest: P-A position

Diseases can change tissue density in human body. When this change reaches a certain degree, it can make the normal black-white image change in X-ray films. Therefore, pathological changes with different tissue density can produce corresponding pathological X-ray images.

Section 2 Equipment of X-ray and property of radiography

X-ray examination has been constantly improved with the development of science and technology. In particular, the past three decades have witnessed the digitization of X-ray imaging. Nowadays X-ray examination has more diverse applications.

1 Conventional X-ray and imaging performance

Conventional X-ray includes general radiography, gastrointestinal machine, angiography, mobile X-ray, mammography, and dental radiography, during which the X-ray penetrates the human body and displays the findings on films. It has many advantages: a) high spatial resolution of image; b) showing the whole structure tissue in a wide range; c) low X-ray radiation; and d) economically affordable. However, it also has many limitations: a) strict radiographical conditions; b) low density resolution of image; c) organizational structures overlapping each other in the image, which has some impact on displaying the pathological change; d) the black-white degree of images is connected with the radiographical condition, therefore makes it difficult to display tissues of different densities at the same time; and e) inconvenient to utilize and manage the X-ray films.

2 Digital X-ray equipment and X-ray properties

Based on technical principles, digital X-Ray equipment includes computed radiography (CR), which can be combined with conventional equipment, and digital radiography (DR), which includes universal, gastrointestinal, mammary, and mobile machines.

However, when taking pictures, X-ray penetrating human body must be pixelized and digitized before computer processing. Unlike CR, which uses image plates (IPs) as carrier for information of X-ray penetrating human body instead of films, DR uses flat panel detectors. The advantages of digital radiography are as follows: a) the requirements of taking pictures are not limited, thus reducing X-ray radiation dose; b) it improves the quality of images; c) it has many image post-processing functions such as measurement, edge sharpening, and subtraction; d) the digital data can be printed into films or be visible on the monitor screens, or be saved in computers. The disadvantages of CR include: a) its slow imaging makes X-ray examination impossible; and b) it is not highly efficient. However, DR can not only greatly shorten the time of imaging in X-ray examinations, but also further improve efficiency, thereby reducing exposing dose; DR can perform more image processing, such as volume rendering (multi-plane tomographic image of any thickness in the projected position can be obtained by performing one scan), automatic mosaic (large-scale such as full spine DR seamless image after mosaic can be achieved by one scan) and so on.

3 Digital subtractive angiography system and X-ray imaging performance

Digital subtractive angiography (DSA) system is a combination of computer technology and conventional angiography. The image acquisition system of DSA was composed of X-ray image intensifier and high-resolution video camera at first. Since the framework of DSA looks like a "C", it is also known as C-arm X-ray machine. DSA can be divided into single C-arm and double C-arm or suspension type and floor type according to the installation method. There are also mobile DSA and fixed DSA in hybrid operation rooms.

DSA can be used in cardiovascular system imaging and interventional therapy. In the past, imaging for the blood vessels was extremely difficult since they were surrounded by bones and soft tissues. Now DSA can display cardiovascular system more clearly and completely. Among the digital subtraction methods, the most common algorithm using digital radiographic systems is temporal subtraction method, which can provide legible blood vessel images without being affected by bone tissues and soft tissues by subtracting the radiographic image obtained without a contrast agent from an image taken with a contrast agent by computer-assisted techniques (Fig 1-1-2). Blood vessels of 200um or above in diameter can be obtained clearly by this method. So far, DSA is still a golden standard in diagnosing cardiovascular diseases as well as an indispensable imaging approach in endovascular interventional treatment.

A. mask image; B. angiogram; C. DSA image. After pixel and digital transformation, the digital subtraction of both mask image (A) and angiogram (B), the digitals of bones and soft tissues offset and only intravascular contrast media digital remains. After digital/analog conversion, finally we will obtain a

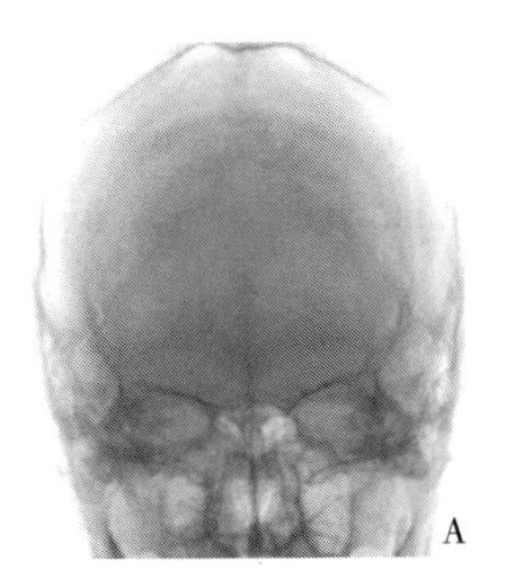

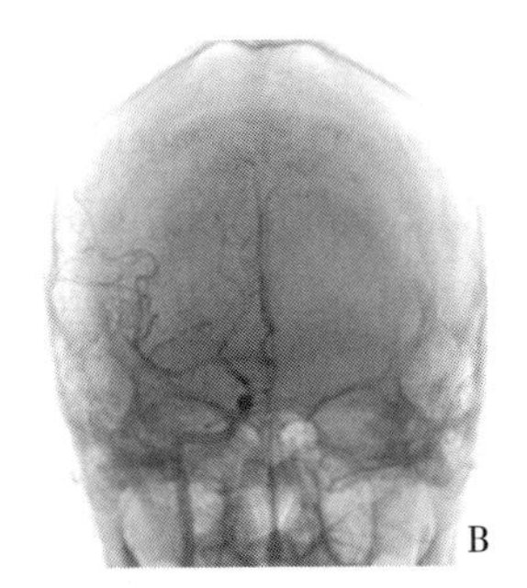

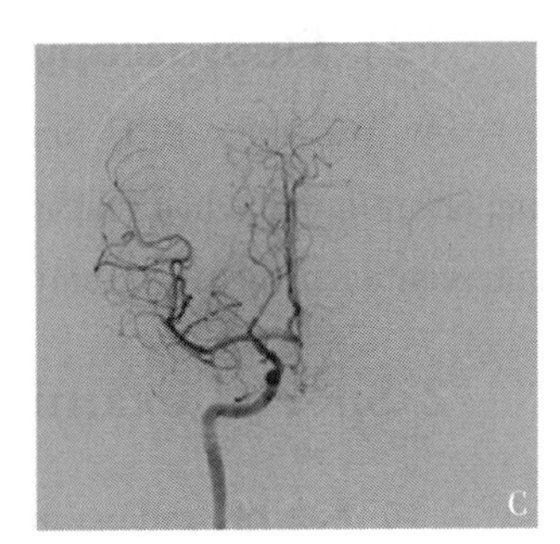

Fig 1-1-2 The principle of DSA

digital subtraction vascular image (C)

Section 3 X-ray examination techniques and characteristics of images

The differences in the density and thickness of human tissues are the basis for producing X-ray image contrast, namely natural contrast. Plain film is an image that depends on this natural contrast. As for tissues or organs lacking natural contrast, higher or lower contrast media are deliberately introduced into these structures to produce contrast between them, which is called artificial contrast. The examination by means of artificial contrast is called X-ray contrast examination.

1 Conventional examinations

(1) Radiography

Radiography is applied broadly in checking various parts of human body. Generally speaking, it is necessary to take two different orientations such as normotopia and mediolateral in order to figure the lesion out better and display its feature and location. For instance, it can display angulation displacement fracture of one bone in one orientation, which can not be shown in another orientation.

(2) Fluoroscopy

At present, FPD and image enhancement television system are two important approaches that are widely applied in gastrointestinal barium imaging, interventional therapy, and reduction of fracture and so on.

2 Special examinations

(1) Soft ray radiography It is used for the examination of soft tissues (especially the breast) based on molybdenum target or rhodium target.

(2) X-ray subtraction technique It can provide pure soft tissue image or bone tissue image with CR or DR subtraction function. For example, one subtraction chest pure soft image will enhance the positive proportion of the diagnostic results for tiny non-calcified pulmonary nodules.

(3) Volume tomography

With this DR technique, we can obtain multi-dimension images in any depth and thickness. For example, it is possible for us to figure out the bone destruction through observing the continuous structures of centrums and vertebral arches when checking vertebral column, which is difficult to display in plain films.

3 X-ray angiography

(1) The types and applications of contrast agents

a) medicinal barium sulfate, just used in esophagus and gastrointestinal tract contrast radiography; and b) water-soluble organic iodine contrast agent: ionic and non-ionic, mainly used in angiography, intravascular interventional therapy, urography, hystero-salpingography, contrast fistulography, and T-tube cholangiography.

Water-soluble organic iodine contrast agent injected into the vessel may cause adverse reactions, which can be severe in some cases. The pervasive application of contrast agent is non-ionic for less and light degree of adverse reactions, whereas ionic contrast agent has been obsolete. Besides, water-soluble organ iodine contrast agent should be used with caution (or even forbidden) in the patient with liver and/or kidney dysfunction, hyperthyroidism, cachexy, and allergies or in the infants and the elderly.

(2) Methods of introducing contrast agents

a) Direct entry: oral medication, such as upper gastrointestinal radiography; perfusion method, such as barium enema, retrograde urography, hystero-salpingography; puncture, such as angiography and percutaneous transhepatic cholangiography; and b) indirect entry: intravenous pyelography.

4 Characteristics of X-ray images

X-ray images have the following characteristics: a) Black-white gray scales of X-ray images reflect the density of tissues. The low, moderate, and high densities of X-ray images mean low-, moderate-, and high-density tissues during the diagnosis. For example, pulmonary tissue with gas shows low density in X-ray images because of its light quality. b) X-ray images are the overlapping ones of human tissues with the neighbouring. It is usually difficult to identify the pathological changes because of the overlapping images; for example, the images of the soft tissue of chest wall, bone tissue of thorax, lung tissue, heart, and great vessels may cover each other, and thus the pathological changes of the lungs behind the heart and beside the spine can not be displayed clearly in X-ray images. When we take digitized X-ray images, the use of subtraction techniques and multi-dimensional volumetric imaging techniques can reduce the impact of overlapping images and improve the detection rate of pathological changes.

We usually identify X-ray images by the features of X-ray images: a) X-ray images show white as high density tissues such as bones, especially bone cortex, gray as moderate density tissues such as muscle and parenchymal organs, black as low density tissues such as fat and air. b) Tissue structures in the X-ray images are overlapping. For example, vertebrae and pedicle of vertebral arch in X-ray images are overlapping, which is the characteristic of spine radiographs in anteroposterior or oblique (Fig 1-1-3-A/B). The identification of X-ray radiography images is similar to this, and the difference lies in the fact that the tissues or organs contain high density contrast agent.

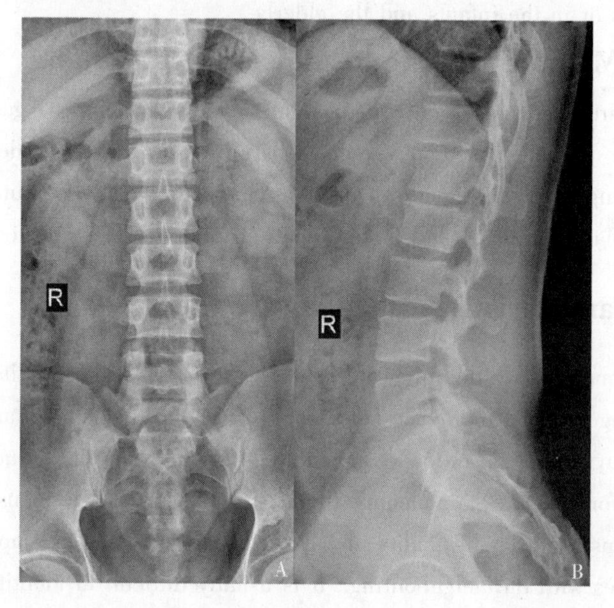

Fig 1-1-3-A/B Lumbar spine film (A) and lumbar lateral film (B)

Section 4 The security of X-ray examination

X-ray can lead to radioactive damage due to its biological effect. Thus, the indications of X-ray examination must be strictly mastered, avoiding unnecessary exposure, especially for pregnant women and children. X-ray examination should be a taboo in the early pregnant stage. Aslo, we must comply with the following three basic protection principles to avoid unnecessary harm to patient health: a) Shield protection means an object with X-ray absorption placed between the X-ray source and the operators, such as lead glass and concrete; b) Distance protection means the operators must be as far away from the X-ray source as possible; and c) Time protection means that people must reduce the time staying at an X-rays room, or exposing to X-rays.

Lesson 2 Computed Tomography

Computed tomography (CT) was designed by British engineer Hounsfield and has been clinically applied since 1972. The use of CT has dramatically improved the observation of pathological changes and the accuracy of diagnosis, marking a major advance in medical imaging. In 1979, Hounsfield was awarded the Nobel Prizes in Physiology or Medicine.

Section 1 The principles of computed tomography

In a broad sense, CT belongs to digital radiography. CT imaging can be summarized into three continuous steps:

1 Collect the digitized information of scanning slice

CT detectors receive X-rays that pass through the transverse section of human body with certain thickness using highly collimating X-ray and convert these X-ray signals into digitized information.

2 Obtain the X-ray absorption coefficient

Obtain the X-ray absorption coefficient of each voxel in the scanning slice, which can be divided into innumerable cubics or cuboids named voxels (Fig 1-2-1). The digitized information is the super-position of X-ray absorption coefficient

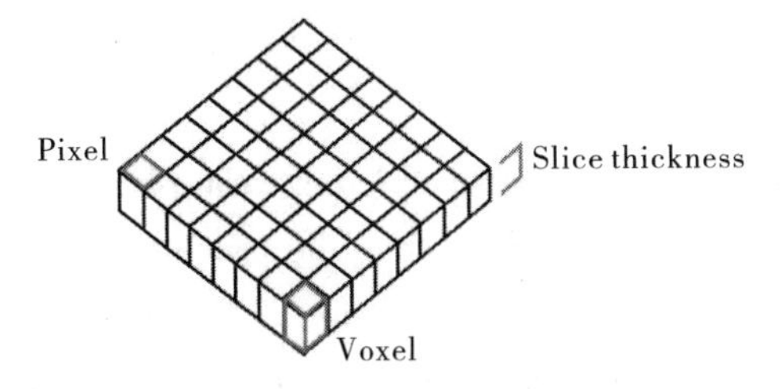

Fig 1-2-1 Pixel and voxel

of each scanning direction before inputted into a computer, and then the X-ray absorption coefficient of each voxel of this scanning slice can be obtained through different algorithms by computer, which will be displayed into digital matrix according to their original position.

3 Gray-scale image of CT

The gray-scale image of CT actually composes of many small units whose gray scale values are determined by the discretion of the numerics in the matrix. These basic units are known as pixels.

Although the principles of CT differ from those of conventional radiography, CT is also based on the principle that each slice of human body has different density and thickness. CT has two characteristics: a) the cross-sectional imaging of the human body with a certain thickness; and b) the cross-sectional images undergo digital transformation. On CT, the pathological changes can be described as high-density lesions, low density lesions, or mixed density lesions when a specific disease changes the density of tissues in human body.

Section 2 CT scanner and the imaging performance of CT

1 CT scanner

CT scanner has undergone a rapid development and renewal. Now multi-slice spiral CT (MSCT) has become the mainstream model of CT, which includes 2-, 4-, 8-, 16-, and 64-slice MSCT. The newest models include 256-slice, 320-slice, dual source CT (DSCT), and spectral CT.

(1) MSCT

MSCT is designed to use the taper X-ray wiring harness and multi-detector-row on the Z axis, which is different from the prime CT that scans step by step. So MSCT is also known as multi-detector row CT (MDCT). When MSCT works, X-ray tube and multi-detectors make a continuous rapid synchronous rotation and scan around the inspection area; meanwhile, the examination table translates with constant speed along the longitudinal axis, so the multi-level images will be obtained by reconstruction. MSCT collects not a transverse section but a certain volume of digital information, so it is called volume CT. Besides, MSCT has remarkably improved scanning speed and layer thickness: the entire 360-degree scanning time can be as short as 0. 27 to 0. 4 seconds and the layer thickness can be as thin as 0. 5 to 0. 625 mm.

(2) Dual source CT

DSCT belongs to MSCT. It has two X-ray tubes and two groups of detectors in the same equipment. DCST can perform spectral imaging.

(3) Energy spectrum CT

Energy spectrum CT is an MSCT that has a completely new function of energy spectrum imaging. Using the data obtained from the two groups of X-ray absorption figures, it may attain the spatial distribution density values of different materials. Energy spectrum CT is particularly valuable in detecting pathological changes and making qualitative diagnosis.

2 The performance of CT

(1) The main advantages of CT imaging

1) High density resolution

The density resolution of CT is 10 to 20 times higher than that of conventional X-ray. Thus, CT can clearly display soft tissue structures and organs such as brain, mediastinum, and organs in enterocoelia and pelvic cavity. It also can identify lesions such as hematencephalon.

2) The quantitative analysis of density

As a digital approach, CT images not only can be described as high-, moderate-, and low-density but also can be expressed using CT values, with Hu being its unit. The scope of CT value in human tissues and lesions is 2, 000 HU (-1000-1000) (Fig 1-2-2). Different widow settings including window level and window width should be applied to observe images on screen in order to improve visualization of detailed tissue structures and differentiate two tissues in which the CT value difference is small. For example, lung widow (widow level is-700 Hu and widow width is 1, 500 HU) enables the perfect visualization of lung tissue and lesion, whereas mediastinal widow (widow level is +35 HU and widow width is 400 Hu) provides perfect visualization of mediastinum and lesion.

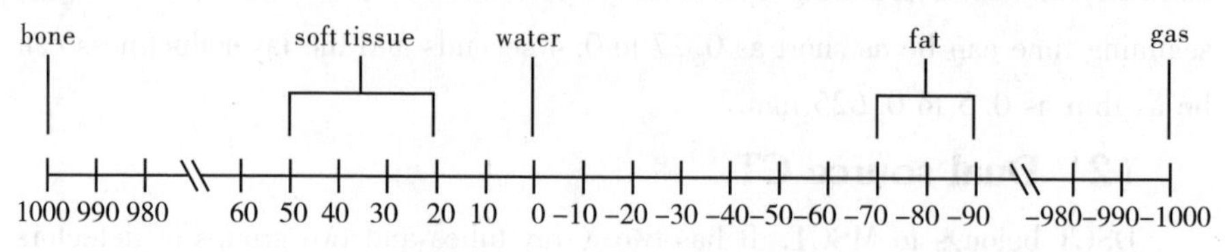

Fig 1-2-2 CT values (unit: Hu)

3) Images without overlapping

There is no overlapping for organ structures and pathological changes, which helps to improve the detection rate of lesions.

4) Images post-processing techniques

The digital images can be reconstructed into two-dimensional and three-dimensional images by computer software. In this way, the application fields of CT are further expanded and the diagnosis value of CT is improved.

(2) The limitations of CT imaging

1) CT images can not display organ structures and lesions as a whole.

Routine cross-sectional CT images can not display organ structures and pathological changes. Application of three-dimensional display techniques can overcome the limitation, but it will increase the post-processing time.

2) Many images are not convenient for quick observation.

CT scan will obtain many cross-sectional images, which are not suitable for quick, comprehensive and careful observation. It will speed up the observation process with movie pattern or multi-planner reconstruct (MPR) on the screen.

3) Partial volume effect

If there are two different density objects in the same slice, the CT value represents their average value, which can not reflect the CT value of any object. This phenomenon is called partial volume effect, which will affect the display of small lesions. It can be overcome by using thinner-slice scan and reconstruction.

4) X-ray radiation

The X-ray radiation dose of CT is tens of times, even hundreds of times higher than that of conventional X-ray. So we should strictly master the indication of CT examination and pay attention to the protection.

Section 3 CT examination techniques and characteristics of images

There are many methods in CT examination, which must be selected according to clinical needs in actual use.

1 Plain scan

It refers to the scan without contrast agent excluding taking orally contrast agent when gastrointestinal scanning. It is a routine examination method. Just using plain scan, some pathological changes can be diagnosed, for example, acute cerebral hemorrhage, bronchiectasis, liver cyst and kidney stones. But some pathological changes can not be diagnosed with plain scan, and in some cases CT images can not show the pathological changes.

2 Contrast enhancement examination

It refers to the scan using CT contrast agent, which is water soluble organic iodine injected through ulnar vein. Enhancement examination is necessary when the plain CT scan shows the pathological changes but fails to diagnose them or the plain CT scan shows normality but other examinations indicate disease. It can improve density of normal tissues and pathological tissues, thanks to iodine contrast agent. It is often helpful to qualitative diagnosis by recognizing whether the pathological changes strengthen or not, enhancement degree, the mode of enhancement, and so on. Contrast enhancement CT scans can be divided into four kinds: a) Ordinary contrast enhancement CT scan is often used to diagnose diseases of brain. b) Multiphase contrast enhancement CT scan is useful in qualitatively diagnosing diseases by observing the changes of the lesions and is mainly used to diagnose the disease of enterocoelia and pelvic cavity. c) CT angiography (CTA) is also named spiral CT angiography, and is often used to diagnose vascular diseases such as pulmonary embolism, aortic dissection, and so on. And d) CT perfusion imaging: The basic principle is to perform rapid dynamic scanning of a selected slice during the first pass of contrast agent and obtain sequential dynamic images, and then analyze the density change of each voxel corresponding to every pixel during the first pass of contrast agent and obtain parameters reflecting blood perfusion to make new digital matrix, which can be visualized in corresponding gray scales or colors. Perfusion imaging can reflect the vascularity and blood perfusion of tissues, and it belongs to the scope of function imaging. At present, CT perfusion imaging is used in acute cerebral infraction diseases such as cerebral infraction and can also be used in researching the diagnosis and the malignant degree of tumors.

3 Image post-processing techniques

It means to utilize volume data from spiral CT to perform various image post-processing under the support of relative workstation software in order to observe and analyze diseases from a new way. Explicitly, it should be chosen according to the clinical needs: not all patients need the image post-processing techniques.

(1) 2-D display multiplanar reconstruction

It can improve spatial resolution greatly and help to observe small spherical pathological changes.

1) Multiplanar reconstruction (MPR):

It includes images of coronal view, sagittal view, and random direction view, and is useful in determining the location of pathological changes and the relationship with adjacent organization structures.

2) Curved planar reconstruction (CPR):

It can display bending structures integrally, for example coronary artery.

(2) 3-D display techniques

1) Maximum intensity projection (MIP):

It can observe high density structures integrally such as enhanced blood vessels. Minimum intensity projection (minIP): It can observe low density structures integrally such as bronchial trees.

2) Surface shaded display (SSD) and volume rendering (VR):

They can 3-D display general views of complex constructions. VR can realize the structure pseudo color and transparent process, realistic imaging. They are used to 3-D display cardiovascular system, bone system and their relationship with adjacent structures.

(3) The examination of energy spectrum CT

The examination of energy spectrum CT can provide: a) The CT images of various monoergic scanning planes; b) The spectral HU curve; c) The CT density images of the scanning plane which is called physical separation technology. Energy spectrum can provide more information for the diagnosis and detection of the pathological changes.

(4) Other post-processing techniques

These may include: CT virtual endoscopy (CTVE); various separation techniques of structures; analysis techniques of pulmonary nodules, bone mineral density, cardiac function, coronary artery, and so on.

4 The characteristics of CT images

The main characteristics of CT images: a) Black-white gray scale on the image reflects the density of tissues. It is the same as X-ray images: both of their parameters are the density of tissues. b) General cross-sectional images. CT can display anatomical relationship without overlapping. c) The contrast of black-white gray scale can be affected by window techniques. Different contrast gray scale images can be obtained by using different window techniques on the same image. d) Contrast enhancement examination can change the tissue density because of the different iodine content in the tissue. e) Image post-processing techniques can change the display mode of cross-sectional images.

5 The characteristics of CT image are the basis of identifying CT images:

Identifying the images of plain scan must be based on the following two points: a) Conventionally displayed are cross-sectional images, which are clear to identify organizational structure without overlapping. b) High density tissue CT images show white such as bone, especially bone cortex. Moderate density tissue CT images show gray such as muscle and parenchymal organs. Low density tissue CT images show black such as fat. Contrast enhancement CT images can display vessels and organs with rich blood supplying enhancement, namely increased density.

MPR images show different display orientation. CPR images can display bending structures integrally. MIP images can display bones with high density or/and enhanced vessels; MinIP images can display low density structures with air; SSD and VR have the stereoscopic effect similar to portraits; CTVE can reconstruct the surface cubic images of cavity organs similar to fibre edoscopy.

Section 4 The security of CT

We should pay attention to protection when taking CT examinations because the accepted X-ray is much higher than conventional X-ray. In addition to the indications of CT examinations that must be strictly mastered, three basic principles of radiation protection should be strictly followed. Now how to reduce the accepted X-ray when taking CT examinations has been the focus of the medical imaging field. It should be pointed out that we should not pursuit the quality of images merely by increasing the radiation dose arbitrarily during CT examinations. Besides, some measures have been adopted to reduce accepted X-ray on the design of CT and data processing, including auto voltage, auto milliampere technique, iterative reconstruction algorithm, and so on. For example, we can still obtain images of the same or even higher quality while reducing 60%~80% dose of radiation using iterative algorithm.

Lesson 3 Magnetic Resonance Imaging (MRI)

Magnetic resonance imaging (MRI) provides a method showing the human body's anatomic images with high soft-tissue resolution in vivo. Of the four major clinical imaging modalities, magnetic resonance imaging is the one developed most recently. The first image was acquired in 1973 by Paul Lauterbur, who shared the Nobel Prize for physiology and medicine in 2003 with Peter Mansfield for their contribution to the invention and development of MRI. MRI does not use ionizing radiation. It is considered safer than many other techniques. MRI is a versatile technique able to generate great variety of image contrasts for a wide range of clinical and research applications.

Section 1 The basic theory of MRI

1 Human body in the strong external magnetic field produces longitudinal vector and ^{1}H precession.

Nuclei with unpaired protons or neutrons possess a property called quantum spin, which makes them "MRI active". The most common of these "MRI active" nuclei is ^{1}H. There are a lot of ^{1}Hs in the human body, which are commonly used in MRI. ^{1}Hs that are spinning can be thought of as spheres spinning on their own axis. Usually the protons are randomly arranged in the human body, while in the presence of an external magnetic field they will become aligned. Nuclei align either parallel or antiparallel to the magnetic field due to the fact that protons can occupy multiple energy states. Low-energy protons line up parallel to magnetic field while high-energy protons line up antiparallel. In the presence of magnetic field the protons do not simply line up; they actually precess or "wobble" around the magnetic field axis. This is analogous to the motion of a spinning top, which spins around its own axis, meanwhile precessing around its surface point of contact. The precessional frequency is proportional to the magnetic constant.

2 Launch of a specific radiofrequency induces magnetic resonance phenomenon.

Launch a specific radiofrequency (RF) pulse to the human body in the magnetic field, the frequency of which equals to proton (^{1}H) precession. RF energy is transmitted as an electromagnetic wave and its magnetic component (the β_1 field) can interact with the magnetic moments of spinning protons. The β_0 field is assumed to be in the z direction and then a perpendicular RF pulse is in the x-y plane. On transmission of a resonant RF pulse, protons, which were previously precessing around the z-axis, will line up and start precessing around the axis of the$\beta 1$ field (Fig 1-3-1-A/B). This leads to two important changes. The first, the absorbed energy of proton is arranged anti-magnetic field, causing longitudinal vector become small and disappear. The second, proton is synchronous, moving in the same speed and phase precession, producing transverse magnetic vector.

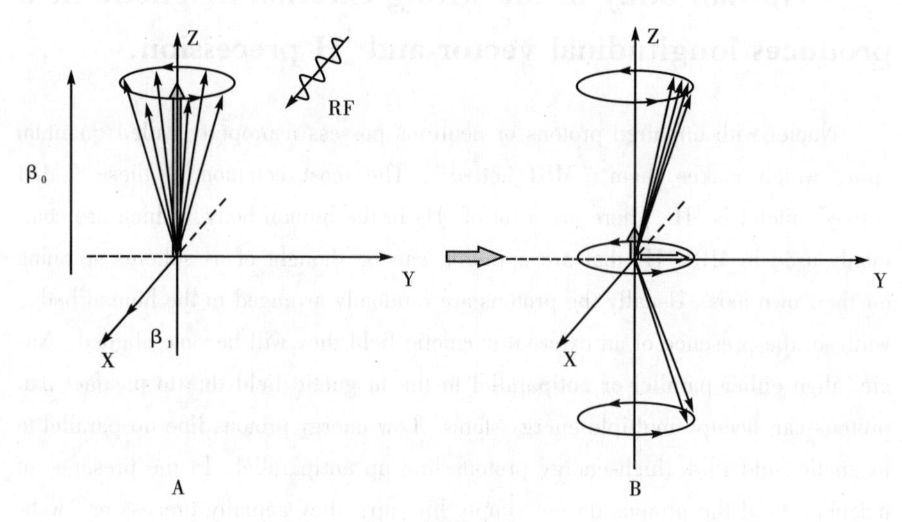

Fig 1-3-1-A/B

3 Stop the RF pulse, and proton returns to its previous state and generates magnetic resonance signals.

Relaxation is the process by which magnetization returns to its resting state after RF excitation. The time of relaxation process is relaxation time. There are two processes involved, both of which are dependent on the atomic arrangement within tissues. Thus, the rate of relaxation is tissue specific and can be used to develop. Longitudinal magnetic vector recovery time is longitudinal relaxation time, also known as T1 relaxation time. The other relaxation process is transverse relaxation. The transverse magnetic vector attenuation and disappearance time is transverse relaxation time, also known as T2 relaxation time. The process of resonance ^{1}H relaxation produces MR signals which represent T1 and T2 values.

4 Acquire and process MRI signals and reconstruct MRI images

The MRI signals of T1 and T2 values that reflect human body tissue structures can be reconstructed into MRI gray scale images through acquisition, coding, computing and other complicated processings.

MRI image gray contrast reflects the difference between tissue relaxation time. MRI has two kinds of basic images. One reflects the tissue difference of T1 values, which is called T1WI (T1-weighted imaging). The other reflects the difference of T2 values, which is called T2WI (T2-weighted imaging). T1 and T2 relaxation time of the tissue are the most common sources of contrast in the clinical applications of MRI. T1 contrast is usually used to generate anatomical images of various organs and tissues in the human body, while T2 contrast is used to identify pathological tissues, such as tumor or edema. The gray scale MRI image is called signal intensity. The white scale is called the high signal, ash is called secondary signal, and the black scale is called low signal. In T1WI, the high signal representing the tissue's T1 relaxation time is short, called short T1 signal, such as fat tissue; low signal representing the tissue's T1 relaxation time is long, often called long T1 signal, such as cerebrospinal fluid. On T2WI high signal representing the tissue's T2 relaxation time is long, often called long T2 signal, such as cerebrospinal fluid; low signal representing the tissue's T2 relaxation time is short, often called short T2 signal, such as cortical bone (Table 1-3-1).

Table1-3-1 The signal intensity of several normal tissues in T1WI and T2WI

		alba	ectocinerea	water	muscles	fat
T1WI	signal intensity	high	moderate	low	moderate	high
T2WI	signal intensity	moderate	high	high	moderate	high

Section 2 MRI performance

MRI does not use ionizing radiation and therefore is considered safer than many other techniques. MRI generates images with excellent soft tissue contrast and thus is particularly useful for neurological, musculoskeletal, cardiovascular, and oncological imaging. Although not as sensitive as PET or SPECT, or as fast as CT, MRI is a very versatile technique able to generate great variety of image contrasts for a wide range of clinical and research applications. The main advantage of MRI are as following:

1 Multile parameter sequence imaging

Magnetic resonance imaging has the advantages of high resolution, multiparameter and multiple imaging sequence, such as spin echo sequence, inversion recovery sequence, gradient echo sequence etc. Different pathological tissues with different signal intensity characteristics use different magnetic resonance sequence examination techniques. It's very helpful for the detection and diagnosis of both clinical and differential lesions.

2 MRI hydrography

The heavy T2WI sequence can display organs and gaps filled with liquid without contrast agent. This kind of MRI method is called MRI hydrography, including magnetic resonance cholangiopancreatography (MRCP), magnetic resonance urography (MRU), magnetic resonance myelography (MRM), and so on.

3 Magnetic resonance angiography

It displays the whole vessel through the time of light or the phase contrast method by making use of the liquid flow effect without contrast agent, and the images are similar to the angiographic. This kind of MRI method is called MRI angiography (MRA).

4 Magnetic resonance spectroscopy

Biochemical analysis of tissues and lesions of metabolites in vivo using magnetic resonance imaging is called magnetic resonance spectroscopy. ^{1}H resonance frequency is varying in different biochemical components, which can detect the biochemical composition and content of metabolites in vivo tissues and lesions.

5 Function MRI

Function MRI includes the followings: a) Diffusion weighted imaging (DWI) and diffusion tensor imaging (DTI). Diffusion weighted imaging (DWI) can reflect the diffusion movement of hydrone in the tissues and lesions and its limitation degree. Diffusion tensor imaging (DTI) can show anisotropic specific of hydrone diffusion, and therefore can realize albaimaging. b) Perfusion weighted imaging (PWI): the value of perfusion can reflect the perfusion parameters of the tissues and lesions. c) The location of the brain function imaging: this kind of imaging method is a technique to determine which areas of the brain are involved in specific cognitive tasks as well as general brain functions such as speech, language and sensory motion. The basis for the method is that the MRI signal intensity changes depending upon the level of oxygenation of the blood in the brain, a phenomenon termed the blood oxygen level dependent (BOLD) effect.

Section 3 MRI examination techniques and characteristics of images

1 MRI plain scan

(1) Plain MRI scan

Plain MRI scan is common in patients without special requirement. It includes T1WI and T2WI sequence transverse view imaging; the coronal, sagittal or images in other directions may be provided if necessary.

(2) Special plain scan

1) Fat suppression technique

Fat suppression technique is a special magnetic resonance scanning sequence, which can help to identify the fatty tissue in the lesions and facilitate the detection of fat containing lesions.

2) The same and reverse phase T1WI by gradient echo

The same and reverse phase T1WI technique can facilitate the diagnosis of fatty lesions, such as adrenal adenoma.

3) Free water suppressed T2WI magnetic resonance scanning sequence

Free water suppressed T2WI magnetic resonance scanning sequence is useful in diagnosing the lesions on the side of brain ventricle and sulcus, such as brain infarction.

4) MRI susceptibility weighted image

MRI susceptibility weighted image is a special image reflecting interstitial magnetic susceptibility differences and displaying the small vein, micro-bleeding, iron deposition within the lesions. It is mainly used in the diagnosis of intracranial venous malformation, cerebral diffuse axonal injury, endometrial cyst, and so on.

2 Contrast-enhanced MRI

Contast-enhanced MRI is a kind of T1WI or T2WI scanning after intravenous injection of MRI contrast agents. In many clinical scans, there is sufficient contrast-to-noise in the appropriate T1WI, T2WI or proton density-weighted image to distinguish diseases from healthy tissues. However, in certain cases such as the detection of small lesions, where partial volume effects occur within the slice, the CNR may be too low to make a definitive diagnosis. In this case, MRI contrast agents can be used to increase the CNR between healthy and diseased tissues. There are two basic classes of contrast agents of MRI: paramagnetic and super-paramagnetic, which are also called positive and negative agents respectively. In addition to lesion detection, positive agents are also often used in combination with TOF angiography. Paramagnetic contrast agents shorten the T1 relaxation time of the tissue in which they accumulate, and are therefore referred to clinically as positive contrast agents since they increase the MRI signal on T1-weighted scans. All the agents are based on a central gadolinium ion, which is surrounded by a particular chemical chelate. The Gd^{3+} ion has seven unpaired electrons, and the interaction between water protons and these electrons produces a very efficient T1 relaxation and so reduces the T1 relaxation time of the tissue. Gd-based paramagnetic contrast agents are most often used in the diagnosis of central nervous system disorders, such as the presence of tumors, lesions, gliomas and meningiomas. All the agents are intravascular and extracellular in nature. The second general class, namely super-paramagnetic MRI contrast agents, acts primarily as negative contrast agents, i. e. they reduce the MRI signal in the tissues in which they accumulate. They are used for liver diseases, specifically for confirming the presence of liver lesions or focal nodular hyperplasia. These agents consist of small magnetic particles containing iron oxide with a biocompatible coating. Ultra-small super-paramagnetic iron oxides (USPIOs) have a core which is less than 30nm in diameter, whereas super-paramagnetic iron oxides (SPIOs) have diameters between 30nm and 100nm. According to the delayed scanning time, the enhanced MR scanning is divided into ordinary enhanced scan and multi-phase dynamic contrast-enhanced scan. Ordinary enhanced scan is mainly used for the diagnosis of brain diseases. Multi-phase dynamic contrast-enhanced scan can observe the lesion's signal intensity changes in dynamic process and is mainly used for the diagnosis of abdominal, pelvic, mammary gland, pituitary diseases.

3 Magnetic resonance angiography (MRA)

MRA is mainly used for the diagnosis of vascular diseases. MRA is divided into ordinary scan and enhanced scan. The enhanced MRA requires the intravenous injection of contrast agents (Gd-DTPA). The displaying effect of small blood vessels is superior to the ordinary MRA.

4 Magnetic resonance water imaging

Magnetic resonance cholangiopancreatography (MRCP) is mainly used for pancreatic duct and bile duct disease diagnosis, especially for biliary obstructive diseases. Magnetic resonance urography (MRU) is mainly used for the diagnosis of urinary tract obstruction.

5 Magnetic resonance spectroscopy (MRS)

Magnetic resonance spectroscopy is routinely applied in studying the molecular content of various chemicals. The same technique can be used to identify a range of metabolites in human bodies in vivo by acquiring spectra of a wide range of NMR-active nuclei. The utility of magnetic resonance spectroscopy (MRS) in providing biochemical information in vivo relies on the ability to localize the MRS signals within a specific region in the body. ^{1}H magnetic resonance spectroscopy (^{1}H-MRS) is mainly used in clinical work. MRS is predominantly a research tool, but advances in hardware development and pulse sequence designs by the commercial MRI scanner manufacturers have led to increased interest in using MRS techniques in clinical applications in the brain, prostate, heart, and other organs.

6 Functional magnetic resonance imaging

(1) Diffusion weighted imaging (DWI) and diffusion tensor imaging (DTI)

DWI is widely used, and commonly in the super acute cerebral infarction. It can also be used for differential diagnosis of tumors. Whole body DWI is used for diagnosis of primary tumors and metastases. DTI is used for cerebral white matter imaging. It can display cerebral white matter shift, destruction and disruption caused by lesions clearly.

(2) Perfusion weighted imaging (PWI)

PWI is mainly used for the diagnosis of ischemic diseases and differential diagnosis of neoplastic diseases.

(3) The location of cerebral function imaging

The location of cerebral function imaging is used for brain tumor operation scheme, which can help to avoid injury of the important cerebral functional area.

7 The characteristics of MRI image

The main characteristics of the MRI image include: a) Black and white gray scale of the MRI image represents signal intensity and human body tissue relaxation time. b) MRI images of human body tissue structures are usually multi sequence and plane without overlapping. c) The image signal strength of human body tissue structures is related to imaging sequence and technology. d) Black and white gray scale contrast is related to window image width and level settings. And e) MRI enhancement scanning can change the signal intensity of T1WI and T2WI images.

Section 4 The security of MRI

Ferromagnetic objects must not be brought into the MRI examination room, because the strong magnetic field may attract such objects toward the center, which will destroy the coil and may seriously do harm to the patient inside the coil. The medical workers must make sure that all the materials and equipment (e. g. artificial respirator, scissors, hair pins, paper clips) brought into the MRI examination room are MR-compatible absolutely. Non-ferromagnetic metallic compounds are safe. Metallic objects inside the body are not unusually seen (e. g. dental fillings, heart valves, pacemakers, and surgical clips). Patients with heart valves, pacemakers or recent surgical clips (present for less than 3 months) must not undergo MRI examination. However, the implants in recent years are always safe for scanning. The metallic foreign body in the eye or the metallic intracranial aneurysm clip will move in the magnetic field, which may cause hemorrhage, to which we should pay more attention. Patients with implanted devices, such as magnetic or electronic activation should not be examined by MRI in principle. MRI contrast agents (Gd-DTPA) used in enhancement MRI scanning may cause nephrogenous systemic fibrosis (NSF). The use of gadolinium is forbidden in patients with renal insufficiency.

Lesson 4 Ultrasonography (US)

Sound pressure wave with frequency of 20, 000Hz or higher is called ultrasound, as its frequency is beyond the limit of human hearing range. With rapid development of diagnostic ultrasound technique, ultrasonography, as an important branch of medical imaging, has been widely used and playing a more important role in clinical diagnosis.

Section 1 Basic principles

1 The physical principle of ultrasonic imaging

(1) Wavelength and Frequency

The distance between corresponding points on the time-pressure curve is defined as the wavelength and the time to complete a single cycle is called the period. The number of completed cycles in a unit of time is the frequency of sound. Frequency and period are inversely related. If the period is expressed in seconds, then $f = 1/T$ or $f = T \times sec^{-1}$. The unit of acoustic frequency is hertz (1 Hz = 1 cycle per second). High frequencies are expressed in kilohertz (kHz; 1kHz = 1000Hz) or megahertz (MHz; 1MHz = 1, 000, 000Hz). Sound frequency used for diagnostic applications typically ranges from 2 to 15 MHz.

(2) Propagation of sound

Most clinical applications of ultrasound use brief bursts or pulses of energy that are transmitted into the body where they are propagated through tissues. It is possible for acoustic pressure waves to travel in a direction perpendicular to the particles being displaced (transverse wave). But in tissues and fluids, sound propagation is following the direction of particle movement (longitudinal waves). In the body, the propagation velocity of sound is assumed to be 1540m/sec. This value is calculated based on the average of measurements obtained from normal tissues. Although this is a value representative of most soft tissues, some tissues, such as aerated lung and fat, have propagation velocities significantly less than 1540m/sec, and others, such as bone, have greater velocities. The propagation velocity of sound is related to frequency and wavelength by the following simple equation: $c = f\lambda$. Frequency of 5 MHz can be shown to have a wavelength of

0.308 mm in tissue: $\lambda = c/f = 1540\text{m sec}^{-1}/5,000,000 \text{ sec}^{-1} = 0.000308\text{m} = 0.308\text{mm}$.

(3) Acoustic impedance

Current diagnostic ultrasound scanners rely on the detection and display of reflected sound or echoes. When sound passes through a totally homogeneous medium, there is no reflected sound, and the medium appears anechoic or cystic. At the junction of tissues or materials with different physical properties, acoustic interfaces are present. These interfaces are responsible for the reflection of variable amounts of the incident sound energy. Thus, when ultrasound passes from one tissue to another or encounters a vessel wall or circulating blood cells, some of the incident sound energy is reflected.

Interfaces with large acoustic impedance differences, such as interfaces of tissues with air or bone, reflect almost all of the incident energy; interfaces composed of substances with small differences in acoustic impedance, such as a muscle and fat interface, reflect only part of the incident energy, permitting the remainder to continue. Like propagation velocity, acoustic impedance is determined by the properties of the tissues involved, and is independent of frequency.

(4) Directivity

Ultrasonic waves are different from ordinary sound waves, due to the high frequency, wavelength and the pattern of a straight line in the medium. Therefore, ultrasonic waves have good directivity. The ultrasound examination for different structures is the basis of the detection of human organs.

(5) Reflection

It refers to the change of direction of sound wave at a boundary of two different media with different acoustic impedance. In this situation, a part of incident sound wave does not enter the second medium. It occurs at the interface where the dimension of the interface is much larger than the wavelength. The angle of incidence is equal to the angle of reflection.

(6) Refraction

A change in direction of sound when crossing a boundary is called refraction. There are two requirements for refraction to occur:

a) Oblique incidence; and b) Different propagation speeds on either side of the boundary. Refraction is important, because if it occurs, the lateral position shows the artifacts on image.

(7) Scatter

The reflecting object is comparable in size, if the object is smaller than the wavelength, or if a larger object does not have a smooth surface, the incident sound will be scattered in all directions. Scatter is the basic of Doppler ultrasound, which is an extremely important method of blood flow in many clinical diagnostic protocols.

(8) Absorption and attenuation

As an ultrasound beam passes through the body, its energy is attenuated by a number of mechanisms including reflection, scatter and absorption. The net effect is that signals received from tissue boundaries deep in the body are much weaker than those from boundaries which lie close to the surface.

(9) Doppler Ultrasound

Echoes produced by moving objects have different frequencies than the pulse sent into the body. This is called the Doppler effect, which is put to use in detecting and measuring tissue motion and blood flow.

If boundary is flowing towards the transducer, the detected frequency is higher than the transmitted frequency and vice versa.

2 Clinical diagnostic scanning modes

There are three basic modes of diagnostic "anatomical imaging" using ultrasound, namely A-mode, M-mode and B-mode. Depending on the particular clinical application, one or more of these modes may be used.

(1) A-mode

Amplitude (A) -mode scanning acquires a one-dimensional "line-image" which plots the amplitude of the backscattered echo vs time. The major application is ophthalmic corneal pachymetry, which is a non-invasive technique for measuring corneal thickness.

(2) M-mode

Motion (M) -mode scanning acquires a continuous series of A-mode lines and displays them as a function of time. The brightness of the displayed M-mode signal represents the amplitude of the backscattered echo. It is one-dimensional image showing movement as a function of time. Several thousands of lines can be acquired per second, and so real-time display of dynamic movement is possible. M-mode scanning is used most commonly in cardiac and foetal cardiac imaging.

(3) Two-dimensional B-mode scanning

Brightness (B) -mode scanning is the most commonly used procedure in clinical diagnosis and produces a two-dimensional image, through a cross-section of tissues. Each line in the image is an A-mode line, with the intensity of each echo being represented by the brightness on the two-dimensional image. In B-mode ultrasound scanning, we divide the echo features into five levels.

①***Echo-free or echogenic*** (***no reflection***): all liquid, including blood, urine, ascites and pleural effusion.

②***Hypoechogenic or low-level echo*** (***less reflection***): such as renal cortex and lymph node. Medium level echogenicity (less reflection): in relatively homogeneous organs, such as liver, spleen, testis and thyroid gland.

③***Hyperechogenic or high level echogenicity*** (***more reflection***): such as heart valves, vessel wall and renal sinus.

④***Echogenic or strong echo*** (***all reflection***): such as air, bone and stone.

(4) Doppler-mode (D-mode)

1) Spectral-Doppler

Two types of Spectral-Doppler instruments are used for Doppler direction of flow in the heart and blood vessels: continuous-wave (cw) and pulsed-wave (pw). PW is transmitted in pulses of ultrasound into body with good depth resolution, but it can not measure high velocity of blood flow. CW can measure high velocity of blood flow.

2) Color flow Doppler imaging (CDFI)

Color flow Doppler imaging uses a color map to display information based on the detection of frequency shifts from moving targets. Backscattered signals from red blood cells display red color when they move toward the transducer and blue color when they move away from the transducer. The degree of the saturation of the color is used to indicate the relative velocity of the moving red cells. It can show blood flow directly and clearly. So it can play a very important role in diagnosis of heart and vessel diseases. It also can help to diagnose malignant tumors through detecting their rich supply of blood flow.

Section 2 Ultrasound instrument

1 Ultrasound instrument

The ultrasound waves are generated by a piezoelectric transducer which is capable of changing electrical signals into mechanical waves (ultrasound waves). The same transducer can also receive the reflected ultrasound and change it back into electrical signals. Transducer is both a transmitter and a receiver of ultrasound.

The transducers (also called probes) are of different shapes and sizes. They are divided into three types: linear array transducers, sector transducers, and convex transducers. The linear array transducers with high frequency are generally used for superficial organs and blood vessels. The convex transducers are usually for scanning of abdomen in obstetrics and gynecology. The sector transducers are mainly for echocardiographic scanning.

Now the ultrasound equipment used clinically mainly includes two types: B-mode ultrasound equipment: the basic ultrasound equipment with function of B-mode and M-mode, with or without PW and CW, but it does not have the function of CDFI. The color equipment has been widely used. Except for CDFI, the color equipment is usually allocated with high frequency transducer, which is used to scan superficial organs and peripheral blood vessels with high resolution.

2 Advantages and disadvantages of ultrasonic imaging performance

(1) Advantages

①Ultrasonic belongs to the mechanical wave without radioactive injury.

② Ultrasound can dynamically display organ movement function and abnormal hemodynamic condition. Ultrasound can realize real-time imaging of the body arbitrary bearing section, thus can obtain information on the function and morphology.

③Ultrasound is widely used in clinical settings due to its relatively low cost, high portability, non-invasiveness, and relatively high sensitivity. Ultrasound is the only modality to provide high frame-rate real-time imaging. It is also the only modality that is routinely used during pregnancy.

(2) Disadvantages

①Ultrasound can not be used in diagnosis of lung and bone diseases. The diagnostic value of ultrasound in stomach and intestine remains controversial.

②Ultrasound examination shows limited scope of anatomy, and it is difficult to show whole larger organs. Compared with CT and MRI examination, ultrasound is less effective to show organs and pathological changes.

③The accuracy of ultrasonic examination results, in addition to related equipment performance, to a large extent, depends on the operation technology and experience of the physician.

Section 3 Techniques and characteristics of images

1 Two-dimensional B-mode scanning

Two-dimensional ultrasound is able to display real-time dynamic images for viscera morphological condition, anatomic level and surrounding structures, as well as the distribution of blood vessels and other tubular structures. It is currently the most widely used method of ultrasound and is mainly used for examination of abdominal and pelvic viscera, eye, thyroid, breast and salivary gland, such as small organs, the heart and vessels.

2 M-mode

M-mode is used to examine the heart and vessels. By evaluating the distance-time curve, it can detect atrial, ventricular and aortic diameter line, left and right ventricular walls and inter-ventricular septum thickness, valve moving range and speed, as well as left and right ventricular systolic function. The main characteristic of M-mode:

①Distance-time curves based on multiple images represent multi-layer interface echoes of locomotor organs (heart, vessels).

②Images record the motion range and speed of the locomotor organs (heart, vessels).

3 D-mode

(1) Spectral Doppler

It is used to obtain information about tissue and organ structures and the pathological changes of blood flow, including blood flow direction, speed, and pressure. It can provide guidance on qualitative and quantitative analysis about the heart, blood vessels and blood flow of the viscera lesions.

The main characteristic of PW: a) Images based on spectrum show the peak frequency value that is in the position above or below the baseline, which reflects blood flow velocity and direction. b) Images record real-time blood flow information of a certain period of time.

(2) CDFI

Because of its sensitivity, it is used to track blood flow to the heart, blood vessels and organs, through the color change of abnormal blood flow, and it can be used for precise quantitative analysis. The main characteristics of CDFI include:

①The different color signals represent flow directions, and the brightness of the color reflects the blood flow velocity.

②Real-time imaging of hemodynamic information.

4 New techniques of ultrasonic imaging

(1) Tissue Doppler imaging

It is the application of Doppler technique, and is used to access myocardial function by spectrum quantitative analysis of local myocardial motion.

(2) Color Doppler energy (CDE)

It produces images through parameters of blood flow signals corresponding to the scattering energy, and it is mainly related to red blood cells quantity, therefore providing important information for assessing the blood vessels and blood perfusion in the lesions.

(3) Contrast enhanced sonography

Contrast enhanced sonography is the application of ultrasound contrast medium to traditional medical sonography. Ultrasound contrast agents rely on the different ways in which sound waves are reflected from interfaces between substances. This may be the surface of a small air bubble or a more complex structure. Commercially available contrast media are gas-filled microbubbles that are administered intravenously to the systemic circulation. Microbubbles have a high degree of echogenicity, which is the ability of an object to reflect the ultrasound waves. The echogenicity difference between the gas in the microbubbles and the soft tissue surroundings of the body is immense. Thus, ultrasonic imaging using microbubble contrast agents enhances the ultrasound backscatter, or reflection of the ultrasound waves, to produce a unique sonogram with increased contrast due to the high echogenicity difference. Contrast enhanced sonography can be used to image blood perfusion in organs, measure blood flow rate in the heart and other organs.

(4) Acoustic quantification (AQ)

①The brightness of light spots in the images (from black to white) represents the looseness and density of the organizational structures.

②The images are unable to show larger organs and lesions.

③Acoustic imaging examination has changed the echo of the organizational structure in the image.

④Echocardiographic automated border detection (ABD) is a new way for non-invasive acoustic quantification (AQ) of heart function.

Chapter 2

Imaging of the Central Nervous System

The central nervous system (CNS) includes the brain and spinal cord. They are located in cranial cavity and spinal canal surrounded by the bone. There are limited ways for general examination and medical imaging is an important one. Many complicated diseases happen in the central nervous system, including congenital abnormality, tumor, trauma, vascular, infectious, pathological, demyelinating and mental disorder. The treatment plans to the diseases are totally different. Medical imaging can help to make an accurate diagnosis and evaluate the prognosis. All imaging techniques can be used in the examinations of central nervous system and we should master the advantages, disadvantages and different scope of each one.

Lesson 1 Brain

Section 1 Examination techniques

1 Radiography

(1) Plain skull films

Plain skull films are not commonly used today, as they show only the bone structures, intracranial calcifications, and pneumocephalus.

(2) Cerebal angiography

DSA technology is applied in the clinical practice broadly, which includes carotid arteriography and vertebral arteriography. It is used to evaluate the cerebral and vascular lesions. It is the gold standard to the diagnosis of cerebrovascular diseases. At the same time, cerebral angiography is an important part of interventional treatment.

2 CT

(1) Plain CT

Plain CT scan is a conventional method of brain detection. It is used to diagnose acute traumatic brain injury, acute cerebral hemorrhage and congenital malformation.

(2) Enhanced CT

If we find intracranial lesions, usually we should use enhanced CT. We have to use different examination methods with different clinical manifestations.

1) Enhanced CT

It can be used in the diagnosis of most brain diseases like tumorigenicity, vascular disorder and infection. It can make definite diagnosis by the ways and levels of the enhancement of the lesions.

2) CTA

CTA can be used for diagnosing cerebrovascular cerebral arterial stenosis, intracranial aneurysm, arteriovenous malformation and so on.

3) CT perfusion

CT perfusion can show both parenchymal microcirculation and perfusion. It is mainly used for the diagnosis of acute cerebral ischemia and brain tumor.

3 MRI

(1) Plain scan

1) Common plain scan:

It is the routine examination, which includes axial T1-and T2-weighted images. When necessary, coronal and sagittal images are also needed. T1-weighted imaging is better in showing the anatomic structures, while T2-weighted imaging is more sensitive in finding the lesions.

2) Special plain scan

It includes FLAIR, SWI and fat-suppression sequence, and so on.

①***FLAIR***: FLAIR can susceptibly find the diseases that happened in brain ventricle, cortical sulci and cistern, which T2WI can not.

②***Fat suppression technique***: Fat suppression technique can find the diseases of brain tissues which have fat, such as the pimeloma of the corpus callosum, the dysembryoma of pineal body, and so on.

③***SWI***: SWI can find the diseases like small lesions of hemorrhage which happened after diffuse axonal injury as well as abnormalities of cerebral venule which CT and MRI can not discover.

(2) Enhanced scan

It should be used usually. The indications of enhanced scan are: a) lesions which plain scan can find but can not make sure of the size, amount and property of them. b) diseases that are highly considered as cerebral diseases by clinical but show no abnormality on plain scan.

(3) MRA

MRA can find the diseases of the brain but the showing effectiveness is not as good as CTA.

(4) ^{1}H-MRS

^{1}H-MRS can analyze the changes of the metabolism of cerebral pathological changed tissues, and diagnose and deferentially diagnose them, especially tumors.

(5) fMRI

fMRI can show the changes in brain function, which are caused by diseases, and reach the destination for the diagnosis and differential diagnosis of the diseases. Meanwhile, fMRI is a very important examination of mental imaging (a new branch of medical imageology).

(6) DWI&DTI

DWI is mainly used for the early diagnosis of acute cerebral infarction, diagnosis, and differential diagnosis of brain tumors, and assessment of the pathology stage. DTI white matter imaging can show a normal tract of white matter fiber and display whether the constitution is complete or not. It also can show the compression, displacement, damage, or interruption of the white matter. DTI white matter imaging also can show the value for the diagnosis, treatment, and evaluation of prognosis of the diseases.

(7) PWI

PWI is an examination mainly used to show the cerebral ischemic diseases. Meanwhile, it can show the value to evaluate the ischemic penumbra of acute cerebral infarction. It also can be used for the diagnosis, differential diagnosis, and pathological evaluation of the astrocytomas.

(8) Brain function positioned examination

Brain function positioned examination can locate the cortical functional areas by BOLD. It also can help to make the scheme before the cerebral surgery. This helps to avoid the damage of cortical functional areas. In addition, it can be used for the location of the epilepsy lesions before the surgery.

Section 2 Normal imaging findings of brain

1 CT scan

Normal brain plain CT appearances are shown in Fig 2-1-1-A/B/C/D/E.

(1) Skull

Skull shows high density on plain CT scan, while on the layer of skull base the foramen jugulare, foramen ovale, foramen lacerum and so on can show low density. Paranasal sinuses and the air in mastoid show extremely low density on plain CT scan.

(2) Brain

The brain can be divided into frontal lobe, temporal lobe, occipital lobe, parietal lobe, cerebellum and brain stem. The cortex shows higher density than the medulla and the boundary is clear.

(3) Ventricular system

It includes both sides of lateral ventricles, third ventricular and fourth ventricle. The cerebrospinal fluid flowing in the ventricular system shows water-liked uniform density.

(4) Subarachoid

It includes anfractuosity, schizencephaly and cistern. The cerebrospinal fluid is flowing in them, showing water-liked uniform density.

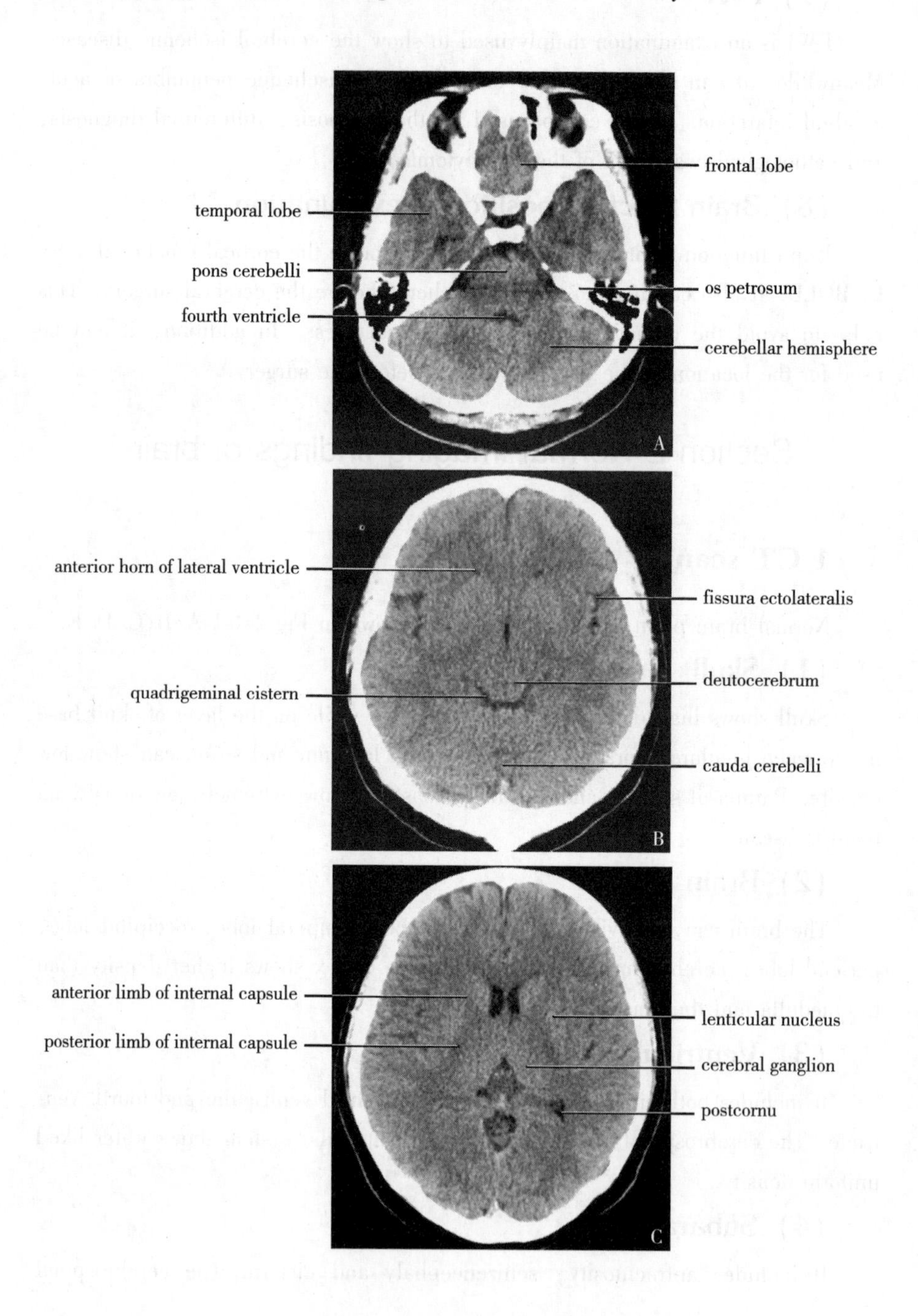

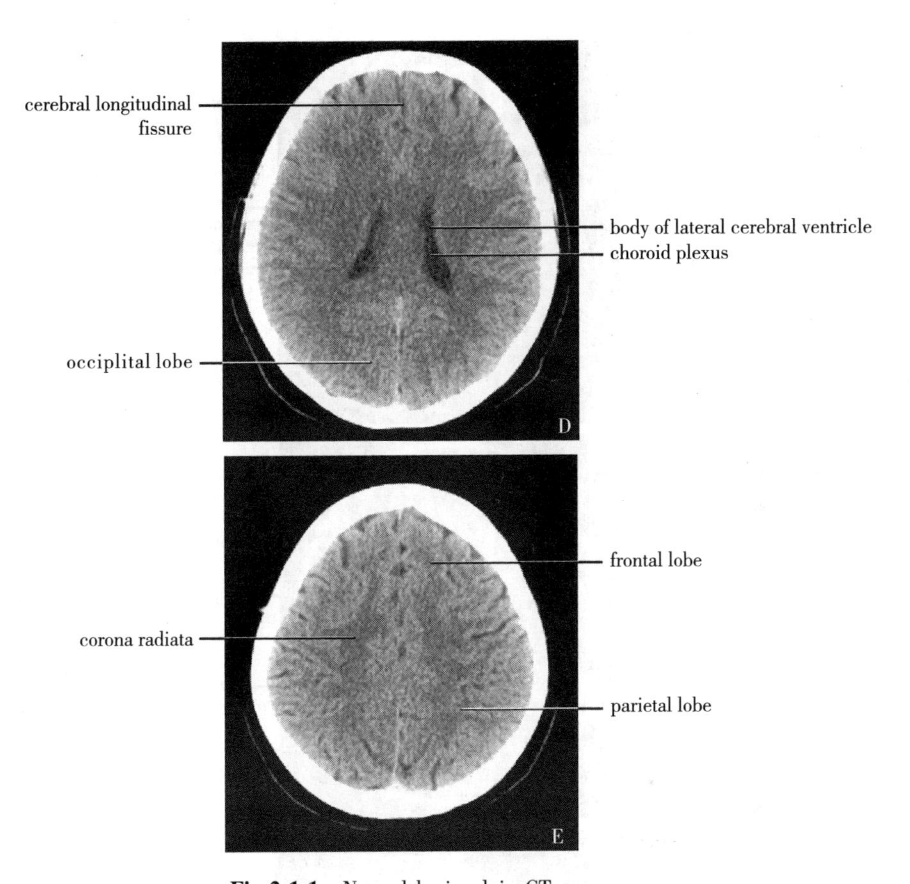

Fig 2-1-1 Normal brain plain CT appearances

A: pons cerebelli level, B: deutocerebrum level, C: cerebral ganglion level, D: body of lateral cerebral ventricle level, E: top of lateral cerebral ventricle level

2 MRI

The normal brain appearances of T1-and T2-weighted images are shown in Fig 2-1-2-F/G/H.

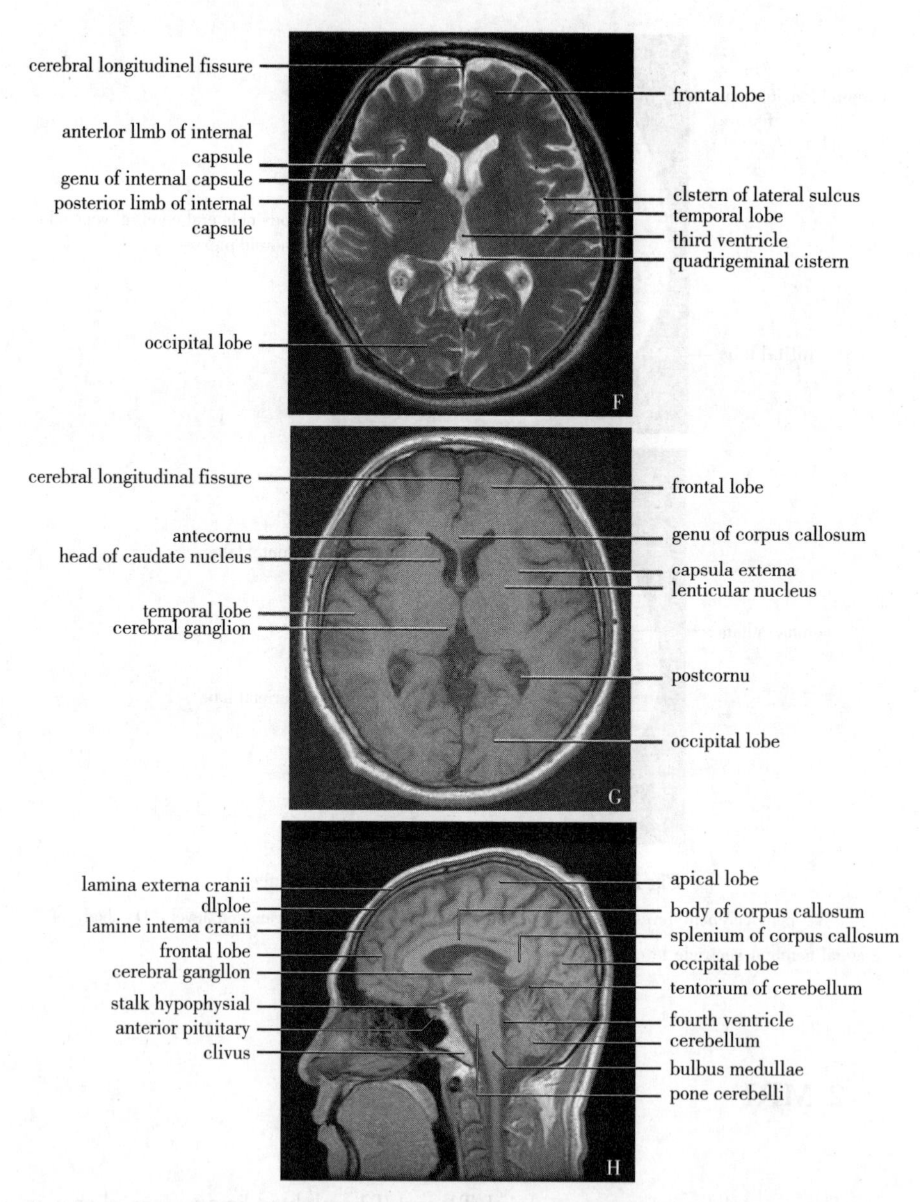

Fig 2-1-2 Normal brain appearances of T1-and T2-weighted images

F：axial plane of T1WI，G：axial plane of T2WI，H：sagittal plane of T1WI

Section 3 Techniques and characteristics of images

1 Radiography

The DSA of cerebral vessels: The occlusion of the cerebral vessels stenosis can always be seen on cerebral antherosclerosis. The circumscribed cerebral vessel protrusion will always be the intracranial aneurysm. Abnormal thickening, increase, and circuity of the circumscribed cerebral vessels are the appearances of intracranial arteriovenous malformation. The appearances of compression, gathering or separation, and straightness or angulation can always be seen on intracranial space occupying lesions.

2 CT

(1) Plain CT

1) The change of density

a) The high density lesion: It can always be seen on newly happened hematoma and calcification. b) The iso-density lesion: It can always be seen on intracranial neoplasms and the absorption period of hematoma. c) The low density lesion: It can always be seen on some kinds of intracranial neoplasms, inflammation, and infarct. d) The mixed density lesion: It can always be seen on some kinds of intracranial neoplasms, cerebral vascular disease and abscess, and so on.

2) The change of brain structure:

a) Mass effect: It happened because of the intracranial space occupying lesion and peripheral edema. The mass effect can be shown like the circumscribed cerebral sulci, cistern and cerebral ventricles being compressed, narrowing and occlusion. At the same time the midline structures move to the opposite side. b) Encephalanalosis: It can be circumscribed or diffuse atrophy of pallium, showing the thickening of cerebral sulci and schizencephaly. It also shows the expansion of cistern. While the encephalon atrophy shows the expansion of cistern. c) Hydrocephalus: When it comes to the hydrocephalus, the enhanced

CT scan shows the general expansion of ventricular system and the cerebral cistern. As for obstructive hydrocephalus, the proximal side of obstruction can show the expansion of cerebral cistern but the cortical sulci and ventricles show no expansion.

(2) Enhanced CT

1) The general enhanced CT:

a) Homogeneously enhanced: It can always be found in meningioma and metastatic tumors, and so on. b) Non-homogeneously enhanced: It can always be found in glioma and vascular malformation, and so on. c) Ring enhanced: It can always be found in cerebral abscess and metastatic tumors, and so on. d) Non-enhanced: It can always be found in encephalitis cysts and edema, and so on.

3 MRI examination

(1) Plain scan

1) The change of signal

The signal of the lesion is related to the property and tissue components.

①***Tumor***: The tumor that contains a high quantity of water shows long T1- and long T2-weighted signal changes. The fat-containing tumor shows short T1- and long T2-weighted signal changes. The melanoma that contains paramagnetic material shows short T1-and short T2-weighted signal changes. The tumor that contains calcification and ossification shows long T1-and short T2-weighted signal changes.

②***Cysts***: The cysts which contain water show long T1-and long T2-weighted signal changes. While the cysts which contain mucoprotein and adipoid show short T1-and long T2-weighted signal changes.

③***Oedema***: It is shown as long T1-and long T2-weighted signals.

④***Hemorrhage***: The signal may vary during different periods. a) Acute hemorrhage: It shows iso-signal or low signals in T1-weighted images and it is always hard to detect. b) Subacute hemorrhage: The area around the hematoma shows raising signals in T1-weighted images and T2-weighted images and impels to the center of the hematoma. c) Chronic hemorrhage: It shows high signals in both T1-and T2-weighted images and low signals of hemosiderin circle around it. d) Cystic degenerating period: It shows low signals in T1-weighted images and high signals in T2-weighted images, and the low signal circle is more clear.

⑤***Infarction***: a) The early stage of cerebral infarction (super acute cerebral infarction): It can show normal signals in both T1-and T2-weighted images. b) Acute and chronic period: Because of the edema, necrosis and cystic degenerate of brain, it can show long T1-and long T2-weighted signals.

(2) Enhanced scan

The analysis of cerebral lesions on enhanced MRI is similar to CT.

(3) ^{1}H-MRS

The abnormal peak value of metabolin is always seen on brain neoplasms, cerebral infarction and cerebral abscess.

(4) DWI and DTI examination

The abnormal appearance on DWI is high signal. It can be seen in all diseases which lead to the change of water molecule within the tissue, such as super acute cerebral infarction, brain neoplasms and cerebral abscess.

Section 4 Diagnosis of diseases

1 Brain tumor

(1) Astrocytic tumors

Astrocytic tumors are the most common brain tumors.

[**Pathology and clinical manifestations**]

The tumors can be divided into four grades. On histology, low grade astrocytomas are characterized by proliferation of well differentiated astrocytes that demonstrate only mild nuclear pleomorphism. Cystic degeneration and hemorrhage can be present, but necrosis is absent. Peripheral edema usually surrounds the tumor.

The main clinical manifestations are epilepsy, movement disorders, and the signs of increased intracranial pressure.

[**Imaging appearances**]

1) CT

Grade Ⅰ tumors are of iso-or hypo-density compared to adjacent brain on plain CT. Grade Ⅱ ~ Ⅳ tumors are of mixed density. The margins are poorly delineated. Surrounding edema is typically minimal or absent. When slowly growing masses involve the cortex, pressure erosion of the adjacent skull may occur. Enhanced CT can show no or mild to moderate enhancement. Grade Ⅱ ~ Ⅳ tumors typically enhance strongly but nonuniformly. Irregular rim enhancement is common.

2) MRI

Grade Ⅰ tumors are of iso-to hypo-intensity compared to adjacent brain in T1-weighted images and homogeneous hyper-intensity on T2-weighted images. Grade Ⅱ ~ Ⅳ tumors show heterogeneous signals on T1-weighted images. A common appearance in T2-weighted images is a central core of hyper-intensity surrounded by an iso-intensity rim with peripheral fingerlike high intensity projections secondary to vasogenic edema. Grade Ⅰ tumors may show no or mild enhancement. Grade Ⅱ ~ Ⅳ tumors may show marked but irregular peripheral ringlike enhancement (Fig 2-1-3-A/B).

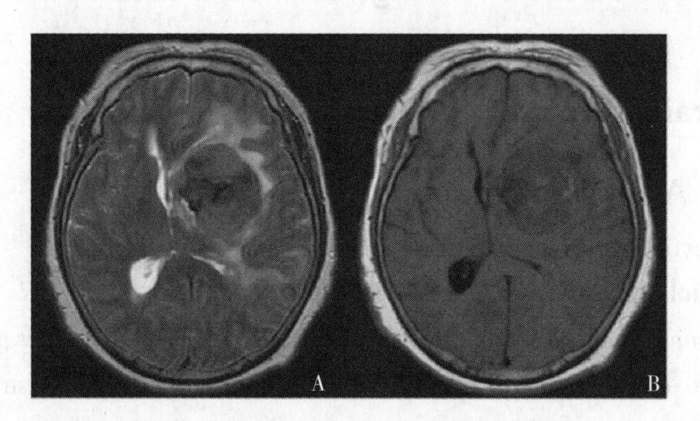

Fig 2-1-3 MRI of tumors

A: T2WI shows heterogeneous signals with surrounding edema,

B: T1WI shows heterogeneous signals.

[**Diagnosis**]

CT and MRI can demonstrate the type and location of tumors. It is easy to diagnose.

(2) Meningioma

Meningioma accounts for 15% ~ 25% of brain tumor and is mainly seen in populations aged 40 to 60 years.

[**Pathology and clinical manifestations**]

Meningiomas are the most common intracranial extra axial neoplasm, which typically occur along intradural venous sinuses, at the confluences of multiple cranial structures, or at other sites where arachnoid granulations and arachnoid cell rests occur. The common sites include parasagittal region, convexity, sphenoid ridge, olfactory groove, parasellar region, and posterior fossa. Cystic changes, necrosis or gross hemorrhage are uncommon.

[**Imaging appearances**]

1) CT

Plain CT scans show a sharply circumscribed round or smoothly lobulated mass that abuts a dural surface, usually at an obtuse angle. They are homogeneously of hyper-density or iso-density relative to adjacent brain. Enhanced CT scans show intense, relatively uniform enhancement.

2) MRI

Most meningiomas are of iso-or slightly hyper-intensity relative to cortex in T1-weighted images and iso-or slightly hyper-intensity in T2-weighted images. Nearly all meningiomas enhance rapidly and intensely following contrast administration. The dura adjacent tumor can show liner enhancement, which is so-called dural tail sign. The dural sign is suggestive but not specific to meningioma (Fig 2-1-4-A/B/C).

[**Diagnosis**]

Most meningiomas can be confirmed by most predilection sites combined with CT and MRI.

(3) Pituitary tumors

Pituitary adenomas are the most common type. Pituitary adenomas account for approximately 10% of all primary intracranial tumors.

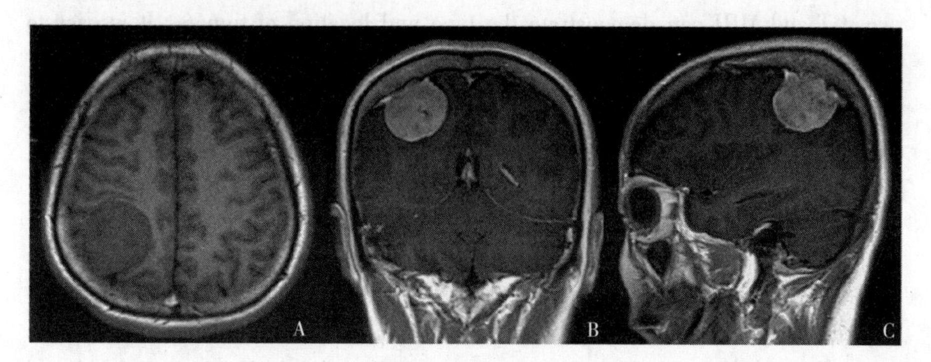

Fig 2-1-4-A/B/C

A：tumors with isointensity relative to cortex on T1WI;

B/C：enhanced MRI show uniform enhancement mass and dural tail sign

[**Pathology and clinical manifestations**]

Pituitary adenomas show a spectrum of hormonal activities. They can be divided into functional adenomas and nonfunctioning adenomas. There are two types of pituitary adenomas：macroadenomas and microadenomas. Microadenomas are defined as pituitary adenomas that are 10 mm or less in diameter, while macroadenomas are larger than 10 mm in diameter. Necrosis, hemorrhage, and cyst formation are common in large adenomas. The main clinical manifestations are pituitary dysfunction and visual field defect.

[**Imaging appearances**]

1) CT

Microadenomas uncomplicated by hemorrhage or cyst formation are typically of isodensity with the adjacent normal pituitary gland and may be invisible on plain CT scans. Enhancement following contrast administration occurs but is usually delayed compared to the immediate, intense enhancement of the normal pituitary gland. Macroadenomas are typically isodensity or hyperdensity on plain CT scans. Enlargement of the sella turcica can be seen. Enhanced CT shows obvious enhancement.

2) MRI

Microadenomas enhance less rapidly than normal pituitary tissues and therefore appear relatively hypointensity in rapid-sequence contrast-enhanced T1-weighted images. Macroadenomas can bulge superiorly, often extending through the diaphragma sellae into suprasellar cistern (Fig 2-1-5-A/B). Combined intra- and suprasellar pituitary adenomas have a characteristic figure "8" appearance on imaging. Lateral extension into one or both cavernous sinuses is common. Dorsum erosion can also occur.

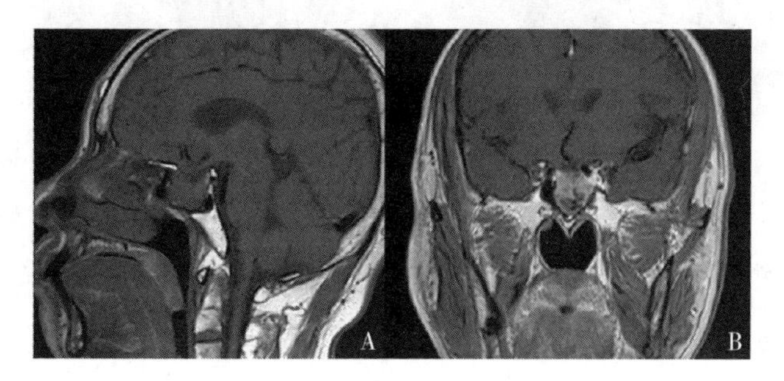

Fig 2-1-5-A/B

Tumor bulges superiorly and extends through the diaphragma sellae into suprasellar cistern

[**Diagnosis**]

Pituitary tumors can be confirmed by endocrine examination combined with CT and MRI.

(4) Acoustic neurinoma

Acoustic neurinoma is the common type of posterior fossa tumor in adults, which accounts for approximately 8~10% of intracranial tumors.

[**Pathology and clinical manifestations**]

Acoustic neurinoma mainly locates in the cerebello-pontine angle (CPA). Necrosis, hemorrhage, and cyst formation are common. The main clinical manifestation is hearing impairment.

[**Imaging appearances**]

1) CT

The lesion is located in the CPA. The tumors are typically of isodensity, hypodensity or mixed density on plain CT. The enlargement of internal auditory canal with a cone shape will appear on bone window of CT scan. Enhanced CT shows obvious enhancement.

2) MRI

The findings on MRI are similar to CT. Enhanced MRI can detect tumors of 3mm in diameter (Fig 2-1-6-A/B/C).

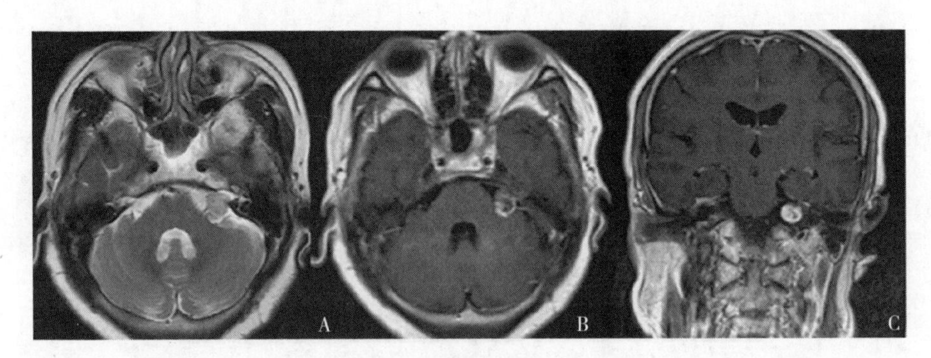

Fig 2-1-6-A/B/C

A: Isointensity mass locates in the CPA on plain MR;

B/C: Enhanced MRI shows obvious enhancement.

[**Diagnosis**]

The tumors can be confirmed by the characteristic position combined with CT and MRI.

(5) Craniopharyngioma

Craniopharyngioma accounts for approximately 2% ~ 6% of intracranial tumors. It is common in children.

[**Pathology and clinical manifestations**]

It belongs to benign tumors, and mainly locates in the suprasellar region. The main clinical manifestation is growth retardation, visual changes and hypopituitarism.

[**Imaging appearances**]

1) CT

The lesion is located in the suprasellar region. The tumors are mainly cystic and solid lesions with hypodensity on plain CT. The radiography findings of shell pattern of calcification may occur. Enhanced CT shows obvious enhancement of cystic walls and solid lesions.

2) MRI

The tumors can show hyperintensity in T2-weighted images and heterogeneous signals in T-weighted images. Enhanced T1-weighted images show obvious enhancement of cystic walls and solid lesions.

[**Diagnosis**]

The tumors can be confirmed by the characteristic calcification combined with CT and MRI.

(6) Metastatic Tumors

Metastatic tumors account for approximately 20% of intracranial tumors. They are usually present in middle and old aged patients.

[**Pathology and clinical manifestations**]

The most common primary tumors to metastasize to brain are lung, breast, and kidney cancer and so on. Extensive periphery edema often occurs. The main clinical manifestations are headache, nausea, vomiting, ataxia, and papilla e-dema.

[**Imaging appearances**]

1) CT

Typically well-defined circumscribed nodules can be seen. Most metastases are of isodensity or hypodensity on plain CT. Edema associated with metastases can be shown. Both solid and ringlike patterns of enhancement can be seen on enhanced CT.

2) MRI

The tumors can show hyper-intensity in T2-weighted images and hypo-intensity in T1-weighted images. The findings in enhanced M-weighted images are similar to enhanced CT.

[**Diagnosis**]

The tumors can be confirmed by the primary tumor history combined with CT and MRI.

2 Head trauma

Head trauma is a very serious craniocerebral impairment. Acute head trauma leads to a high mortality. Ever since the utilization of CT and MR, the diagnosis of head trauma is improved, and the rates of mutilation and mortality decrease obviously.

[**Pathology and clinical manifestations**]

Because of different positions that have been compressed and the different sizes, directions, and strength, the external force may cause different types and degrees of craniocerebral impairment. For instance: Contusion and laceration of brain, intracerebral and extracranial hematoma, and so on. Extracranial hematoma also includes epidural hematoma, subdural hematoma and subarachnoid hemorrhage.

[**Imaging appearances**]

(1) Cerebral contusion

The pathologies of cerebral contusion are scattered cerebral stigmas, venous congestion and brain swelling. If there are meningeal, cerebral and vascular lacerations combined with the cerebral contusion then it should be called cerebral laceration. But cerebral contusion is always combined with cerebral laceration so they are collectively referred to as contusion and laceration of brain.

1) CT

On the plain CT scan, there are intracerebral hematoma with high density hematomas, extensive cerebral edema with low density edema, or scattered high density hematoma within the edema with space-occupying sign.

2) MRI

Cerebral edema can show iso-signal or low signal in T1-weighted images and high signal in T2-weighted images. The signal intensity of hemorrhage shows relevance to the duration of the bleeding. In the advanced stage, encephalomalacia and cerebral atrophy can be shown.

(2) Intracerebral hematoma

Intracerebral hematoma is often located in the stressing points or hedging position of the brain tissue. Intracerebral hematoma mainly occurs in frontal lobe and temporal lobe. It is different from the hypertensive intracerebral hemorrhage which mainly occurs in basal ganglia and thalamic.

1) CT (plain scan)

Acute intracerebral hematoma shows a clear boundary round lesions with high density.

2) MRI (plain scan)

The signal intensity of hematoma shows relevance to the duration of the bleeding.

(3) Epidural hematoma

Epidural hematoma, most common in the middle meningeal artery, is mainly caused by the damage of the meningeal vascular. The blood gathered in the epidural space and, because duramater and the internal lamia adhere closely, the hematoma can be circumscribed and fusiform-like.

1) CT (plain scan)

It shows that the fusiform and semicircular like high-density lesion below the skull plate is mainly located near the fractures and does not cross cranial sutures (Fig 2-1-7).

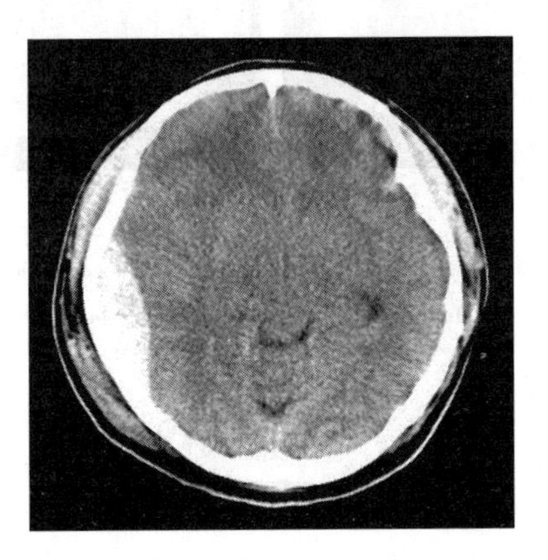

Fig 2-1-7

fusiform like high-density lesions below the skull plate

(4) Subdural hematoma

Subdural hematoma is mainly caused by the damage of veins of pons or the sins venosus. The blood gathers in the subdural space and is widely distributed along the surface of the brain.

1) CT (plain scan)

①***Acute stage***: It shows the high-density of crescent or half moon under the skull plate, and is always combined with intracerebral hematoma or contusion and laceration of the brain. It can clearly show the cerebral edema and occupying lesions (Fig 2-1-8-A).

②***subacute or chronic hematoma***: It shows slightly high-density, low-density or mixed-density lesions (Fig 2-1-8-B).

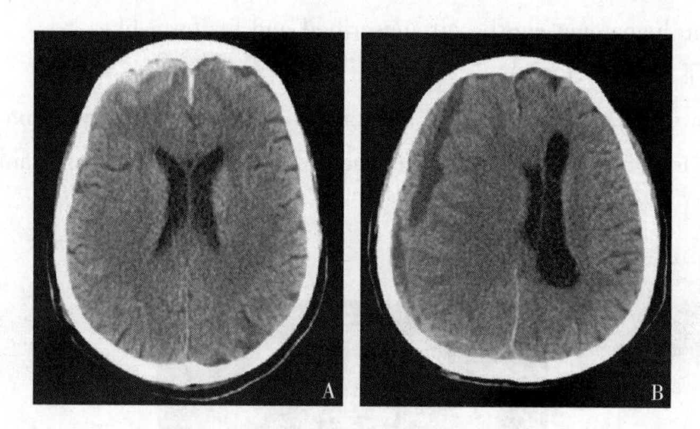

Fig 2-1-8-A/B

A: acute subdural hematoma: high-density of crescent under the frontal skull plate; B: chronic subdural hematoma: half moon like mixed-density lesion below the skull plate

2) MRI (plain scan)

The signal intensity of subdural hematoma shows relevance to the duration of the bleeding. But the iso-signal showed on plain CT scan clearly shows high signal in T2-weighted images and T1-weighted images.

(5) Subarachnoid hemorrhage

Subarachnoid hemorrhage can always be found in children with traumatic brain injury. The typical clinical symptoms of this disease are severe headache, meningeal irritation sign and hematodes cerebrospinal fluid. The bleeding is always located in cerebral longitudinal fissure and interhemispheric cistern. CTA and MRA can find the reason to this disease,

1) CT (plain scan)

It shows the increased (high) density in anfractuosity and cistern which is like a casting mold. The bleeding can always be found in interhemispheric cistern, and it shows narrowband shaped longitudinal high-density lesion which is located in midline area. The bleeding can also be found in ambient cistern, suprasellar cistern, superior cerebellar cistern and cistern of lateral sulcus (Fig 2-1-9-A/B). Subarachnoid hemorrhage can be absorbed in about 7 days, which can not be shown on CT.

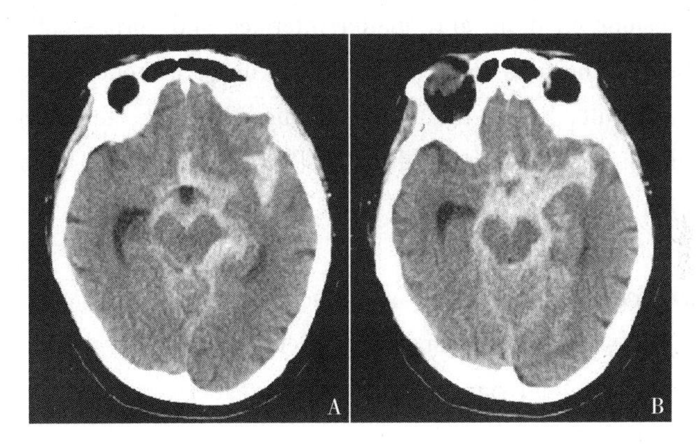

Fig 2-1-9-A/B Subarachnoid hemorrhage

High density lesions in ambient cistern, suprasellar cistern and cistern of lateral sulcus

2) MRI (plain scan)

Acute subarachnoid hemorrhage can hardly be shown in MRI. But when the bleeding is absorbed and hard to be seen on CT, high signals can be shown on MRI.

(6) Diffuse axonal injury

Diffuse axonal injury happens when the head gets sudden acceleration or deceleration force. Alba and ectocinerea may experience relative displacement because of the different inertial velocities and this causes damage of axis cylinder and corresponding brain tissues, or even serious brain disorder.

Diffuse axonal injury always happens on both sides of the brain, and the predilection sites are brain gray matter interface, corpus callosum, internal capsule, basal ganglia and dorsolateral of brain stem. The mild clinical expressions are headache, dizziness and the serious one is coma. Pathologically speaking, diffuse punctate bleeding and subarachnoid hemorrhage can be observed with naked eyes, and with the aid of microscope, we can see damage and fracture of axis cylinder which may flinch to a ball.

1) CT (plain scan)

The results of first examinations are mostly negative. Short-term reexamination: punctiform hemorrhage lesions can be seen. Typically it shows punctate high density lesions on brain gray matter interface and corpus callosum and the lesions can be seen on both sides of the brain with or without subarachnoid hemorrhage. As a result, when the clinician suspects that the disease might be diffuse axonal injury but the result of the first CT examination is negative, follow-up visits are necessary.

2) MRI

①***plain scan***: The typical expressions of the plain scan are scattered spots, slices and strips like lesions of different sizes which show low signals in T1-weighted images, high signals in T2-weighted images or negative in both T1- and T2-weighted images.

②***SWI***: SWI is very sensitive in showing the micro hemorrhage lesion of the diffuse axonal injury. It can show irregular but clear frontier spotted, striped and conglomerate low signal lesions.

3 cerebrovascular diseases

(1) Intracerebral hemorrhage

Intracerebral hemorrhage belongs to cerebrovascular disease, and can always be seen in quinquagenarians with high blood pressure and people who have arteriosclerosis.

[**Pathology and clinical manifestations**]

Autogenous hemorrhage may secondary happen in high blood pressure, aneurysm, intracranial vascular malformation, hematologic diseases and brain neoplasms. It secondary happens mainly in high blood pressure. High blood pressure mainly happens in basal ganglia, thalamus, pons and cerebellum and the blood always gets into brain ventricle. Hematoma and the combined brain edema always lead to compression, necrosis and malacia of the brain. The succession of the hematoma is divided into acute phase, absorbing phase and cystic change phase, and the period is related to the size of hematoma and the age of the patient.

[**Imaging appearances**]

1) CT (plain scan)

a) Acute phase: Hematoma shows clear frontier kidney form, abnormal form and similar circle like high-density (Fig 2-1-10). The width of the edema belt is varied, and the part of the brain ventricle is compressed and displaced. When the blood gets into the brain ventricle it can show high density. b) absorbing phase: It happens 3~7 days after the intracerebral hemorrhage. It can show

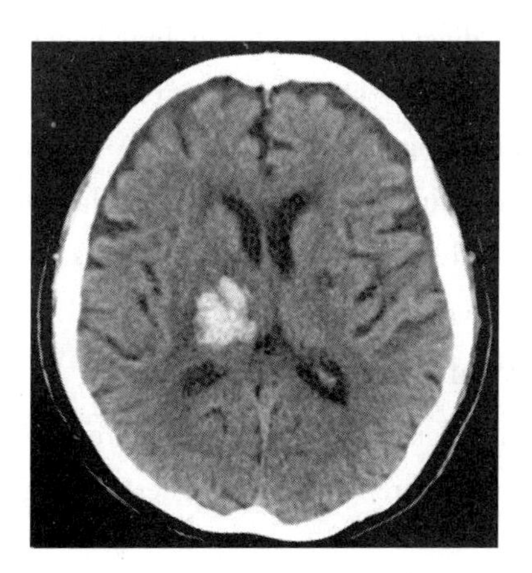

Fig 2-1-10

On plain CT, a circular high density lesion in right dorsal thalamus the size and density decrease of the hematoma. The peripheral zone of the hematoma gets dim and the width of the edema belt increases. The tiny size of hematoma can be absorbed. c) cystic change phase: After 2 months of the intracerebral hemorrhage after the absorbing of major size hematoma, there always leave some slit-shaped capsular spaces of different sizes and cerebral atrophy of different levels.

2) MRI (plain scan)

It can show diverse signals of the intracerebral hemorrhage in different periods of the hemorrhage.

a) Acute phase: The hematoma shows iso-signals in T1-weighted images and low-signal in T2-weighted images but not as clearly as the CT scan. b) Subacute phase and chronic phase of the hematoma: It can show high signals in both T1-and T2-weighted images. c) Cystic change phase: When the cysts are completely formed, it can show low-signal in T1-weighted images and high-signal in T2-weighted images. The peripheral zone of the lesion can show low signal circular which is the deposit of hemosiderin. In this period the MRI is more sensitive than CT.

[**Diagnosis and differential diagnosis**]

Depending on the typical CT and MRI findings and the accidental clinical symptoms, it is easy to diagnose the intracerebral hematoma. CT and MRI are complementary to the diagnosis of the intracerebral hemorrhage and it is very helpful for the differential diagnosis of the disease. When the intracerebral hemorrhage shows no obvious clinical symptoms during the cystic change phase, the CT scan may show iso-density and therefore it is necessary to differential diagnosis it from brain neoplasms.

(2) Cerebral infarction

Cerebral infarction belongs to ischemic cerebrovascular disease. The incidence rate of the cerebral infarction is the highest among cerebrovascular diseases.

[**Pathology and clinical manifestations**]

Cerebral infarction is the ischemia and necrosis of the brain tissues due to the occlusion of the cerebral vessels. The causes of the disease are: cerebral thrombosis forms and secondary happens after cerebral arteriosclerosis, brain aneurysm, vascular malformation and inflammatory or non-inflammatory arteritis; cerebral embolism (e. g. thrombus, air and fat embolism); hypotension; and thrombin condition. Pathologically, cerebral infarction can be divided into ischemic, hemorrhagic and lacunar cerebral infarction.

[**Imaging appearances**]

For Ischemic infarction

1) CT (plain scan)

It is hard to show the lesion in 24 hours, but after 24 hours it can show low-density. The region and the range shown on plain CT scan are accordant to the obliterated vessel. The cortex and the medulla can be affected at the same time and show sector form on CT. The space-occupying lesion can also be seen but it is very slight. Enhancement CT: The perfusion imaging can find something abnormal on the first day the disease happens and it can show the obvious decrease of the cerebral blood flow in the diseased region. Then it can show cerebriform reinforcement on the normal enhancement CT. After 1 ~ 2 months it can form clear frontier low-density capsular space, which won't be reinforced any more.

2) MRI

MRI is very sensitive to the cerebral infarction and can show it when it just happens. It can show regional gyrus swelling and distension, and cortical sulci narrowing an hour after the cerebral infarction happened, and then may show long signals in T1-and T2-weighted images. The examination of DWI can find cerebral ischemic lesion earlier and can show high signals.

3) MRA

MRA can show the obliteration of major arborization of cerebral arteries (Fig 2-1-11-A/B/C/D).

For Hemorrhagic infarction (it always happens a week after ischemic infarction).

1) CT (Plain scan)

It can show abnormal macular lesions, lamellar hemorrhage lesions and obvious mass effect in cerebral infarction.

2) MRI (plain scan)

High signals are shown in the infarction zone in T1-weighted images.

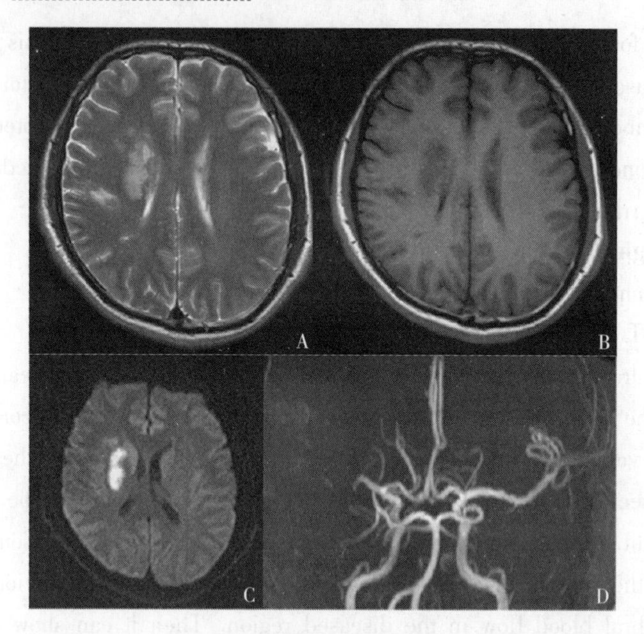

Fig 2-1-11-A/B/C/D

A/B：Long signal on T1WI and T2WI，C：high signal on DWI，
D：MRA can show the obliteration of right middle cerebral artery.

For Lacunar infarction：It happens when the deep part of perforating branch arteries are blocked. The size of the ischemic lesion is about 10～15mm and it can always be found on basal ganglia，thalamus，cerebellum and brain stem in middle and old aged people.

1）CT（plain scan）

24 hours after the disease happened，it can show on deep part of the brain lamellar low-density region without mass effect.

2）MRI

The early DWI can show lacunar infarction，which can be expressed like tiny high signal region. After that it can show low signals in T1-weighted images and high signals in T2-weighted images. The realignment of DTI can show the destruction of corticospinal tracts.

［**Diagnosis and differential diagnosis**］

According to the aforesaid CT and MRI findings and combining them with the case history, it is easy to make conclusive diagnosis. When the CT and MRI can not show typical expressions, it is necessary to identify cerebral infarction from astrocytic tumors and viral encephalitis. Astrocytic tumors can show more serious mass effect than cerebral infarction and mainly show abnormal reinforcement. Viral encephalitis is always accompanied by fever, the lesions of viral encephalitis show bilateral symmetry, and the heterolog antibodies of the cerebrospinal fluid are active.

(3) Intracranial aneurysm

Intracranial aneurysm can always be seen in middle and old aged people, in particular in women.

[**Pathology and clinical manifestations**]

Intracranial aneurysm often happens in cerebral artery and is always the reason for subarachnoid hemorrhage. The lesions are always capsular and of different sizes. There may be thrombus in the tumor cavity.

[**Imaging appearances**]

1) Radiography

On DSA examinations intracranial aneurysm and the artery of the intracranial aneurysm can be shown intuitively.

2) CT

a) Direct sign: The intracranial aneurysm should be discussed in 3 different sizes: The intracranial aneurysm without thrombus can show nearly circular size high density lesion on plain CT scan. While on the enhancement CT, the lesion can show homogeneous enhancement. The intracranial aneurysm with manipulus thrombus can show central or eccentric size high density lesion on plain CT scan. While on the enhancement CT the central and the parietal of the aneurysm can be reinforced but the thrombus between them can not be reinforced, and this sign can be called the target sign. The intracranial aneurysm with thrombus can show iso-density lesion with arcuated or spotted size calcification. While on enhancement CT the parietal of the aneurysm can show annular reinforcement. b) Indirect sign: When the intracranial aneurysm broke, CT examinations always can not show the aneurysm, but the secondary subarachnoid hemorrhage, intracerebral hematoma, cerebral edema, hydrocephalus, cerebral infarction and some other expressions can be found on CT.

3) MRI

The tumor cavity of the intracranial aneurysm can show circular flow void phenomenon signals in T1-and T2-weighted images. The thrombus of the intracranial aneurysm can show high and low miscellaneous signals. In addition, CTA and MRA can three-dimensionally display the relation between intracranial aneurysm and the artery of the aneurysm.

[**Diagnosis and differential diagnosis**]

According to the typical expression and the position of the lesion on CT and MRI, or what can be seen on DSA, CTA and MRA, the diagnosis of intracranial aneurysm is easy to make. Among all these examinations CTA is the first choice but DSA can find the intracranial aneurysm that can not be shown on CTA, and can be used in the interventional therapy.

(4) Intracranial vascular malformation

Intracranial vascular malformation can happen at any age and is more often seen in men than in women.

[**Pathology and clinical manifestations**]

The intracranial vascular happens because of the malformation of the embryo stage. The malformation can be arteriovenous malformation (AVM), venous and capillaries malformation, great cerebral vein tumor, and cavernous hemangioma. Among all these malformations AVM happens the most common. AVM always happens in the supply area of anterior and middle cerebral arteries, and is formed by the blood supply arteries, malformation vascular mass, and the draining veins.

[**Imaging appearances**]

1) Radiography

DSA can show clearly the full picture of intracranial arteries and veins malformation, including blood supply arteries, malformation vascular mass and the draining veins. The interventional therapy can be done with the help of DSA.

2) CT

a) direct sign: The plain scan can find high and low abnormal lesions, part of which are accompanied with calcification and mass effect but without cerebral edema. The enhancement CT can show spotted and arc size calcification. b) Indirect sign: The secondary subarachnoid hemorrhage, intracerebral hematoma, cerebral atrophy can be found on CT.

3) MRI

Plain scan can show dilating flow empty vascular mass malformation. The miscellaneous or low signal which happens adjacent to the brain parenchymal is the expression of iterative hemorrhage (Fig 2-1-12-A/B). In addition, CTA and MRA can both directly show the malformation of the vascular mass, blood supply vascular and draining vein.

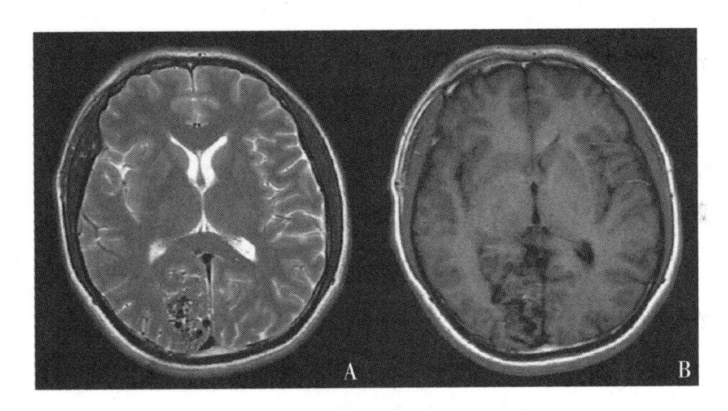

Fig 2-1-12-A/B

MRI reveals dilating flow empty vascular mass malformation over right occipital lobe

[**Diagnosis and differential diagnosis**]

Based on the typical CT and MRI findings of AVM, the diagnosis is usually easy to make. DSA, CTA, and MRA can show the full expression of AVM, among them CTA is always the first choice while DSA is mainly used in interventional therapy.

4 Cerebral Infection

(1) Brain Abscess

Brain abscess is caused by inflammation and collection of infected materials that come from local or remote infectious sources and further develop into abscesses.

[**Pathology and clinical manifestations**]

Cerebral abscesses result from pathogens growing within the brain parenchyma, initially as cerebritis and then eventually demarcating into cerebral abscesses. Direct extension from sinus or scalp infections was the most common source. Brain abscesses usually occur in the temporal lobe and cerebellum. Symptoms may develop slowly, over a period of 2 weeks, or they may develop suddenly. Symptoms may include: fever and chills, headache, changes in mental status, confusion, stiff neck, vomiting and symptoms of systemic infection.

[**Imaging appearances**]

1) CT

①***Acute inflammation period***: On plain CT scan, the lesion is presented as a large low-density area with ill-defined edge and mass effect. On enhanced CT, the lesion isn't enhanced.

② ***Maturation period***: Irregular rim enhancing lesion with hypodense center

③***Abscess formation period***: Well-defined rim enhancing mass; an outer hypodense and inner hyperdense rim (double rim sign)

2) MRI (plain scan)

Central part of abscess demonstrates low intensity in T1-weighted images and high intensity in T2-weighted images. DWI scan shows high signals within the abscess. Gd-DTPA enhanced scan demonstrates thin-walled ring enhancement.

[**Diagnosis**]

Ring enhancement on CT or MRI contrast scan may also be observed in cerebral hemorrhages (bleeding) and some brain tumors. However, in the presence of the rapidly progressive course with fever, focal neurologic findings (hemiparesis, aphasia etc.) and signs of increased intracranial pressure, the most likely diagnosis should be brain abscess.

(2) Tuberculous meningitis and encephalitis

Tuberculous meningitis and encephalitis is the fifth type of tuberculous, the extrapulmonary tuberculosis. Tuberculous meningitis has a peak incidence in childhood and adolescence.

[**Pathology and clinical manifestations**]

Tuberculous meningitis is caused by *Mycobacterium tuberculosis*. The infection spreads hematogenously from a distant focal point, usually pulmonary tuberculosis. It can rupture into the subarachnoid space, forming an exudate. This purulent material is primarily located in vicinity of basal cisterns, superior cerebellum and floor of the fourth ventricle, from where infection spreads to interpeduncular cisterns, around optic chiasm and to pontomesencephalic, ambient and suprasellar cisterns.

Complications include arteritis, which may result in ischemic infarcts. In addition, obstructive hydrocephalus is common.

[**Imaging appearances**]

1) CT

①***Tuberculous meningitis***: Perhaps no abnormality is found in the early time. When there is much exudate in interpeduncular cisterns, the density will rise. Granuloma formation will make adjacent cistern occlusive. Enhanced scan manifests wide strengthening of meninge and nodular enhancement with irregular shapes.

②***Cerebral tuberculoma and tuberculous abscesses***: Plain CT scan shows equal or low density lesions. On enhanced scan, lesions show ring or nodular enhancement.

2) MRI

①***Tuberculousmeningitis***: Plain MRI scan demonstrates the structure of basal cisterns unclearly with hyperintense on T1WI and higher signal on T2WI. On T2-FLAIR, the range and shape of lesions appear clearer. MRI enhanced scan findings are similar with CT enhanced scan.

②***Cerebral tuberculoma and tuberculous abscesses***: On plain MRI scan, the lesions show slightly low-intensity on T1WI and low, equal or high mixed intensity on T2WI with mild edema. Enhanced MRI scan findings are similar with CT scan.

[**Diagnosis**]

Combining the imaging performance with the clinical proof, the diagnosis is not difficult to make.

(3) Viral encephalitis

Viral encephalitis is a condition in which a virus infects the brain and produces an inflammatory response. Viruses that can cause encephalitis include enteroviruses such as poliovirus and echovirus, herpes simplex virus, varicella-zoster virus, Epstein-Barr virus, cytomegalovirus, adenovirus, rubella, measles, Murray Valley encephalitis (MVE) virus, Kunjin virus and Japanese encephalitis virus.

[**Pathology and clinical manifestations**]

The symptoms of viral encephalitis include high temperature, headache, consciousness and mental disorders. In cerebrospinal fluid, lymphocytes increase significantly and virus-specific antibodies are positive. On gross examination, variable degrees of meningitis, cerebral edema, congestion, and hemorrhage are observed in the brain. Microscopic examination confirms a leptomeningitis with round-cell infiltration, small hemorrhages with perivascular cuffing, and nodules of leukocytes or microglial cells.

[**Imaging appearances**]

1) CT

①***Plain CT scan***: The lesions show flake-like low density areas with slightly mass effect.

②***Enhanced CT scan***: Encephalitis lesions show irregular enhancement.

2) MRI

MRI is sensitive in the early stages of viral encephalitis although rarely it may be normal in this condition.

①***Plain MRI scan***: Encephalitis lesions show low signals in T1-weighted images and high signals in T2-weighted images.

②***Enhanced MRI scan***: The lesions show punctate, flake or Gyrus-like enhanced areas. However, the results of CT or MRI may be negative sometimes.

[**Diagnosis**]

Combining virus-specific antibodies in CSF with clinical manifestations, the diagnosis of viral encephalitis is not difficult. CT and (or) MRI is helpful for evaluating the extent of diseases. Viral encephalitis should be distinguished with bacterial encephalitis and early brain abscess.

5 Cerebral cysticercosis

Cerebral cysticercosis, also known as neurocysticercosis, is the most common infection disease in human brain. Cerebral cysticercosis accounts for about eighty percent of cysticercosis.

[**Pathology and clinical manifestations**]

Cerebral cysticercosis is a common neurologic disorder caused by the encysted larva of the tapeworm Taenia solium. It can affect any organ, but the most common site of involvement is the central nervous system.

Cerebral cysticercosis has been classified according to locations and disease stages. With respect to location, it has traditionally been classified into meningeal, brain parenchymal, and brain ventricle types.

The number of lesions of cerebral cysticercosis can be different in each individual. The cyst is round and the average diameter is about 4 ~ 5mm. After the death of cysticercosis it becomes a calcification spot.

[**Imaging appearances**]

(1) Brain Parenchymal type

1) CT scan

Cerebral cysticercosis appears as multiple hypodense cyst. It is frequently seen near the gray matter-white matter junction. In the cyst, the punctate densification area represents the scolex.

2) MRI

MRI is sensitive for the diagnosis of cerebral cysticercosis. The major part of cyst appears low intensity lesion in T1-weighted images and high intensity lesion in T2-weighted images. Eccentric nodules in cyst demonstrate hyperintense in both T1-weighted images and T2-weighted images. On enhanced MRI scan, the capsule of cyst and the scolex show slight enhancement. For the calcifications, CT scan is more sensitive than MRI. A typical hydatid disease may involve single big cyst, granuloma, infarction and encephalitis.

(2) Brain ventricle type

Intraventricular cysticercosis often leads to obstructive hydrocephalus and ventriculitis, with the fourth ventricle being the most common site. CT or MRI can demonstrate the enlarged ventricles and hydrocephalus. Sometimes, the cyst wall and the scolex show sight enhancement.

(3) Meningeal type

Subarachnoid-cisternal neurocysticercosis involves the subarachnoid spaces and adjacent meninges. CT and MRI findings are similar with the brain ventricle type. Cistern dilatation, meningeal enhancement and adjacent brain parenchyma smooth compression can be found in this type.

[**Diagnosis**]

Typical cases can be diagnosed by combining the clinical performance, laboratory diagnosis and imaging findings. A typical hydatid disease should be distinguished with granuloma, infarction and encephalitis.

6 Demyelinating diseases

Demyelinating diseases are characterized by lesions that are associated with loss of myelin of axons. There are many types of diseases that damage myelin of axons. a) myelin dysplastic white matter disease: adrenoleukodystrophy. b) demyelinating diseases: multiple sclerosis, devic syndrome. In this section, we will only introduce multiple sclerosis (MS). Multiple sclerosis is one of the most common demyelinating diseases as well as a common cause of non-traumatic disability of teenagers.

[**Pathology and clinical manifestations**]

The causes of MS are still unclear and may be associated with heredity, virous infection or environment factors. There is good evidence that the body's own immune system is at least partially responsible. Acquired immune system cells called T-cells are known to be present at the site of lesions. Other immune system cells called Macrophages (and possibly Mast cells as well) also contribute to the damage. The lesions mainly involve the brain, the cerebellum, brainstem, spinal cord and optic nerves, and both cerebral gray matter and white matter may be involved. Pathology mainly demonstrates demyelination, axonal damage and inflammation.

MS usually occurs among young people. It is slightly more prevalent in women than in men. The clinical performance of MS can be complicated. Focal neurologic deficits, seizures, and/or aphasia are often found in MS. The clinical pattern appears in three main types: relapsing-remitting multiple sclerosis (RRMS), secondary progressive MS (SPMS), and primary progressive MS (PPMS). In CSF, the performance of Oligoclonal bands is often positive.

[**Imaging appearances**]

1) CT

① ***Axial plain CT scan***: multiple hypodensity area without mass effect.

② ***Enhanced CT scan***: Active MS lesions show enhancement while chronic MS lesions show no enhancement.

2) MRI

① ***Plain MRI***: MS lesions usually occur in the next lateral ventricles, semi-oval center, corpus callosum, brainstem and cerebellar with patch shape. The lesions are perpendicular to the lateral ventricle, which is the characteristic performance. The lesions appear hypointensity in T1-weighted images and hyper-intense in T2-weighted images.

② ***Enhanced MRI***: Enhanced MRI can be used to assess lesion activity just like contrast-enhanced CT (Fig 2-1-13). Either nodular or ringlike en-

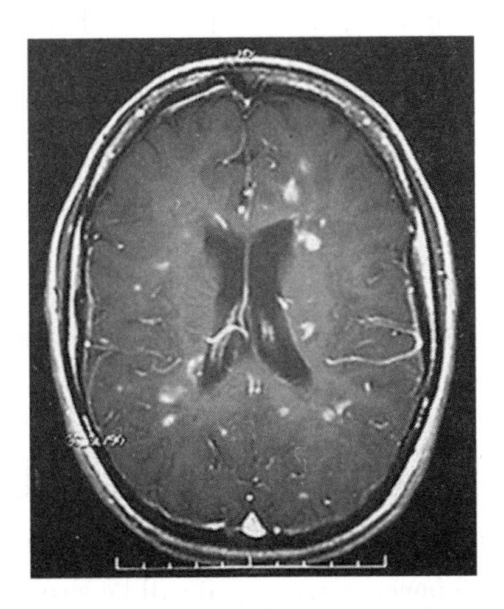

Fig 2-1-13 Patchy enhancement lesions in the next lateral ventricles on enhanced MRI

hancement may be seen early after contrast injection, but the central areas tend to fill in and become more homogeneous on delayed scan. Immediate postcontrast scan is most sensitive to detect MS, and delayed scan is not necessary. Contrast-enhanced MRI can be used to follow up the progression of disease and to assess the response to therapy.

[**Diagnosis**]

The diagnosis of MS needs the lesions to have the characteristics of temporal and spatial variation. Before making the final diagnosis, multiple MRI examinations are necessary. Also, MS needs to be distinguished with Neuromyelitis and Multi-infarct.

7 Cerebral malformations

Chiari malformation, sometimes known as tonsillar herniation or tonsillar ectopia, is caused by congenital malformation.

[**Pathology and clinical manifestations**]

It consists of a downward displacement of the cerebellar tonsils through the foramen magnum (the opening at the base of the skull), sometimes causing non-communicating hydrocephalus as a result of obstruction of cerebrospinal fluid (CSF) outflow. The common symptoms include headaches, fatigue, muscle weakness in the head and face, difficulty in swallowing, dizziness, nausea, impaired coordination, and, in severe cases, paralysis, caused by the hyper pressure in skull.

[**Imaging appearances**]

1) CT (plain scan

The main findings are supratentorial hydrocephalus and abnormal soft tissues in the upper cervical spinal canal, which are the herniation of the cerebellar tonsil.

2) MRI

MRI is the primary diagnosis method for Chiari malformations. On sagittal scan: a) the cerebellar tonsil gets sharpened. If the lower pole of the cerebellar tonsil is 3mm under the foramen magnum, it will be suspicious. If the lower pole of cerebellar tonsil is 5mm or more under the foramen magnum, Chiari malformation can be diagnosed. b) the fourth ventricle and medulla usually become deformed and shift down. c) syringomyelia and supratentorial hydrocephalus can also be found by MRI examinations.

[**Diagnosis**]

Diagnosis is made through combination of patient history, neurological examination, and imaging examination. MRI is considered the best imaging modality for Chiari malformation.

Lesson 2 Spinal Cord

Spinal cord is a part of central nervous system in mankind and vertebrates. It's accommodated in canalis vertebrates, the upper part connecting the medulla oblongata and there are pairs of nerves on both sides, which will be distributed in arms and legs, body walls and internal organs. The spinal cord is the center of many simple reflexes, and it is the bridge between brain and organs to some extent. So the diagnosis of diseases of the spinal cord is a very important part among the discipline of image diagnostics.

Section 1 Examination techniques

1 Radiography

(1) Radiography

It is mainly used for checking some changes caused by spine itself and lesions and spinal canal diseases, including changes of bone, intervertebral space, bony vertebral pipe diameter line, and intervertebral foramen size. Regularly, spine anteroposterior and lateral films will be enough, but when observing intervertebral foramens, oblique films are necessary.

(2) Spinal angiography

It is used, as a kind of gold standard of diagnosis, for checking the vascular malformation in spinal canal, and can be used in interventional therapy as well.

2 CT

(1) Plain CT scan

CT scan is often used as a preliminary examination in spinal canal lesions. It can be used for estimating bone changes of vertebral column and lesions of intervertebral disc, measuring the bony vertebral pipe diameter line and sectional area, and showing the abnormity of the soft tissues beside the spinal canal. In these aspects, CT scan is better than the conventional radiography.

(2) Enhanced CT scan

It is used to examine the spinal canal tumor and vascular diseases. CTA examination has a high value of finding spinal canal vascular malformation.

3 MRI

MRI is the first choice and main image examination technique in checking various intraspinal diseases including spinal cord abnormity.

(1) Plain MRI Scan

MRI scan is a routine examination method in finding spinal cord lesions, and it can fully observe anatomical structures and lesions of spinal cord, and find lesions sensitively. Priority is given to sagittal position T1-weighted images and T2-weighted images, and, if necessary, coronal and axial positions. Occasionally, fat-suppression T1-weighted imaging and T2-weighted imaging will be used to check and diagnose the lesion that contains fat.

(2) Enhanced MRI Scan

The enhanced MRI is always used to distinguish lesions in spinal cord or spinal canal.

(3) Magnetic resonance angiography (MRA)

It is very helpful in finding and diagnosing vascular malformation in spinal canal.

(4) Magnetic resonance myelography (MRM)

MRM can help obtain spinal subarachnoid cerebrospinal fluid imaging. It is helpful in locating lesions in spinal canal, but it is seldom used.

Section 2 Normal imaging findings of Spinal cord

1 Radiography

(1) Radiography

On the conventional plain radiography, the structure associated with the spinal cord is bony spinal canal. On the frontal film, vertebral pedicles on both sides are symmetrical, and the medial margin ligatures of up and down adjacent to vertebral pedicles constitute the two sides of the bony spinal canal, which are smooth and sequential. On the lateral film, trailing edge ligatures of all centrums stand for antetheca of bony spinal canal, which are very smooth and in line with spine curvature.

(2) Spinal angiography

This method can display more than one blood supply artery and their branches, among which the thickest one stretching like a hairpin is called Adamkiewicz Artery.

2 CT

(1) Bony spinal canal

Axial position is suitable for observation of the size and morphology of spinal canal: a) In the vertebral pedicle level, there is a bony circle consisting of trailing edge of centrum, vertebral pedicles, vertebral plate and spinous process, which is the transect of the bony spinal canal. Under normal circumstances, the lower anteroposterior diameter limit of bony spinal canal is 11.5mm, the lower transverse diameter limit is 16mm, and the lower width limit of lateral recess is 3mm. Sizes less than the lower limit indicate narrow bony spinal canal. b) In the intervertebral disc, as well as the upper and lower levels, it shows that centrum and vertebral plates are not conjoint, and the space between them is intervertebral foramen, where there are vessels and spinal nerves.

(2) Spinal canal soft tissues

Dural sac is located in spinal canal, and it is round or oval in shape, probably surrounded by a kind of low density fat clearance. Spinal cord and dural sac are both shown as intermediate density. In the upper cervical vertebra, subarachnoid space is much wider, and the space between cervical cord and dural sac is filled with low density cerebrospinal fluid. But in other levels it is difficult to distinguish spinal cord and dural sac. Ligamentum flavum is in the inner side of vertebral plate, and its normal thickness is about 2~4mm.

3 MRI

On midsagittal plane of T1-weighted images, spinal cord is shown as a belt with moderate signal, clear border and uniform signal, and is located in the center of the spinal cord. The fat in the intervertebral foramen is shown with high signal, while nerve root is low. On midsagittal plane of T1-weighted images, spinal cord is still shown with equal signal, while cerebrospinal fluid is shown with high signal. On the axial plane, the relationship between spinal cord, spinal nerves and the surrounding structures is shown clearly (Fig 2-2-1-A/B/C).

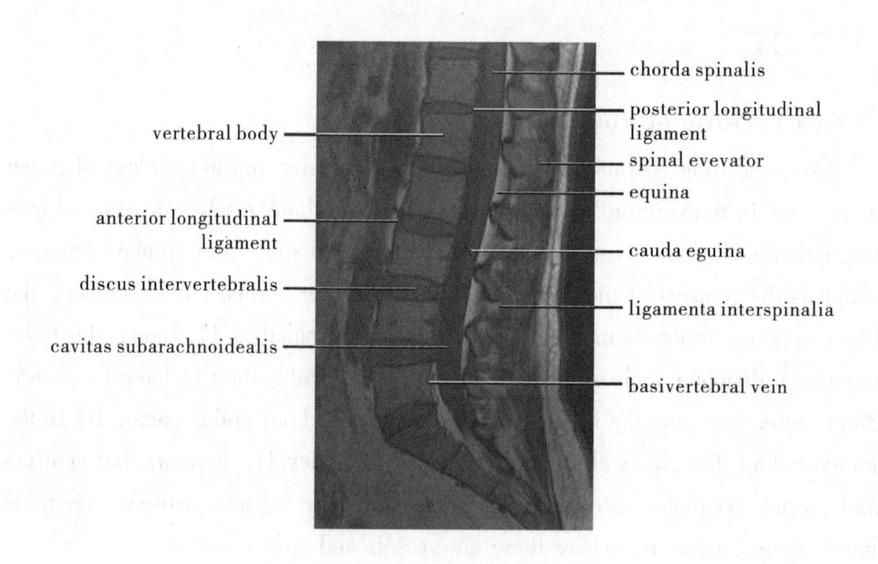

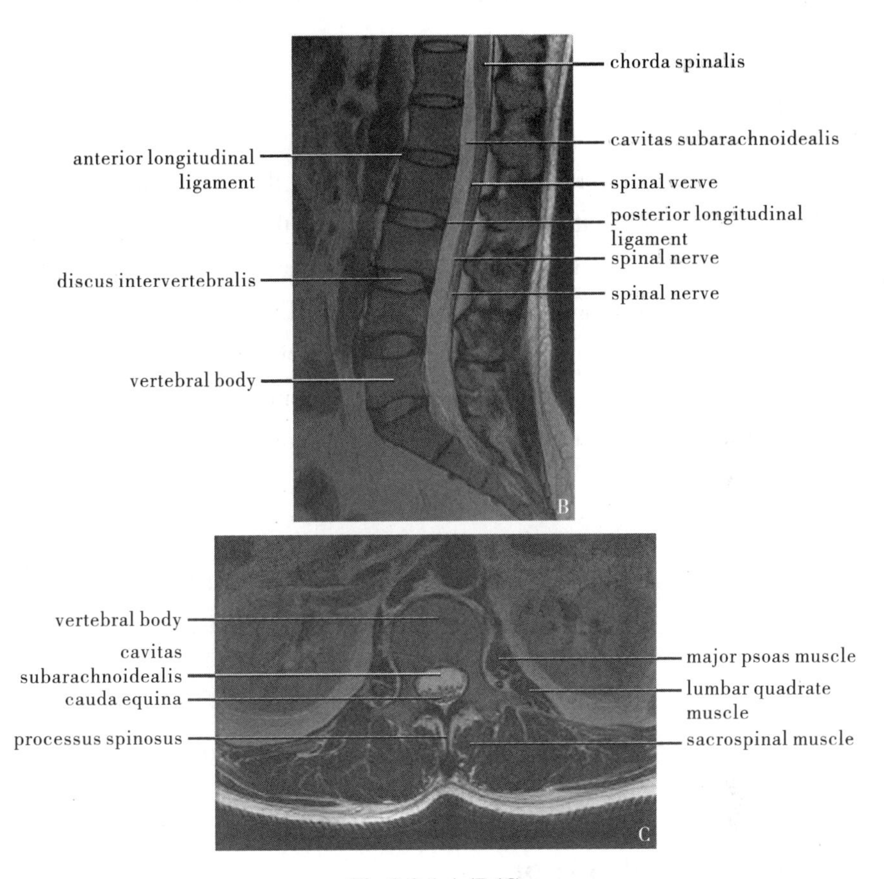

Fig 2-2-1-A/B/C

A: sagittal T1WI, B: sagittal T2WI, C: axial T2WI

Section 3 Imaging signs of spinal cord diseases

1 Radiography

Space-occupying lesions in spinal canal can cause the expansion of bony spinal canal. This circumstance can always be seen in neurogentic tumors. Destructions of bone and surrounding soft tissues may be caused by spondylocace or malignancy.

2 CT

In the level of intervertebral disc, CT can check the protrusion of intervertebral disc, and find if the dural sac is compressed by the protruding intervertebral disc or not. At the same time, CT value can help to analyze the ingredient which may be contained in various tissues and lesions. Enhanced CT scan can be helpful in knowing the condition of blood supply of some lesions like tumor, and in distinguishing benign or malignant tumors. The application of CTA makes the diagnosis of vascular abnormity easier and more accurate.

3 MRI

Basic pathological changes of spinal cord on MRI mainly include hemorrhage, mass, shape changes and necrosis. The appearance is similar to brain MRI.

Section 4 Diagnosis of diseases

1 Intraspinal tumor

[**Pathology and clinical manifestations**]

Intraspinal tumors include a variety of tumor-like lesions arising from different tissues like spinal cord, notochord membrane, and even vertebra bone. According to the location they can be divided into intramedullary tumors which are always seen in ependymoma and astrocytoma; intradural extramedullary tumors, most common of which are neurogenic tumors and spinal meningioma; and epidural tumors which are always metastatic tumors. Clinical presentation normally shows dyskinesia, dysesthesia and nerve radicular pain.

[**Imaging appearances**]

(1) MRI

MRI is a major imaging method of intraspinal tumor. It can clearly show the anatomy of spine. Even without enhanced scan, MRI can also locate the tumor. a) Intramedullary tumor: spinal cord thickens and subarachnoid space narrows or blocks symmetrically. b) Intradural extramedullary tumor: the subarachnoid space broadens on the affected side, and tumor may compress the spinal cord to the contralateral side. c) Epidural tumor: subarachnoid space narrowing and spinal cord being compressed are always the features. In T1-weighted images tumor often shows medium or low signals, while in T2-weighted images often it shows medium or high signals. On Gd-DPTA enhanced scan, different types of tumors can show enhancement of different degrees and modalities (Fig 2-2-2-A/B).

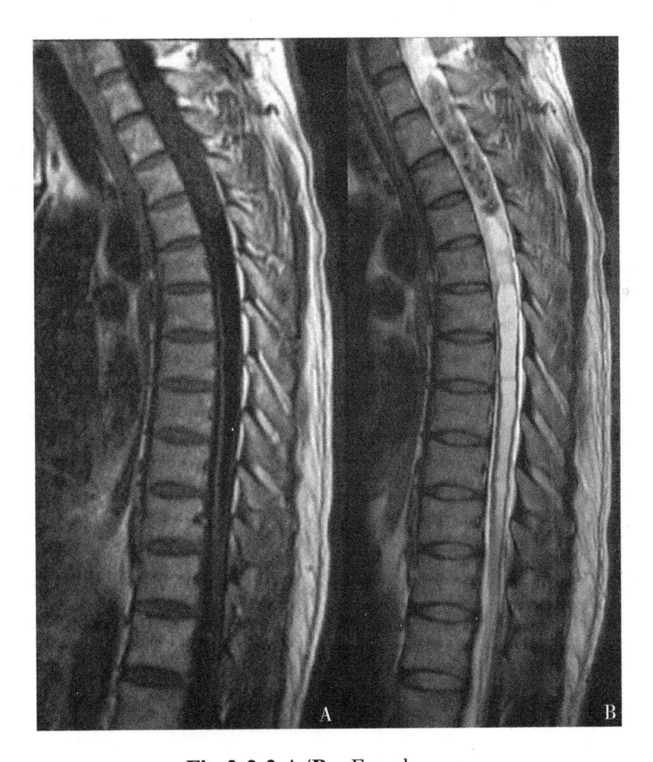

Fig 2-2-2-A/B Ependymoma

Thoracic spinal cord thickening, mass within low signal in T1WI and high signal in T2WI

[**Diagnosis**]

As for intraspinal tumor, according to special clinical presentation, MRI appearances and location, diagnosis is not difficult to make.

2 Spinal cord injury

Spinal cord injury is the most serious complication of spinal injury, and often results in serious physical dysfunction.

[**Pathology and clinical manifestations**]

Spinal cord injuries can be divided into hemorrhagic injuries and non-hemorrhagic injuries. The latter just presents spinal cord edema, swell and prognosis is good. Spinal cord transverse injuries can be divided into two types: partial and complete. Post-injury complications include myelomalacia, atrophy, cystic degeneration and arachnoid adhesions etc.

[**Imaging appearances**]

(1) Radiography and CT

Radiography and CT can find fracture and spondylolisthesis, while CT can also estimate the compression of spinal cord from fracture pieces, and find the hemorrhage.

(2) MRI

MRI can show traumatic spinal canal stenosis, type, location, scope and degree of spinal cord injury directly. a) Hemorrhage: In T1-and T2-weighted images it is always shown as high signal. b) spinal cord edema: It is shown as medium or low signal in T1-weighted images, and obviously high signal in T2-weighted images. c) Myelomalacia, cystic degeneration, cavitation and adhesive cyst can be shown as low signals in T1-weighted images and high signals in T2-weighted images. 4) Spinal cord atrophy is shown as diffuse or localized narrowing of spine and may be accompanied with abnormal signals.

[**Diagnosis**]

It is not difficult to make a diagnosis with definite trauma history and typical MRI appearances.

3 Neuromyelitis optica (NMO)

NMO, also called Devic syndrome, is a kind of demyelinating disease which often occurs in Asians. The optic nerve and spinal cord can be damaged simultaneously or successively. Brain tissues can also be affected. It often causes monocular or binocular blindness.

[**Pathology and clinical manifestations**]

Characterized by the acute onset, serious symptoms and poor prognosis, NMO can both happen in men and women, but more common in women. And the age of onset is 20 to 40. The lesion principally affects optic nerve, optic chiasma and spinal cord (common in cervical segment thoracic segment) and causes monocular or binocular blindness. The main pathological appearances of NMO are demyelination, sclerosis plaque and necrosis, and there can be the infiltration of perivascular inflammatory cell. The spinal cord can be with necrosis and cavity in the end. In blood, NMO-IgG is generally positive, which is a specific indicator of NMO.

[**Imaging appearances**]

(1) CT

The diagnostic value is not that obvious.

(2) MRI

MRI is a very important method to diagnose NMO. a) Changes of optic nerves: The lesion is shown as high signal in fat-suppression T1-weighted images. On the enhanced scan, the lesion is obviously intensified. b) Changes of spinal cord: The lesion always affects more than 3 vertebral segments.

[**Diagnosis**]

MRI examination plays a very important role in diagnosing NMO. In the clinical work, the diagnosis should be based on the following factors: Both optic nerve and spinal cord should be affected, and the affected segments of spinal cord are always more than 3 vertebral segments, but the brain tissues are rarely involved. And in blood NMO-IgG is always positive. This disease should be distinguished with multiple sclerosis: the latter is always seen in brain, the lesion in spinal cord is less than 3 vertebral segments, and NMO-IgG is usually negative.

4 Syringomyelia

Syringomyelia is a kind of chronic progressive spinal degenerative disease. The lesion is always located in cervical cord, and can also affect medulla oblongata.

[Pathology and clinical manifestations]

This disease can be congenital and secondary, and is widely seen in men. Pathologically, basic lesions are cavity and gliosis. The clinical appearances are dyskinesia and dysesthesia.

[Imaging appearances]

(1) CT

The diagnosis of syringomyelia is limited on CT scan. Plain CT scan may accidentally check cysts of low density in upper cervical spine. And on enhanced CT scan the area of low density can not be strengthened.

(2) MRI

On the sagittal plane of MRI, it is very helpful to define the location or the size of the lesion, and even make clear the cause of syringomyelia. The cavity in T1-weighted images is low signal, but in T2-weighted images it is high signal. If the cavity is linked with subarachnoid space, the pulsation of CSF can create irregular stripe of low signal. T2-Flair sequence can display small cavity even more sensitively.

[Diagnosis]

For this disease, according to the special clinical presentation, MRI appearances, the diagnosis is not difficult to make.

5 Intraspinal canal vascular malformation

Intraspinal canal vascular malformation is a kind of vascular dysplasia of spinal cord during embryonic period. It can occur at any segment of the spinal cord and can affect both internal and external spinal cord at the same time. It can be seen more common in men than women during the ages of 20~60.

[**Pathology and clinical manifestations**]

Similar to cerebrovascular malformation, this disease aslo has many different types, and the most common one is AVM (arteriovenous malformation). According to different sites, it can be divided into peridural and intradural ones. Clinically, intradural AVM is more important, because this type can cause dyskinesia and segmental distribution pain.

[**Imaging appearances**]

(1) Radiography

DSA can show the origin of feeding arteries, malformed vessels, and drain veins and thus provide a path for interventional treatment.

(2) CT

Spotted calcification in lesion can be found on routine plain scan. On enhanced scan, tortuous vessels are enhanced as strips or irregular lumps, and sometimes feeding arteries and drain veins can be shown. CTA can display the outline of AVM.

(3) MRI

On routine plain scan, spinal cord swelling can be observed, and malformed vessels show flow-empty. The drain veins are always located on the back side of spinal cord. On enhanced scan, small AVM can be checked. MRA is similar to CTA.

[**Diagnosis**]

Typical AVM is not difficult to diagnose, while atypical AVM should be distinguished from intramedullary tumor and angiocavernoma.

Chapter 3

Imaging of Head and Neck

Head and neck range from the skull base to the superior aperture of thorax and include eyes, ears, accessory sinus, nasopharynx, oropharynx, and larynx.

Nowadays medical imaging techniques can demonstrate the anatomy of head and neck clearlier. They can show the lesions' location, size and extension. The medical imaging techniques include radiography, dacryocystography, ultrasound, computed tomography (CT), and magnetic resonance imaging (MRI). We can choose one or more different imaging techniques to make the diagnosis.

Lesson 1 Eye

Section 1 Imaging methods

1 Radiography

Dacryocystography is used to show the function and shape of the lacrimal sac and duct.

2 Ultrasound

US has a broad impact on the practice of ophthalmology. Modern ultrasound systems provide real-time, highly detailed images of ocular and orbital structures in a rapid, noninvasive manner, posing no significant threat of tissue damage. Real-time ultrasound images, unaffected by optical opacities, have significantly advanced the diagnosis and management of virtually all ocular and orbital diseases. High frequency (typically 10 MHz) ultrasound can provide the detailed resolution required for ocular and orbital examination. High-frequency (50 MHz) ultrasound biomicroscope provides in-vivo microscopic imaging of the iris, ciliary body, anterior chamber and cornea with unparalleled details.

3 CT and MRI

CT and MRI provide another two major imaging methods, which can show the lesions in multiple directions and they are advanced over the conventional radiography. They are applied in the diagnosis of intraorbital and extraocular masses including congenital diseases, various tumors, vascular malformation, and granulomas.

Eyes can be examined with HRCT and be reconstructed in all directions, such as coronal and sagittal planes. The images should be shown on both soft tissue window and bone window.

MRI is usually used in the differential diagnosis of eye diseases, and meanwhile is the major examination for the cavernous sinus and visual access diseases. The conventional MRI scans include T1-weighted imaging and T2-weighted imaging in axial, coronal and sagittal planes. We choose 3 or 4 millimeters as the thickness. The fat-suppression sequence can make the retrobulbar fat's signal declined, which can contribute to observing the lesion's shape.

In clinical settings, the enhanced CT scan, enhanced and/or dynamic contrast-enhanced MRI are commonly applied to determine the nature of the lesion.

Section 2 Normal imaging findings of eye

1 Ultrasonography (US)

On the sonogram the cornea is the most superficial thin convex echogenic membrane, followed by the anechoic fluid of the anterior chamber. The iris is represented by echogenic linear bands that originate from the edge of the eye. The lens is deep to these bands. It is the convex membrane in the posterior chamber followed by the anechoic space of the vitreous body. The thick echogenic round outer membrane of the eyeball consists of three layers. The inner layer is the retina, the middle layer is the choroid, and the outer layer is the sclera. The three layers are difficult to differentiate in a normal sonogram. There is a hypoechoic shadow representing the optic disc posteriorly, and the optic nerve lies behind it.

The retrobulbar fat is hyperechoic. The optic nerve appears as a sagittal hypoechoic structure which runs from the outer part of the eyeball to the tip of the orbit. The extrinsic muscles that form the intraorbital muscular cone appear as hypoechoic bands with typical longitudinal striations. The oblique muscles are almost never seen. The rectus muscles are assessed usually.

Central retinal and ciliary arteries display low resistance flow typically in the color Doppler. The lachrymal glands occupy the upper outer angle of the anterior orbit with almond shaped echo waves. They are not easily to be differentiated from the neighboring fatty tissues. (Fig 3-1-1)

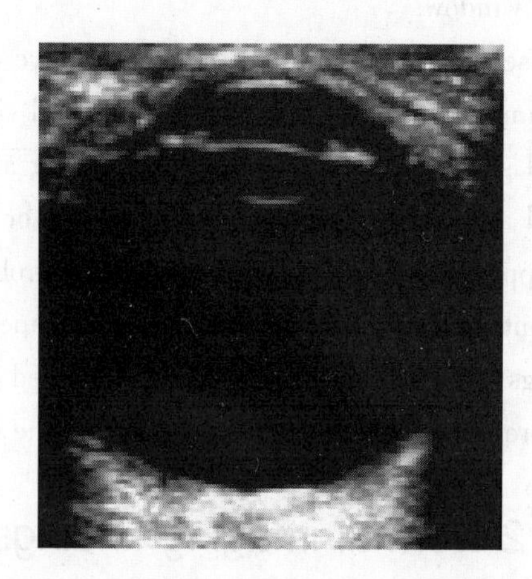

Fig 3-1-1 Normal sonographic appearance of the eye

2 CT

The orbital cavity appears as cone shape and bony density. Eyeball is made up of vitreous body with low density and lens with high density. The wall of eyeball is ring form and homogeneous isodensity, and the three primary layers are difficult to be distinguished. The lachrymal glands lie in symmetric position with isodensity. The retrobulbar fat space is low density. The extraocular muscles are strip-type in the verge and the optical nerve is in the centra of the orbital cavity. The superior orbital fissure and optic canal are the access from orbital apex to cranial cavity. (Fig 3-1-2-A/B)

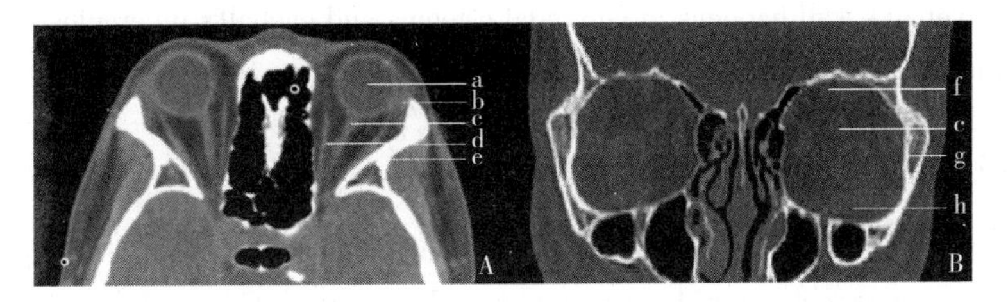

Fig 3-1-2-A/B The normal axial and coronal CT scan

a. eyeball; b. lacrimal gland; c. optic nerve; d. medial rectus; e. lateral rectus; f. superior rectus; g. bone wall of the eye socket; h. inferior rectus

3 MRI

The bony walls of orbital cavity appear as low signal intensiy; extraocular muscles, optic nerve, the eyeball's ring wall and crystalline humor appear as isointensity; corporis vitre appears as lower signal intensity in T1-weighted images and higher signal intensity in T2-weighted images. The orbital fat appears as high signal intensity in T1-weighted images and slight higher signal in T2-weighted images.

Section 3 Imaging signs of eye diseases

Eye's basic lesions include the shape, location, size, echoes, density, and intensity.

1 Eyeball

Eyeball contraction is common in congenital microphthalmus, atrophy of eyeball caused by various reasons. The enlarged ocular bulb is seen in intraocular tumor, the late glaucoma and high myopia. Exophthalmos is seen in the retrobulbar occupying lesions, Graves disease, arteriovenous fistula, orbital hematoma and so on. Enophthalmos happens in the orbital fractures. The local thickness of eye ring protruding into the eyeball is seen in tumors, detachment of retina or choroid. The diffuse thickness of eye ring is seen in inflammation. Calcification of the eyeball's wall happens in choroidal osteoma and eyeball's tuberculosis. Calcification in the eyeball is seen in retinoblastoma.

2 Extraocular muscles

Extraocular muscle atrophy is seen in oculomotor nerve paralysis; hypertrophy of the extraocular muscles happens in inflammation, Graves disease, arteriovenous aneurysm, injure and so on. The eye's inflammation involves the whole extraocular muscles, and the Graves disease involves the extraocular muscles' belly.

3 Optic nerve

Thickened optic nerve is found in the optic nerve glioma, optic nerve sheath meningioma, inflammatory lesions, and intracranial hypertension; optic nerve degeneration appears high signal in T2-weighted images, which can be enhanced or not. Optic nerve becomes thinner in optic atrophy, which can be diagnosed by MRI. But there are not unified diagnosis standards in the industry now. Thickened chiasma opticum and optic tract are seen in glioma, inflammation, or involved by the neighboring lesions.

4 Orbital cavity

The orbital cavity narrows in the craniofacial malformation; the orbital is enlarged by huge tumors and optic nerve fibroma etc. Fractures in trauma can cause the break or displacement of the eye's bone wall. Thickened bone is found in fibrous dysplasia, meningioma of flat type etc. The bone destruction can be caused by malignant tumor. Bone defect happens in optic nerve fibromatosis, dermoid cyst and Langerhans cell histiocytosis. Orbital tumor happens in the orbital muscle cone, such as angiocavernoma, lymphangioma, neurogenic tumor etc.

5 Iacrimal glands

The lacrimal glands can shift forward in old people or orbital tumor. The diffuse enlargement of lacrimal glands is always caused by inflammation and lymphoma. The occupying lesions happen in the orbital lacrimal gland, including benign and malignant pleomorphic adenoma, adenoid cystic carcinoma.

6 Eyelid

The diffuse thickened eyelid is seen in inflammation, Graves's disease, and ophthalmic vein reflux disorder. The eyelid's tumors include capillary hemangioma, carcinoma of basal cell and tarsal gland.

Section 4 Diagnosis of diseases

1 Optical inflammatory pseudotumor

[**Pathology and clinical manifestations**]

The etiology of optical inflammatory pseudotumor remains unclear, although it may be related to abnormal immune function. Optical inflammatory pseudotumor is divided into acute, subacute, and chronic stages. Acute stage: the pathological changes are edema and inflammatory infiltration; the inflammatory cells include lymphocytes, phlogocyte and acidocyte. Subacute and chronic stages: the pathological changes include the form of a large amount of fibrovascular stroma and then fibrous degeneration. Corticosteroid treatment is effective but it is easy to relapse.

The optical inflammatory pseudotumor is divided into seven types by the location: anterior to the orbital septum type, myositis type, dacryoadenitis type, scleritis and around, inflammation of the optical nerve membrane, mass type, and diffuse type.

[**Imaging appearances**]

(1) Ultrasonography

Orbital B-scan ultrasonography in the cases of orbital pseudotumor may show two characteristic types of abnormalities: the inflammatory mass in the orbit and the inflammatory edema of the orbital structures. Most pseudotumors present as hypoechoic areas with irregular outline, infiltrating the retrobulbar fat diffusely. Sound energy is highly attenuated by these masses and usually does not penetrate through them to outline the tumor's posterior extent or the orbital wall clearly. As a result, changes such as inflammatory edema may often be noted acoustically in adjacent orbital structures and indicate the lesion's inflammatory character. The changes may be noted in the optic nerve, the extraocular muscles, or Tenon's space by ultrasound. Oedema of orbital fat may be present, and myositis may be seen as enlargement of the whole extraocular muscle. Oedema in the retrobulbar fascia (Tenon's capsule) tracks along the optic nerve sheath to form the "T" sign. Color Doppler imaging of inflammatory pseudotumor shows no intralesional blood flow.

(2) CT

The eyelid was thickened in the anterior to the orbital septum type. The extraocular muscles get wider from tendon to belly in the myositis type, which is the typical performance and commonly happens in the superior and medical rectus muscles. The scleritis shows the thickening ring of eyeball. The inflammation of optical nerve membrane is manifested as the enlarged optical nerve and the margin of which is ill-defined. The soft mass in orbit happens in the mass type, which is connected to the eyeball's wall with broad base. The dacryoadenitis is manifested as the diffuse enlargement of lacrimal gland. The lesion can be enhanced after intravenous contrast administration.

(3) MRI

The acute lesion shows slightly low signals in T1-weighted images and high signals in T2-weighted images. The chronic lesion shows isointensity in T1-weighted images and hypointensity in T2-weighted images. The lesion can be enhanced moderately or obviously.

[**Diagnosis**]

The following diseases should be differentiated from optical inflammatory pseudotumor: a) lymphoproliferative lesions: multiple structures are involved. The lesions can enwrap the eyeball with homogeneous intensity, which are isointensity or slightly lower than the alba. It should be differentiated from diffuse type of inflammatory pseudotumor. Short-term check after treatment will be helpful. b) metastatic tumor: the extraocular muscle is enlarged with nodular.

2 Ocular tumors

Ocular tumors can origin in all structures of the eye. The orbit can be involved by the neighboring lesions or be transferred from other tumors.

(1) Lacrimal benign mixed tumor:

[Pathology and clinical manifestations]

Lacrimal benign mixed tumor, also known as benign pleomorphic adenoma, is common in adults and the mean onset age is 41 years old. There is no difference between males and females. The tumor occurs in lacrimal gland with round shape. It is slow-growing and can deteriorate.

[Imaging appearances]

1) Ultrasonography

Ultrasonographic appearance of the benign mixed tumor is as round to oval-shaped, isoechoic or hyperechoic lesion with well-defined margin and little attenuation in lacrimal fossa. The tumor's pseudocapsule is smooth, and has a highly reflective anterior surface by ultrasound. The posterior extent and the outline of the tumor are often demonstrated. Ultrasound will reveal a variable pattern within the tumor's interior, depending on the abundance of cystic spaces. Color Doppler imaging of benign mixed tumor may show blood flow signal within the tumor. The mass can not be compressed with probe compression.

2) CT

Plain CT scan: The mass is soft tissue density and smooth margin in lacrimal gland. The calcification is rarely seen. The lacrimal gland fossa is enlarged and the cortical bone is compressed without destruction. The surrounding structures can be pressed. Enhanced CT scan: The mass is obviously enhanced.

3) MRI

The mass appears slightly low signal in T1-weighted images and high signal in T2-weighted images, which are heterogeneous. The mass is obviously enhanced.

[**Diagnosis**]

Benign lacrimal mixed tumor should be differentiated from carcinoma and lymphoma of lacrimal gland. The lesion of lacrimal carcinoma can destruct the bone of lacrimal fossa, the margin of which is irregular. The lacrimal lymphoma is irregular in shape and can enwrap the eyeball.

(2) The optic nerve glioma

[**Pathology and clinical manifestations**]

The optic nerve glioma is originated in the glial cell of optical nerve, and is a common disease in children. It will deteriorate in adults and frequently in females. Fifteen to fifty percent of cases can be combined with neurofibromatosis.

[**Imaging appearances**]

1) Ultrasonography

On ultrasound a fusiform or irregular expansion of the optic nerve can be demonstrated. Secondary changes, such as flattening of the posterior pole of the globe and papilledema, can be shown. The lesion is hypoechoic and shows poor acoustic transmission. Color Doppler imaging of optic nerve glioma may show blood flow within the tumor.

2) CT

Plain CT scan: The optical nerve is thickened with strip or spindle shape and smooth margin, the density of which is homogeneous. The CT value of the lesion is between 40~60HU and will be slightly enhanced in the postcontrast CT image. It can enlarge the optic canal.

3) MRI

The optic nerve glioma is isointensity or slightly low signal in T1-weighted images and high signal in T2-weighted images. The subarachnoid is broadened by the lesion. In the enhanced image, the mass should be enhanced obviously. MRI is the first choice for optic nerve glioma.

[**Diagnosis**]

The differential diagnosis of optic nerve glioma includes the following diseases: 1) optic nerve sheath meningioma: It is mainly in adults. The lesion appears isodensity or slight higher with smooth margin. Calcification can be found in it. The lesion appears isointensity in T1-weighted images and T2-weighted images, which is obviously enhanced and the optical nerve can not be enhanced. It shows the "track sign" . 2) optic neuritis: It is the inflammation of optic nerve sheath and it is difficult to differentiate between them.

(3) Cavernous hemangioma

[**Pathology and clinical manifestations**]

Cavernous hemangioma is a common benign tumor in optical cavity. The mean onset age is 38 years old. Female patient accounts for 52 ~ 70%. It happens in unilateral eye and grows slowly. Vision can be normal in general.

[**Imaging appearances**]

1) Ultrasonography

Ultrasonographic evaluation of the cavernous hemangioma reveals round to oval-shaped, isoechoic or hyperechoic lesion with well defined margin and little attenuation in the extraocular muscle cone. The posterior extent of the tumor and the outline of the wall are often demonstrated. Color Doppler imaging of cavernous hemangioma may show spotty arterial slow flow within the tumor boundaries. Doppler examination results are frequently negative owing to very slow blood flow within the vascular spaces. Calcified phleboliths are seen occasionally. The mass can be compressed with probe compression.

2) CT

The plain CT scan: The tumor is round or oval-shaped with smooth margin, the density of which is homogeneous. The mean CT value is 55 HU. The extraocular muscles, optical nerve, eyeball can be compressed and the optical cavity can be enlarged. On the enhanced CT scan the lesion is progressively enhanced: the lesion is enhanced as a point at first, then extending to the whole. At last the lesion will be enhanced obviously. The enhanced CT scan is very meaningful for the diagnosis (Fig 3-1-3-A /B).

3) MRI

The mass appears as isointensity or slightly low signal in T1WI and high signal in T2WI. The signal is higher with the echo time prolonged in multiple echo sequence (Fig 3-1-3-C/D).

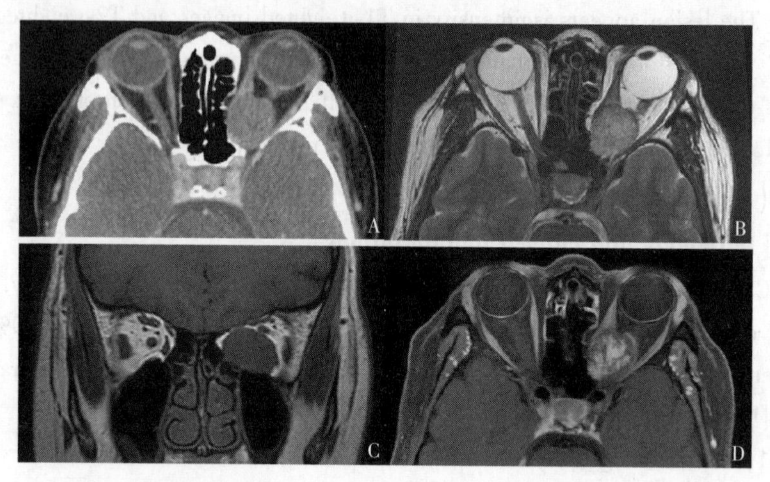

Fig 3-1-3-A/B/C/D Axial CT scan, axial T2WI, coronal T1WI, and axial enhanced T1WI

The cavernous hemangioma is in the left optical cavity. It is isodensity in plain CT images, isointensity in T1WI, and slightly higher intensity in T2WI, which is obviously enhanced.

[**Diagnosis**]

The optical cavernous hemangioma should be differentiated from schwannoma. The latter appears as slightly low density on CT scan, which is heterogeneous. On the enhanced CT scan the lesion should be slightly or moderately enhanced fast.

3 Eye's foreign bodies and injuries

(1) Eye's foreign bodies

[**Pathology and clinical manifestations**]

The disease of eye's foreign bodies is common in clinical settings, which can result in serious complications. The foreign bodies can be divided into metal and nonmetal by nature.

[**Imaging appearances**]

1) Ultrasonography

Ultrasonic detection of orbital foreign bodies depends on their sizes, locations, orientation, and the presence of associated inflammation. Hard materials such as metal, glass or stone are highly reflective and easier to be demonstrated. Small bodies and bodies along the posterior sclera or in the retrobulbar fat are not easy to be recognized by the present ultrasonographic techniques. Following the haemorrhage and/or gas of the foreign body's track penetrating to the vitreous body, we can outline the trajectory and indicate its position.

2) CT

CT shows the foreign body's type, size, number, location, and the relationship to the neighboring structures. The metal body appears high density with radial artifacts. The nonmetal bodies are divided into high and low density: The former includes sandstone, glass and so on, the CT value of which is above 300 HU, and has no artifacts; the latter includes plants, plastics and so on, the CT value of which is between-199 HU and 50 HU.

The CT scan can locate metal bodies, nonmetal bodies with high density, and a few large nonmetal foreign bodies with low density. But it is insensitive to small foreign wooden bodies or other nonmetal bodies with low density (Fig 3-1-4-A/B).

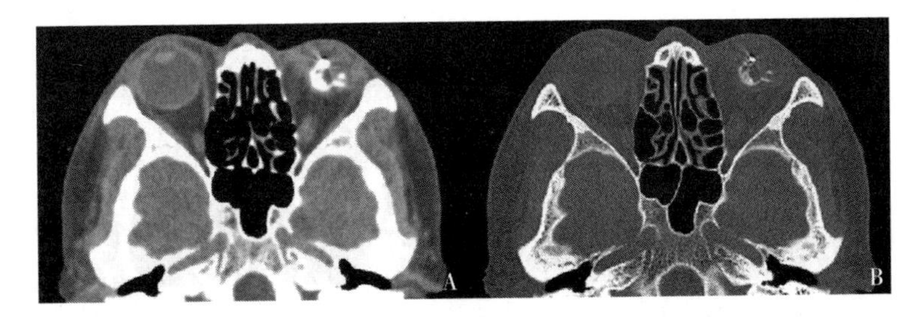

Fig 3-1-4-A/B Axial CT scan (soft tissue window and bone window)

The foreign body has been in the left eyeball for 32 years. It is high density. The left eyeball is atrophied.

3) MRI

The ferromagnetic foreign bodies will move in the high-intensity magnetic field, which can damage the eye again. So MRI is contraindication to metal foreign bodies. Nonmetal bodies contain little oxide protons, which appear as low signal in T1WI and T2WI clearly.

[**Diagnosis**]

The history of trauma is very important for the diagnosis. The differentiations include the followings: eyeball's calcification, calcification in the optical cavity, the artificial crystal and artificial eye.

(2) Fracture of the eye socket and optic canal

[**Pathology and clinical manifestations**]

The fracture of eye socket and optic canal is a common disease in the department of ophthalmology. The medial and inferior orbital walls are involved frequently.

[**Imaging appearances**]

CT

The direct signs include the interruption, crushing and displacement of bone continuity. The indirect signs include the changes of the neighboring soft tissues to the fracture, such as hematoma, the displaced and incarcerated extraocular muscles, the orbital contents inlaid to the neighboring sinus (Fig 3-1-5-A/B).

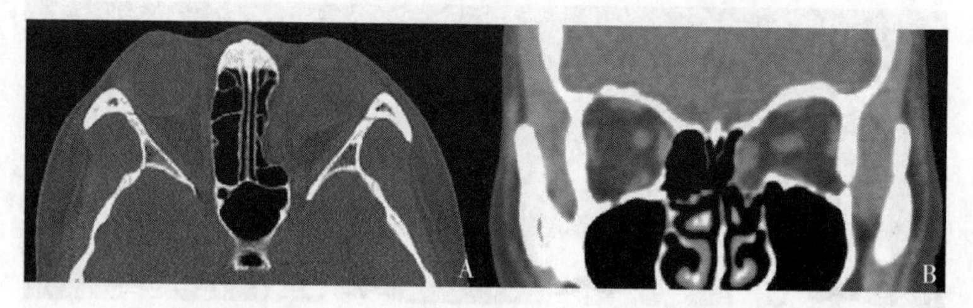

Fig 3-1-5-A/B CT: The left eye socket's inner wall fractures
The medial rectus is protruding into the neighboring ethmoid sinus.

[**Diagnosis**]

CT is the main examination technique for the fracture of eye socket and optic canal.

Lesson 2 Ear

Ear is located in the temporal bone mostly and includes the outer, middle and inner ears. The anatomical structure is clear in the medical imaging. The focus of observation is the structure of bony external auditory canal, the middle ear and inner ear. The related structures can be shown meanwhile, such as the facial nerve canal, the carotid canal, the jugular fossa, the sulcus of sigmoid sinus, the middle cranial fossa and so on, which are related to ear diseases.

Section 1 Imaging methods

1 Radiography

Radiography is used to show the electrode's shape and location after the cochlear implant surgery.

2 Ultrasonography

The application value of US in ear is limited.

3 CT

CT is the main medical examination of ear. The routine inspections include volume scanning, multiplanar reconstruction, and other post-processing techniques, such as SSD, imaging of labyrinthine and ossicular chain. With the development of software, CT virtual endoscopy technique is maturing day by day and is used to observe the tympanum, mastoid antrum, labyrinth and the structure of inner ear.

4 MRI

MRI is an important supplement of CT. The value lies in the demonstrations of auditory nerve, facial nerve, the membranous labyrinth and the soft tissue lesions.

Section 2 Normal imaging findings of ear

1 High-resolution computed tomography (HRCT)

HRCT can show the structure and pneumatization of temporal bone clearly. The temporal bone is composed of squamous bone, tympanic part, mastoid, petrous bone and styloid process (Fig 3-2-1-A/B). The CT scan is useful in showing the anatomical variation.

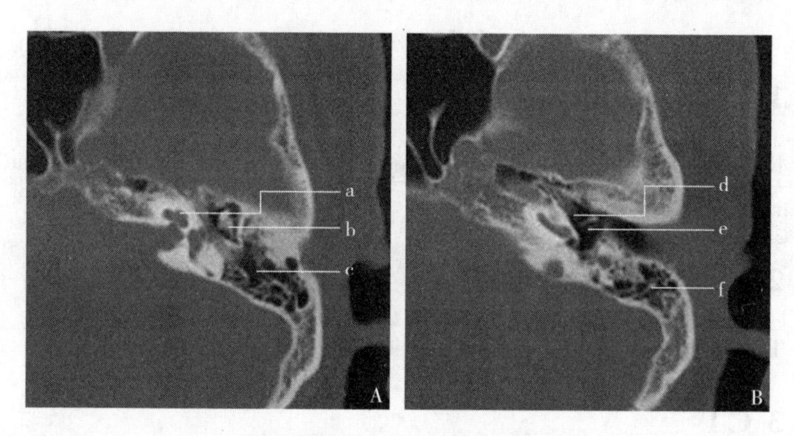

Fig 3-2-1-A/B Axial-CT scan

a. cochlea; b. auditory ossicle (incus); c. mastoid antrum;
d. tympanic cavity; e. auditory ossicle (stapes); f. external auditory meatus

2 MRI

The bone and the gas in the temporal bone are both low signal in T1WI and T2WI. The lymph in the labyrinth and the cerebrospinal fluid that fills the canals of inner ear appear as high signal in T2WI, and low signal in T1WI. The auditory and facial nerves appear as isointensity with strip shape on both T1WI and T2WI.

Section 3 Imaging signs of ear diseases

1 External acoustic meatus

The stricture or atresia of external auditory meatus is common in the congenital malformation. The mass is common in cerumen adenoma, cholesteatoma and carcinoma. The destruction of bone is common in malignant tumors and inflammation.

2 Middle ear

The small tympanic cavity is found in congenital malformation. The enlargement of the tympanic cavity is seen in cholesteatoma and tumors. The soft tissue is common in all inflammations, the hemorrhage after trauma, glomus tympanicum, and glomus jugulare. The ossicular anomalies are always congenitally combined with the malformations of external auditory canal and tympanic cavity. The ossicular chain dislocation or discontinuity happens after the injury and operation. The involvement of ossicular and destruction of middle ear are often seen in the cholesteatoma, malformation and tumor.

3 Labyrinth

The morphological abnormalities of cochlea, vestibule and semicircular canal are seen in the congenial malformation. Broken bones are seen in inflammation, tumor, fibrous dysplasia of bone and Paget disease.

4 Auditory canal

The stricture of auditory canal is found in congenial malformation or fibrous dysplasia of bone, the enlargement of which is found in the acoustic neuroma and facial nerve tumor. MRI can be used to show the malformation of the vestibulocochlear nerve.

5 Sclerosis of the temporal bone

The sclerosis of temporal bone happens in inflammation, fibrous dysplasia of bone and Paget disease etc.

Section 4 Diagnosis of diseases

1 Otomastoiditis

[**Pathology and clinical manifestations**]

Otomastoiditis is a common disease of ear's inflammation. The main clinical manifestations include ear pain, ear secretion and conductive deafness.

[**Imaging appearances**]

(1) CT

a) The typical sign is that medium density lesions fill the tympanic and mastoid instead of air. b) the destruction or sclerosis of bone happens in a few instances. c) there are several complications as follows: There are soft tissues combined with calcification in tympanosclerosis. The soft tissues is obviously enhanced combined with the involvement or destruction of the neighboring bone in cholesterol granuloma, which can not be enhanced in cholesteatoma (Fig 3-2-2).

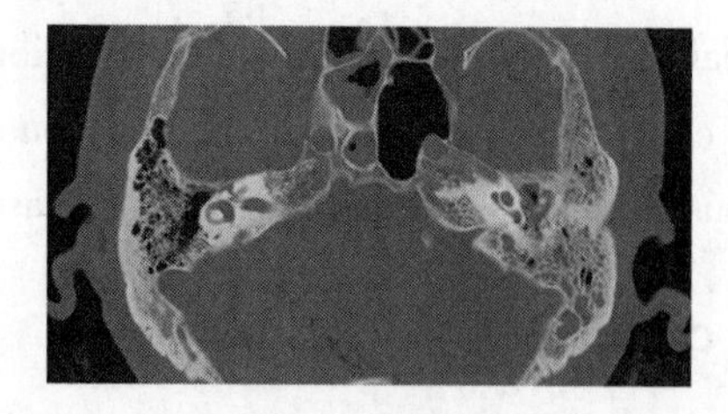

Fig 3-2-2 CT

Cholesteatoma fills in the left middle ear.

The neighboring mastoid process is sclerosis.

(2) MRI

The MRI examination is used to show the involvement in the facial nerve, inner ear and brain.

2 Trauma

[**Pathology and clinical manifestations**]

The temporal bone traumas include fracture and dislocation of auditory ossicles, which can cause conductive deafness and sensorineural deafness.

[**Imaging appearances**]

CT

a) Fractures in the petrous part of temporal bone include longitudinal fractures (account for about 80%), transverse fractures (account for 10% ~ 20%) and mixed fractures. b) The fracture or dislocation of auditory ossicles is characterized by the discontinuity, which is often neglected because of the tiny structures. The 3D display technology has advantage in demonstrating auditory ossicles. The incudostapedial or incudomalleolar joint separation is common (Fig 3-2-3).

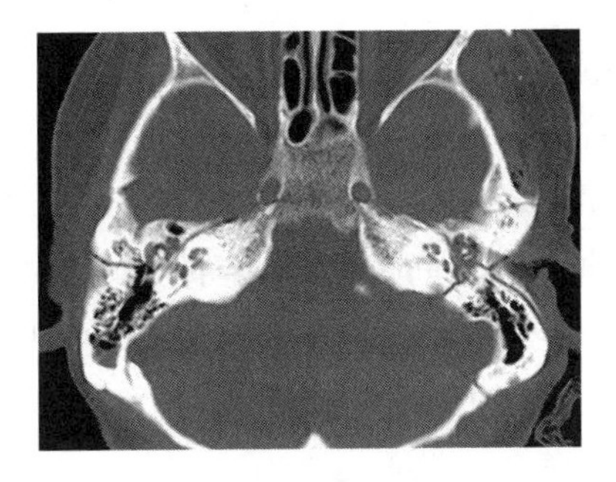

Fig 3-2-3 CT

Temporal bone fracture, which is low density line.

3 Tumor

The secretion and conductive deafness frequently happens in temporal tumors, and the imaging examination has great value in the diagnosis.

(1) Acoustic neuroma

It is discussed in the "Central nervous system" section.

(2) Paraganglioma

[**Pathology and clinical manifestations**]

Paraganglioma includes glomus jugulare and glomus tympanicum. The symptoms contain mainly pulsatile tinnitus and conductive hearing loss. The glomus tympanicum appears purple in otoscopy. It is normal in otoscopy before the glomus jugulare involves in the tympanic cavity.

[**Imaging appearances**]

1) Radiography

The tumor is supported by the external carotid artery in DSA. There are abnormal vessels and tumor staining in the lesion, which is the characteristic of paraganglioma.

2) CT

Glomus jugulare and glomus tympanicum show soft tissues density and the bone involvement is common. The lesion is obviously enhanced. The glomus jugulare enlarges the jugular fossa of the temporal bone, destroys the inferior tympanic wall upward to the hypotympanum and spreads downward to involve in the hypoglossal canal. The glomus tympanicum can grow to fill in the middle ear cavity and cause the bone erosion.

3) MRI

On the non-enhanced MRI, the tumor shows equal signal in T1WI and high signal in T2WI. There are tortuous strip and dot vascular flow void signals in the lesion, which are the typical signs called "salt and pepper syndrome". The lesion is obviously enhanced on the enhanced MRI scan (Fig 3-2-4-A/B/C).

The glomus jugulare in the left jugulare foramen is isointensity on T1WI, high intensity on T2WI, which is obviously enhanced.

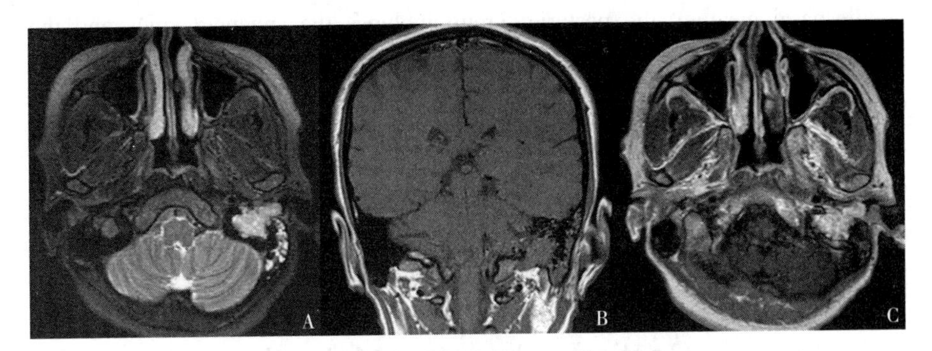

Fig 3-2-4A/B/C Axial T2WI, coronal T1WI, and enhanced T1WI

(3) Carcinoma of the external and middle ears:

[**Pathology and clinical manifestations**]

The carcinoma of the external and middle ears is common among old people. Clinically, the soft tissue fills in the external ear with hemorrhage and exudation.

[**Imaging appearances**]

1) CT

The lesion is manifested as soft tissue in the external ear and tympanic cavity, and the walls are eroded with irregular edge. The lesion can spread and invade the surrounding structures, such as mastoid, the eustachian tube, the jugular fossa, middle and posterior cranial fossa. The focus is obviously enhanced.

2) MRI

MRI has an advantage in displaying the lesions' range. The tumor appears low signal on T1WI and high signal on T2WI, which is obviously enhanced.

Lesson 3 Accessory sinus

Nose and sinus are composed of a plurality of craniofacial bones. The structure of the nasal cavity's lateral wall is complicated, which is made up of superior, middle, inferior conchae, three nasal meatus and sinus openings. The sinus is divided into the former and posterior groups: the former group includes the frontal sinus, maxillary sinus and the anterior ethmoid sinus, which open in the middle nasal meatus; the posterior group includes the sphenoid sinus and the posterior ethmoid sinus, which open in the superior nasal meatus. The anatomy of nasal cavity and sinus is related to individual development, the shape and size of which can be different in different persons. The endoscopic sinus surgery is the conventional operation. The preoperative evaluations are very important, including the lesion's localization and qualitation, the nose and sinus's anatomy and variation. The medical imaging is the indispensable method before surgery.

Section 1 Imaging Methods

1 Radiography

The radiography can be applied in the examination of nose and sinus, but the sensitivity is low. It is less-used at present.

2 Ultrasonography

Application of US in accessory sinus is of limited value.

3 CT

CT is the main examination in the diagnosis of nasal and sinus diseases. HRCT is the routine examination and can be observed in multidimension. The inflammation and tumor can be shown in soft tissue's window. Part of the patients should undergo the enhanced examination. The technique of virtual endoscopy can show the opening and mucous membrane of nose and sinus. CT navigation technology is widely used in all sinus endoscopic operations.

4 MRI

MRI is a complementary technology to CT in nasal and sinus diseases. The axial examination of T1WI and T2WI is conventional; the coronal and sagittal examinations are assistant tests as necessary. The enhanced examination is valuable in the diagnoses and differential diagnoses of nasal and sinus tumors. The MRI technique is used to show the cerebrospinal fluid rhinorrhea.

Section 2 Normal imaging findings of accessory sinus

HRCT can show the normal and abnormal anatomy and the variation of nose and sinus, which is the navigation of the nasal endoscopic operation. HRCT is the routine examination before surgery in order to reduce the postoperative complications.

1 Nose and nasal cavity

The appearances of the nasal cavity's lateral wall include the superior, middle, inferior conchae and nasal meatus. The ostiomeatal complex is in the middle nasal region, including the ethmoidal infundibulum, half crack, the uncinate process, and ethmoidal bulla.

2 Sinus

(1) Maxillary sinus

The maxillary sinus consists of the anterior, posterior, upper and lower walls. When the sinus cavity grows too large, it can spread to the hard palate, the frontal gibbosity, the zygomatic process, the ossa orbitale and the dental process. The sinus cavity narrows when the sinus cavity grows smaller. Sometimes there will be sinus cavities in the bony septum.

(2) Ethmoid sinus

Ethmoid sinus lies in the outside of the top of the nasal cavity. There are air cells on each side. The ethmoid sinus is divided into anterior and posterior groups and opens in the middle and superior nasal meatus respectively. The common variations are as follows: Haller cells, Onodi cells, frontal and ethmoidal bulla etc.

(3) Frontal sinus

The frontal sinus opens in the middle nasal meatus. Some of them can be obsolete and abortive.

(4) Sphenoid sinus

Sphenoid sinus locates in the corpus ossis sphenoidalis. It is divided into several types according to the gasification. It opens in the recessus sphenoethmoidalis. When the sphenoid sinus develops excessively to the other parts of the sphenoid bone, the relative positions of optic canal, foramen rotundum, foramen ovale, pterygoid canal, and carotid canal can move (Fig 3-3-1-A/B).

On the CT scan, the gas in the nasal and sinus cavities appears low density, the bony wall of which appears high density. The normal mucous membrane is too thin to be shown. On the MRI, the gas and the cortical bone appear extremely low signal. The bone marrow in the wall appears high or equal signals. The mucous membrane is linear low signal on T1WI and high signal on T2WI.

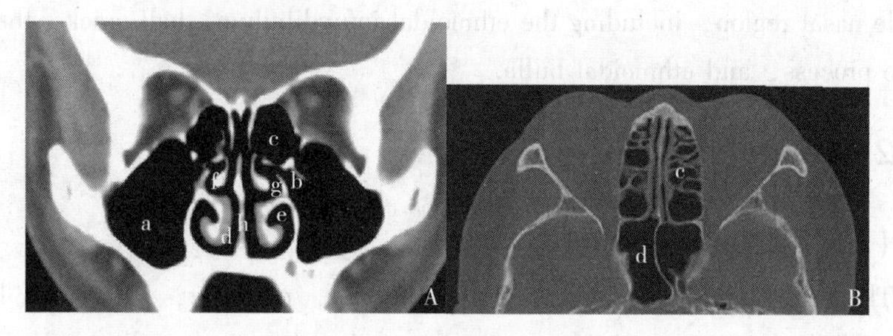

Fig 3-3-1A/B Coronal CT (soft tissue window) and axial CT (bone window)

a. maxillary sinus; b. exit of maxillary; c. antrum; d. inferior concha;
e. inferior nasal meatus; f. middle nasal concha; g. middle nasal meatus;
h. nasal septum

Section 3 Imaging signs of accessory sinus

1 The thickened mucosa

The thickened mucosa is found in all nasal sinusitis. It appears soft tissue density in strips. The thickness is uneven.

2 Sinus cavity effusions

Sinus cavity effusions are manifested as the liquid density or signal, and the air-fluid level is visible. Sinus cavity effusion is common in nasal sinusitis, injures and so on.

3 Tumor

Osteoma and ossifying fibroma are manifested as high density mass with distinct margin. The inverted papilloma appears soft tissue mass in middle nasal meatus. Mucous cyst and nasal polyp present as soft tissue with arch and globular shape in the sinus or nasal meatus. The malignant tumors appear as irregular mass and can invade the surrounding structures.

4 Calcification

Calcification in the sinus cavity can be found in fungal sinusitis.

5 The changes of bone

The destruction of sinus wall is common in all malignant tumors. The sclerosis is found in chronic inflammation. The bony discontinuity is seen in the injury.

Section 4 Diagnosis of diseases

1 Nasal sinusitis

[**Pathology and clinical manifestations**]

The nasal sinusitis is a common disease in clinical settings, which is manifested as stuffy or runny noses, hyposmia and so on.

[**Imaging appearances**]

(1) CT

CT scan is important for determining the types and stages of nasal sinusitis, the performances of which are as follows: a) The mucous membrane is thickened and the sinus cavity's density is increased. The long-term chronic inflammations can cause the bone hypertrophy and the sinus stenosis. b) Calcification in the nasal soft tissue represents the fungal infection. c) The sinus cavity is enlarged and the sinus wall expands. The lesion appears low density in the sinus cavity. The edge of the lesion is enhanced in mucous cyst on the postcontrast CT scan.

(2) MRI

The lesion shows high signal on T2WI. The mucous membrane can be enhanced as ring or lace on enhanced T1WI.

2 Benign tumors of nasal sinus

[**Pathology and clinical manifestations**]

The inverted papilloma is common in the benign tumors of nasal sinus. It is commonly found in men aged 40 to 50 years. The main clinical manifestations include nasal obstruction, rhinorrhea, nosebleeds, anosmia, and epiphora. It can recur after operation. Two percent to three percent of tumors can undergo malignant transformation.

[**Imaging appearances**]

(1) CT

a) On CT scan, the inverted papilloma is manifested as the soft tissue mass in nasal cavity or ethmoid sinus. It can spread to the eye sockets or anterior cranial fossa. The rhinitis secondary occurs to the obstruction of sinus ostia. b) The tumors can be slightly enhanced on the enhanced CT scan, which can contribute to the differentiation between tumor and inflammation. The inflammation is non-enhanced on the enhanced CT scan. c) If the tumor grows quickly and the sclerotin is seriously destroyed, the canceration needs to be considered.

(2) MRI

The lesion appears isointensity or low signal, mixed or high signals on T1WI. It should be enhanced as gyriform on the enhanced T1WI and especially in the sagittal view, which is the characteristic of inverted papilloma.

[**Diagnosis**]

Papilloma should be differentiated from the following diseases: a) chronic sinusitis and nasal polyp: the bone is always normal. b) hemangioma: the lesion is obviously enhanced. c) The mucocele of nasal cavity can cause the enlargement. d) The malignant tumors can destroy the bone, but the qualitative diagnosis depends on histopathology.

3 Malignant tumors of nasal sinus

[**Pathology and clinical manifestations**]

The malignant tumors of nasal sinus are divided into epithelial and non epithelial tumors. The squamous cell carcinoma is common.

[**Imaging appearances**]

(1) MRI

MRI can show the lesion's extent (Fig 3-3-2-A/B/C).

(2) CT

a) On the CT scan, the tumor is manifested as soft tissue mass in sinus. The density is homogeneous generally. The liquefaction necrosis in the large mass appears low density. The calcification is found in part of the lesion, such as the adenoid cystic carcinoma, chondrosarcoma, malignant chordoma etc. The malignant epithelial tumors can progress and involve the neighboring structures. b) On the enhanced CT scan, the tumors are moderately or obviously enhanced (Fig 3-3-2-D).

[**Diagnosis**]

The malignant nasal tumor should be differentiated from the inverted papilloma, nasal polyp, and hemangioma. The differential diagnosis is as follows: the malignant nasal tumor can grow invasively and cause the involvement and destruction of the neighboring structures. It is obviously enhanced.

4 Nasal and sinus injury

[**Pathology and clinical manifestations**]

Facial trauma is a common disease in clinical settings, which can cause the fractures of nasal and maxillary bones.

[**Imaging appearances**]

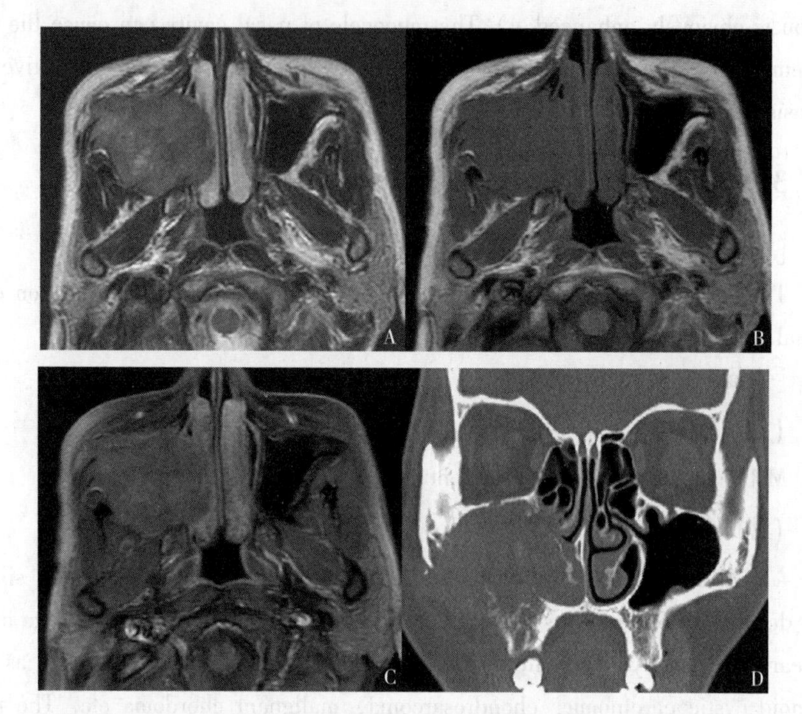

Fig 3-3-2-A/B/C/D Axial T2WI, T1WI, enhanced T1WI, coronal CT scan

Carcinoma of the right maxillary sinus is isointensity on T1WI, slightly higher intensity on T2WI, which is obviously enhanced. On the CT scan the wall of the right maxillary sinus is destroyed.

CT is the main method in the facial fracture's diagnosis. a) nasal bone fracture: it is common in clinical settings, and can involve the lacrimal sac fossa. The separation of sutures is manifested as the broadening of the sutures. b) Sinus fractures are always compound. The walls of the sinus are broken or displaced. The cerebrospinal fluid fistula will happen when the base of the skull and dura mater are involved.

Lesson 4 Pharynx

By the line of epiglottis and soft palate, the pharynx is divided into nasopharynx, oropharynx and laryngopharynx. The pharyngeal tumors are common in nasopharynx. The nasal hemangioma is a common benign tumor, and the nasopharyngeal carcinoma is a common malignant tumor. Because of the invasion to the neighboring structures, the early detection and diagnosis of nasopharyngeal carcinoma are very important. The soft tissue's abnormality can cause the obstructive sleep apnea hypopnea syndrome, which is common in clinical settings.

Section 1 Imaging methods

1 Radiography

Radiography is rarely used in the pharynx.

(1) Pharyngeal angiography

It is used to observe the shape of pharynx and evaluate the swallowing function.

(2) DSA

It has a higher value in the diagnosis of nasopharyngeal angiofibroma.

2 Ultrasonography

US is rarely used in the examination of pharynx. Sometimes it is used to evaluate the lymph nodes metastasis in pharyngeal cancer.

3 CT

CT is the routine examination in nasopharyngeal diseases, which can show the pharynx, pharyngeal wall, parapharyngeal space clearly. HRCT and three-dimensional reconstruction technique have great value in the diagnosis of pharynx, especially in the observation of soft tissue window, coronal or sagittal views. The bone window is used to observe the cranial base. The enhanced examination is used to determine the lesion's nature.

4 MRI

MRI has high-resolution in soft tissues and is the supplement of CT. The sagittal, coronal, axial T1WI and T2WI are the routine examinations. MRI examination is used if necessary.

Section 2 Normal imaging findings of nasopharynx, oropharynx and laryngopharynx

1 Nasopharynx

Nasopharynx is located in the nasopharyngeal posterior, down to the back and trailing edge of the soft palate. Choanal and the trailing edge of the nasal septum compose the front wall. The top wall is composed of sphenoid bone close to the cranial base. The posterior wall is composed of basioccipital region, the first and second cervical vertebras. Ostium pharyngeum tubae auditive, torus tubarius and pharyngeal recess compose the outer wall. Parapharyngeal space and adjacent structures are symmetrical on CT and MRI scans. Besides these, MRI can distinguish the mucosa, submucosa, lateral muscles and parapharyngeal space etc.

2 Oropharynx

The range of oropharynx is from the soft palate to the free edge of epiglottis. CT and MRI images can show the oropharyngeal mucosa, submucous constrictor, parapharyngeal space, tonsil, tongue and the mouth floor.

3 Laryngopharynx

The larynx is from the epiglottic free edge to the lower edge of cricoid cartilage, composed of the lateral wall, sinus piriformis and the gaps around. The axial view of CT and MRI images can show the mucosa, longus colli. The sinus piriformis are symmetrical, the mucosal surface of which is smooth. The upper e-sophagus appears soft tissue density and lies in the back of cricoid cartilage and the trachea.

Section 3 Imaging signs of diseases in nasopharynx, oropharynx and laryngopharynx

1 The stenosis or occlusion of pharyngeal cavity

It is found in the tumors, injuries and obstructive sleep apnea hypopnea syndrome etc.

2 The thickness or asymmetry of pharyngeal wall

It is often seen in inflammations or tumors.

3 The abnormal density, signal or tumor

The abnormal density, signal or tumor of the pharyngeal cavity and parapha-ryngeal space are seen in inflammations or tumors.

4 The abnormality of parapharyngeal space

The displacement or stenosis is often caused by inflammations or tumors.

Section 4 Diagnosis of diseases

1 Pharyngeal abscess

[**Pathology and clinical manifestations**]

The pharyngeal abscess is divided into peritonsillar abscess, retropharyngeal abscess, infection or abscess in the parapharyngeal space. The acute abscess is common in children and is caused by the injury of pharyngeal wall, the piercing of foreign body, ear infections, and purulent lymphadenitis. The chronic abscess is found in cervical tuberculosis, lymphoid tuberculosis. The acute abscess can cause the systemic inflammation, pharyngalgia, dysphagia and dyspnea. The abscess bleeds when the vessel is involved.

[**Imaging appearances**]

(1) CT

On the CT scan, the pharyngeal abscess is manifested as the swelling of pharyngeal soft tissue with low density. On the enhanced CT scan, the mass is edge enhanced with annuliform. The gas or gas liquid plane can confirm the diagnosis. The abscesses in different parts have different appearances: a) Peritonsillar abscess is manifested as the tonsillar enlargement. The surrounding fat gap is fuzzy. The cavum pharyngis is narrowed by the pression. b) The parapharyngeal abscess can be unilateral or bilateral. The parapharyngeal space is pressed. The carotid artery and jugular vein are displaced outward. c) Retropharyngeal abscess is manifested as the strip shadow with slightly low density before the cervical vertebra. The calcification is seen in the wall of tuberculous abscess, combined with the destruction of cervical vertebra, the narrowing of intervertebral space, the enlargement and necrosis of cervical lymph nodes etc.

(2) MRI

On the plain scan, the abscess appears homogeneous low signal on T1WI and high signal on T2WI. The surrounding tissues are compressed and displaced. In the enhanced scan, the wall of abscess is enhanced and the cavity of abscess is non-enhanced. The lesion's range is clearer in the enhanced MRI.

[**Diagnosis**]

It should be differentiated from diseases including traumatic hematoma, pharyngeal cystic lymphangioma, and nasopharyngeal angiofibroma. a) The hematoma is manifested as high density in CT images, and high signal on both T1WI and T2WI. b) The cystic lymphangioma is a common disease in children with large range, which is different with abscess. c) Nasopharyngeal angiofibroma is seen in male adolescents. DSA can show the blood supply. The lesion is obviously enhanced after the injection of contrast medium on CT or MRI scans.

2 Nasopharyngeal tumors

(1) Nasopharyngeal carcinoma

[**Pathology and clinical manifestations**]

Nasopharyngeal carcinoma is one of the common malignant tumors in China. Most of them are poorly differentiated adenocarcinoma in pathology, and are more common in men. The clinical features are as follows: blood in mucus, epistaxis, tinnitus, auditory dysesthesia, nasal obstruction and headache.

[**Imaging appearances**]

1) CT

CT is the preferred examination. a) On the CT scan, the pharyngeal recesses shallow, disappear or swell up. The tumor in the upper, posterior and side walls will protrude into the nasopharyngeal cavity. The deep cervical lymph nodes are tumescence meanwhile. b) On the enhanced CT scan, the lesion can be enhanced homogeneously.

The tumor can extend or invade in different directions with its development. a) The tumor can protrude forward into the posterior nostrils and involve the pterygopalatine fossa, descending lamina of sphenoid bone, maxillary sinus, the posterior wall of the ethmoid sinus to the orbital cavity. b) The tumor can invade back to the musculus longus capitis, the basilar clivus, atlas, and the hypoglossal canal. c) The tumor can invade outward to the tubal torus, tensor veli palatini, levator veli palatini, medial pterygoid, lateral pterygoid and the infratemporal fossa, carotid sheath, styloid process. d) The tumor can invade upward in the cranial base and extend to the intracalvarium and cavernous sinus. e) The tumor can invade downward to the oropharynx and throat.

2) MRI

a) The tumor appears as low or middle signals on T1WI, and middle or high signals on T2WI. There is high signal in the ipsilateral mastoid on T2WI, which is secretory stitis media. b) On the enhanced MRI, the tumor can be enhanced homogeneously. The value of MRI lies in showing the involvement of clivus, cavernous sinus and mandibular nerve sensitively (Fig 3-4-1-A/B/C).

The nasopharyngeal carcinoma appears as thickened mucous membrane in

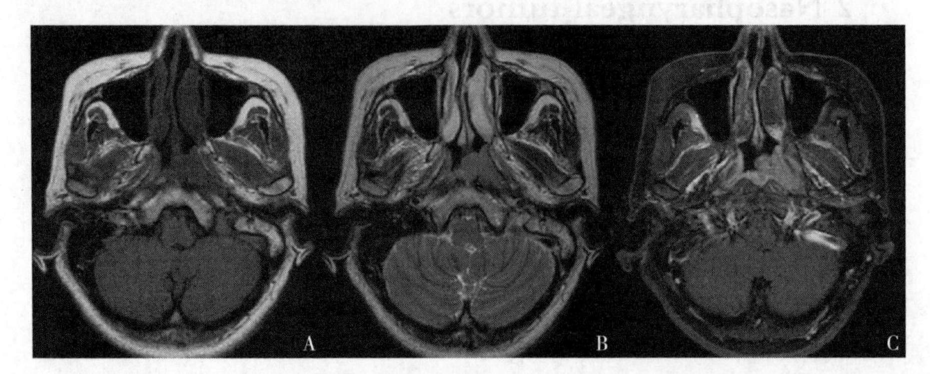

Fig 3-4-1-A/B/C Axial T1WI, T2WI, enhanced T1WI

the left pharynx nasalis, which is isointensity on T1WI and slightly higher intensity on T2WI. It is enhanced obviously.

[**Diagnosis**]

The pharyngeal mucosa lesions of nasopharyngeal carcinoma should be differentiated from the following diseases: a) adenoid hypertrophy: it is common in children and teenagers. The soft tissue in the nasopharyngeal top and posterior wall is thickened symmetrically, the surface of which is smooth or not. The lesion can be enhanced homogeneously. There is a long line enhanced obviously in the deep of the lesion, which represents the complete fascia of nasopharynx. b) nasopharyngeal non Hodgkin's lymphoma: The lymphomas in any other part of the body can enlarge concurrently. c) The malignant tumor of minor salivary gland is difficult to differentiate from the nasopharyngeal carcinoma, the lymph nodes metastasis in which are extremely rare. d) Besides these, the nasopharyngeal carcinoma's involvement in the skull base should be differentiated from the primary malignant tumors.

(2) Nasopharyngeal angiofibroma

[**Pathology and clinical manifestations**]

Nasopharyngeal angiofibroma is common in males aged 10 ~ 25 years. The clinical manifestations include progressive nasal obstruction and intractable epistaxis. The large tumor can create pressure on the neighboring nasal cavity, sinus, ear, and eye, and cause the corresponding syndromes. The pink mass can protrude to the nasopharyngeal cavity in the examination of nasopharynx and cause bleeding easily.

[**Imaging appearances**]

1) Radiography

DSA can show the rich blood vessels and define the feeding arteries and the draining veins.

2) CT

On the CT scan, the nasopharyngeal angiofibroma is manifested as the mass with soft tissue density. The tumor is lobulated, irregular and with distinct border. The nasopharyngeal cavity is deformed and narrow. The tumor can spread to the nasal cavity, sinus, eye sockets, pterygopalatine fossa and infratemporal fossa by the posterior naris. The bone around is pressed and absorbed. The sphenopalatine foramen and infratemporal fossa can be enlarged. On the enhanced CT scan, the tumor is enhanced obviously.

3) MRI

The mass is slightly low signal on T1WI and high signal on T2WI. There is vascular flow void with strip or dot low signal in the tumor, which is characteristically called "salt and pepper syndrome". The lesion is obviously enhanced (Fig 3-4-2-A/B/C).

[**Diagnosis**]

The nasopharyngeal angiofibroma should be differentiated from the adenoid hypertrophy, nasopharyngeal lymphoma, and carcinoma. Nasopharyngeal carcinoma: The mass appears as soft tissue density, the border of which is not smooth. The neighboring structures can be involved combined with the lymphatic metastasis. The differentiation of adenoid hypertrophy and nasopharyngeal lymphoma is discussed in the differentiation of nasopharyngeal carcinoma.

3 Obstructive sleep apnea hypopnea syndrome:

[**Pathology and clinical manifestations**]

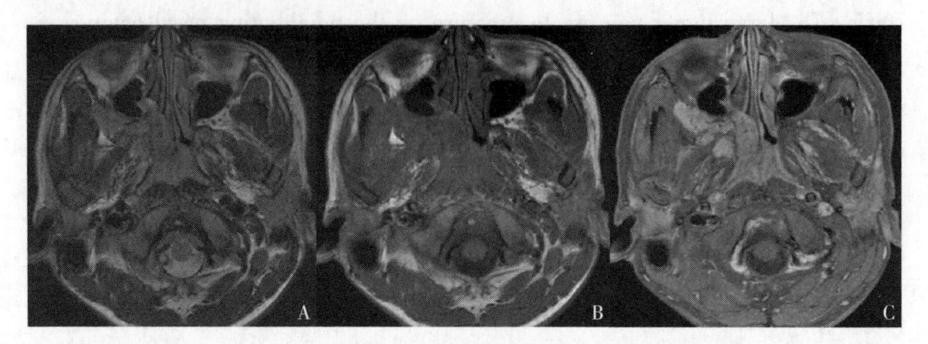

Fig 3-4-2-A/B/C T2WI, T1WI, enhanced T1WI: nasopharyngeal angiofibroma

The lesion is in the pharynx nasalis, which is isointensity on T1WI, isointensity on T2WI. It is obviously enhanced. It is difficult to make the differential diagnosis between nasopharyngeal angiofibroma and nasopharyngeal carcinoma.

The obstructive sleep apnea hypopnea syndrome is caused by the obstruction of upper respiratory tract and is usually combined with a series of clinical symptoms such as apnea, hypoventilation, and snoring. Polysomnography is the gold standard to confirm OSAHS. Imaging examination aims at the location of obstruction.

[**Imaging appearances**]

CT and MRI are used to show the location of obstruction. In adults, the common obstruction is in the pharynx nasalis, pharynx oralis or laryngohypopharynx. All diseases located in the above positions can cause obstruction. In children, the common obstruction is caused by the hypertrophy of tonsil and adenoid. All of these can be manifested in CT and MRI images.

Lesson 5 Larynx

Larynx lies in the throat, from the pharyngeal portion to the trachea. It is divided into supraglottic region, vocal area (ventricle of larynx), and subglottic region by the border of vocal cord.

Section 1 Imaging methods

CT is the main imaging technique in laryngopharyngeal diseases. MRI can show the lesions in all directions, which is a supplement to CT. The enhanced scan is used to make the qualitative diagnosis of the lesions.

Section 2 Diagnosis of diseases

1 Carcinoma of larynx

[**Pathology and clinical manifestations**]

The carcinoma of larynx is one of the common malignant tumors, accounting for 2% of systemic tumors. 93% ~ 95% tumors are squamous cell carcinoma. It is seen mainly in males aged over 40 years. It is mainly located in vocal area, then supraglottic region, but seldom in subglottic region. The main symptoms are as follows: foreign body sensation, laryngalgia, hoarseness, and dyspnea.

[**Imaging appearances**]

1) Ultrasonography

Ultrasonography is valuable in the diagnosis of lymphadenectasis.

2) CT

CT is the main imaging examination in carcinoma of larynx. On the CT scan, the lesion appears as the mass with soft tissue, protruding into the laryngeal cavity. The sinus piriformis is pressed and narrowed. The tumor can extend to the vocal cords on the other side, and invade the para-laryngeal space outward to the thyroid cartilage and muscles. The lymphadenectasis is seen in cervical space. The lesion is obviously enhanced (Fig 3-5-1-A/B/C).

3) MRI

The tumor appears isointensity on T1WI and high signal on T2WI, which is obviously enhanced. MRI has great advantage in showing the tumor's region.

[**Diagnosis**]

The imaging examination is essential before surgery, which can show the le-

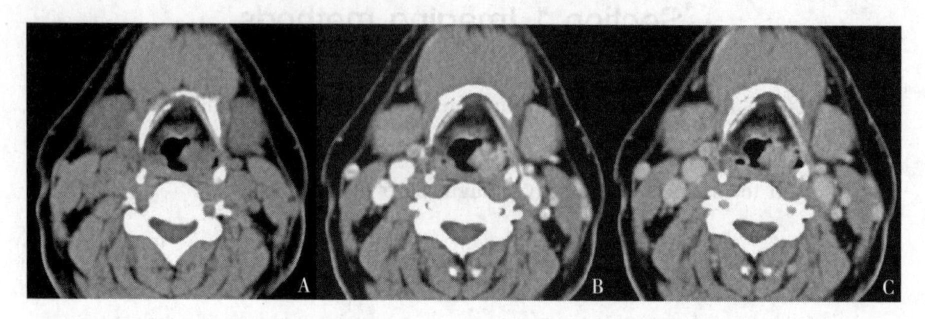

Fig 3-5-1-A/B/C Plain CT, enhanced CT scan: laryngeal carcinoma

The lesion is in the left of the laryngopharyngeal recess. It is isodensity and can be enhanced.

sions' range and cervical lymphatic metastasis. It should be differentiated from laryngeal polyp, papillary epithelioma, laryngophthisis, and amyloidosis of the larynx and so on. The laryngeal polyp and papillary epithelioma locate in the front of vocal cord and are confined to the mucous layer. The laryngophthisis and amyloidosis of the larynx rarely destroy the laryngeal cartilages.

Lesson 6 Oromaxillo-facial region

The imaging methods in oromaxillo-facial diseases include radiography, ultrasound, CT, and MRI. The radiography is used to observe the diseases of teeth and alveolar bone. DSA and ultrasound are mainly used in the diseases of salivary duct. CT is the routine examination. MRI is a supplement to CT, and is the main examination method of tongue and temporomandibular joint.

Section 1 Diagnosis of diseases

1 Parotid tumor

[**Pathology and clinical manifestations**]

90% of parotid tumors are originated in glandular epithelium. The mixed tumor is also known as pleomorphic adenoma, which is a common benign tumor located in the superficial parotid gland. The common malignant tumor is mucoepidermoid carcinoma. The benign tumor manifests as a soft, painless mass with clear border and long-term history. The malignant tumor can involve the nerve, cause pain and facial paralysis. It is difficult to open your mouth when the muscles of mastication are involved.

[**Imaging appearances**]

1) Radiography

Sialography: a) benign tumor: the Stensen's duct is tenuous, straight, or displaced. b) Malignant tumor: the Stensen's duct is pressed to shift, destroyed, or interrupted, and the contrast agent is forced to extravasate.

2) Ultrasonography

The tumor shows low echo. The echo is heterogeneous in large tumors. In the benign tumor, the border is well-defined and there are few blood signals in CDFI. The malignant tumor has an irregular shape and the border of which is ill-defined. There are many blood flow signals in CDFI.

3) CT

a) Benign tumor: In the plain scan, the round or lobulated tumor is iso or slightly high density with clear margin. The tumor can be slightly or moderately enhanced homogeneously. b) Malignant tumor: The mass is slightly high and heterogeneous density with ill-defined border. The mandible can be destroyed. And there are many enlarged cervical lymph nodes. On the enhanced CT scan, the tumor is enhanced obviously (Fig 3-5-2-A/B/C).

4) MRI

The tumor is manifested as isointensity or low signal on T1WI and low to high signals on T2WI. a) Benign tumor: It is round or lobulated mass with clear border, and can be enhanced homogeneously. b) Malignant tumor: It is irregular mass combined with enlarged cervical lymphoma nodes, and can be enhanced heterogeneously. The lymph node metastasis can be homogeneously or ring-shaped enhanced.

[**Diagnosis**]

The parotid tumor should be differentiated from lymphoma, crewels, metastasis, tumors in the ramus of mandible and parapharyngeal space, etc.

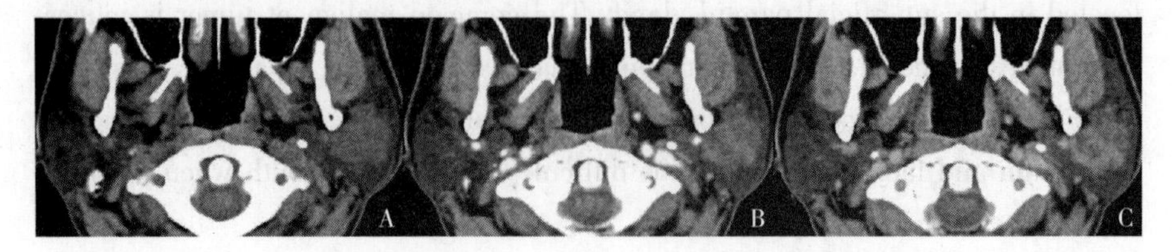

Fig 3-5-2-A/B/C Plain and enhanced CT scans

The pleomorphic adenoma is in the left parotid. The lesion is isodensity and is enhanced heterogeneously.

Lesson 7 Neck

The neck is separated by the deep and superficial fasciae, and encircles the thyroid gland, parathyroid gland, pharynx, larynx, trachea, esophagus and other hollow organs. There are a lot of lymph nodes in the cervical space.

Section 1 Imaging methods

1 Radiography

The radiography is rarely used in neck. DSA is used to show the relationship between the vessels and tumor, and the blood supply to tumor.

2 Ultrasonography

Ultrasonography is applied in the diagnosis of diseases at cervical lymph node, parathyroid gland, and thyroid gland. It is the first and main examination of thyroid gland diseases.

3 CT

CT is the main imaging technique in neck. It is inferior to US in the diagnosis of thyroid diseases. The enhanced CT scan is the routine examination. The lesion should be observed in soft tissue window. The bone window is used to show the cervical vertebrae and the cartilage when necessary. The enhanced CT scan is forbidden in untreated hyperthyroidism.

4 MRI

MRI has high soft tissue resolution and is valuable in diagnosis of cervical diseases, differentiation between cystic lesions, and between postoperative changes and recurrence. MRI is the main supplement to Ultrasound and CT. When the lesion is found, the patient should undergo enhanced MRI.

Section 2 Normal imaging findings of neck

1 Cervical soft tissue and space

DSA can show the respective features of vessels. In the US examination, the normal lymph node is round and small, the medulla of which shows high echo and the cortex of which shows low echo. CT can discriminate the cervical soft tissue: the subcutaneous fat and the fat in cervical space appear as low density. The cervical muscle, vessel, nerve and lymph appear as moderate density. The fascia can not be distinguished from the neighboring structures. The enhanced CT scan is used to show features of cervical vessels. The muscle, nerve and lymph node appear moderate signals on T1WI and T2WI of MR. The artery and vein appear flow void low signals. The fat is high or slightly high signal on T1WI and T2WI.

2 Thyroid gland and parathyroid gland

On the CT scan, the density of thyroid gland is slightly high and homogeneous because of the iodine contained. The thyroid gland is homogeneously and obviously enhanced on the enhanced CT scan. The signal of thyroid gland is slightly higher than the muscles on T1WI and T2WI respectively. The normal thyroid gland is too small to be distinguished in all imaging examinations.

3 Cervical lymph node

The lymph node is round or oval in the cervical space.

Section 3 Imaging signs of cervical diseases

1 The enlarge lymph node

The short diameter of the normal lymph nodes is below 5mm. It is suspicious of enlargement when the diameter of lymph node is between 5 ~ 8mm. The enlarged lymph is confirmed when the diameter is more than 8mm, which is common in inflammation, tubercle, metastasis and lymphoma. The enlarged lymph node appears as round and low echo mass on US image, and is isodensity on plain CT image and locates in the cervical space. The lesion can be enhanced homogeneously, heterogeneously or ring-shaped. The enlarged lymph node appears low signal on T1WI and high signal on T2WI.

2 Soft tissue

The cervical soft tissue is common in all tumors and inflammations. The location, shape, echo, density and signal are varied in different tumors. The carotid body tumor locates at the carotid bifurcation. The neurogenic tumor locates in the carotid space. The cystic lymphangioma can occupy several spaces with no echo, water density or signal intensity. The inflammation can spread to several cervical spaces.

3 The echo, density, and signal intensity in soft tissue space

The abnormalities of echo, density or signal intensity in one or several cervical spaces are common in inflammation, trauma and the lesions after radiotherapy etc.

4 The enlargement of thyroid gland and parathyroid gland

The diffuse enlargement of thyroid gland is found in goiter or chronic inflammation. The thyroid mass is in thyroid adenoma, thyroid carcinoma, lymphoma and multinodular goiter. The enlargement of parathyroid gland is common in parathyroid adenoma, carcinoma and hyperplasia.

Section 4 Diagnosis of diseases

1 Carotid body tumor

[**Pathology and clinical manifestations**]

The carotid body is located above or behind the carotid bifurcation, the diameter of which is about 5mm. The carotid body tumor is paraganglioma in middle-aged women, and is rare in clinical settings. The main clinical manifestations are cervical mass, dizziness, and headache. It can be combined with the vagus nerve and adrenergic nerve compression symptoms.

[**Imaging appearances**]

(1) Radiography

In DSA, the carotid bifurcation is broadened. And there is mass with rich blood supply in the carotid bifurcation.

(2) CT

On the CT scan, the lesion is manifested as round soft tissue with clear border, and is obviously enhanced after administration of contrast medium. CTA can show the compressed and displaced carotid artery and vein. The angle of carotid artery bifurcation is enlarged (Fig 3-7-1-A/B/C).

(3) MRI

The tumor is isointensity or slightly low signal on T1WI and high signal on T2WI. The signal is heterogeneous when the tumor is large enough. There are several flow void low signals in the lesion. The tumor is obviously enhanced.

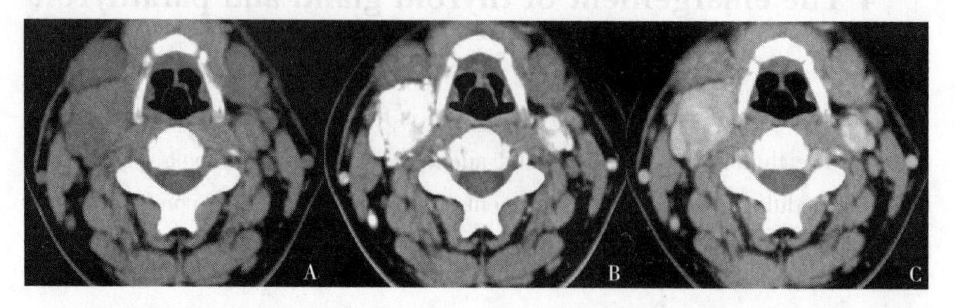

Fig 3-7-1-A/B/C Plain and enhanced CT scans (arterial phase and venous phase): The carotid body tumor in the right carotid bifurcation is isodensity on plain CT scan. It is obviously enhanced in the arterial phase.

MRA can show the enlargement of carotid bifurcation and the dissection between carotid artery and vein.

[**Diagnosis**]

The differential diagnoses include neurofibroma, schwannoma, lymphadenovarix and so on.

2 Thyroid tumor

[**Pathology and clinical manifestations**]

The thyroid tumors include benign and malignant ones. The main benign tumor is adenoma, accounting for 60%. The common malignant tumor is thyroid carcinoma, especially the papillary carcinoma. The benign and malignant tumors are common in females aged from 20 to 40 years old. It can cause hoarseness and dyspnea. The malignant tumor can be combined with the lymph node metastasis.

[**Imaging appearances**]

(1) Ultrasonography

The thyroid tumor appears as mass in the thyroid. The benign tumor has distinct border and homogeneous low echo, and there are few blood flow signals in or around it. The ill-defined border is seen in the malignant tumor, the echo of which is heterogeneous. There are rich blood flow signals around it.

(2) CT

The thyroid adenoma appears as round and oval mass with low density and distinct margin. The adenoma is non-enhanced or slightly enhanced after injection of contrast agent. Thyroid carcinoma has irregular shape and ill-distinct border with low density. There is focal calcification and necrosis with low density. The lesion is ill-defined from the surrounding structures. The cervical lymph nodes can be enlarged. On the enhanced CT scan, the thyroid carcinoma is enhanced heterogeneously. The lymph node metastasis is enhanced as ring-shaped.

(3) MRI

Thyroid adenoma appears as nodular with low, isointensity or high signal on T1WI, the border of which is clear. The follicular adenoma appears as high signal because of the gelatinoid contained. The thyroid carcinoma is heterogeneous hypointensity signal with ill-distinct border on T1WI. The thyroid adenoma and carcinoma appear as homogeneous and heterogeneous high signal on T2WI.

3 Goiter

[Pathology and clinical manifestations]

The goiter is seen in the area short of iodine, which is endemic goiter. But it will be sporadic goiter, too. It is common in the aged females.

[Imaging appearances]

(1) Ultrasonography

The thyroid gland is enlarged diffusely. One or more nodules can be seen in different echoes. CDFI shows the blood echo around the nodules.

(2) CT

a) There are nodules with low density in the diffusely enlarged thyroid gland, the density of which is homogeneous when it is small and heterogeneous when it is large. b) The goiter with multiple nodules can spread downwards to the front mediastinum. Sometimes there are low density nodules in the lesion with marginal calcification. c) Adenomatoid hyperplasia nodules can be enhanced slightly and the neighboring structures will not be involved.

(3) MRI

The swollen thyroid gland appears as heterogeneous high signal on T2WI. The signal appears as low to high on T1WI, which depends on the amount of colloid protein.

4 Parathyroid adenoma

[**Pathology and clinical manifestations**]

The parathyroid adenoma is a common cause of hyperparathyroidism. The adenoma has integrate envelope and rich blood. The first symptoms are as follows: bone-arthrosis pain, fracture after micro trauma, urinary calculus, decreased appetite, abdominal distension, constipation and so on. The characteristic laboratory index is the increased parathyroid hormone. The serum calcium, urinary calcium, and urinary phosphorus are increased and the serum phosphorus is reduced.

[**Imaging appearances**]

(1) Radiography

The plain film of skeletal system: the bone appears as different kinds of low density. The pathological fracture can be concurrent and multiple. The abdominal film can show the renal calculus.

(2) Ultrasonography

The parathyroid adenoma has homogeneous hypo-echo, the border of which is well-defined with intact capsule. There are hemorrhage and cyst formation in the adenoma, which can cause the echo changes (Fig 3-7-2).

(3) CT

a) On the CT scan, the parathyroid adenoma is located in the lower pole of the thyroid gland and the gap by the side of tracheal-bronchus. The lesion is manifested as soft tissue nodule with homogeneous density and distinct border. The diameter of the lesion is 1 to 3cm. A few adenomas are heterogeneous density with single or multiple low densities within the lesion. The wall of the cystic lesion varies in depth, which is cause by the necrosis and remote hemorrhage. b) On the enhanced CT scan, the nodule appears obviously homogeneous or

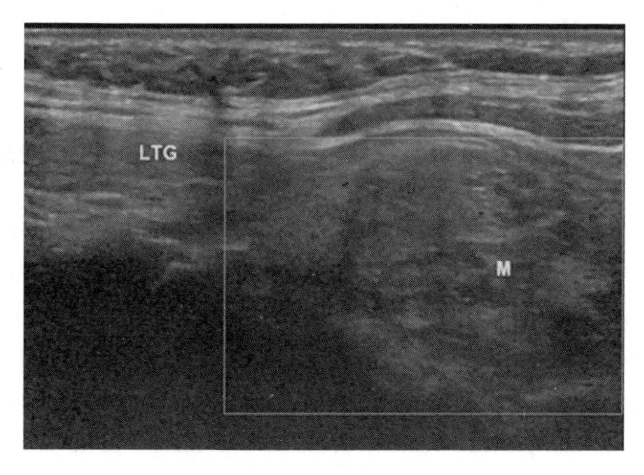

Fig 3-7-2 Adenoma of parathyroid

ring-shaped enhanced.

(4) MRI

The adenoma is isointensity or low signal on T1WI and high signal on T2WI. Some adenomas appear as heterogeneous signals. The enhanced form of the adenoma is similar to CT.

Chapter 4

Imaging of the Respiratory System

The diseases of the respiratory system are common and complex. Imaging methods are very important in diagnosis of the respiratory system. Radiography is the primary examination of chest due to its good natural contrast. Ultrasound is an uncommon technique in the respiratory system because the lung and the skeleton can reflect ultrasonic waves. CT is the most important method for the respiratory system. CT scan can provide detailed cross-section images of the thorax. The images can be electronically modified to display different tissues. Dynamically enhanced CT can show the blood provision of lesion. MRI can usually be used to distinguish masses in the mediastinum and to evaluate the relation between tumor and heart and great vessels. However, MRI has limited usage in the trachea, bronchus, and lung without hydrogen proton.

Lesson 1 Imaging Methods

1 Radiography

(1) Chest radiography

It is the most common examination in chest diseases. The conventional projection position is: a) Posteroanterior and lateral plain films are the most common projection positions. They are often used in the first examination, localization and post-operation re-examination. They are also the most common methods of health examination. b) Oblique position is often used for detection of rib fractures.

(2) Chest fluoroscopy

Chest fluoroscopy is an uncommon method. It can be used for detection of abnormal movement of diaphragmatic muscles.

2 Ultrasonography

Ultrasonography is an uncommon technique in the respiratory system.

3 CT

(1) Plain CT

Plain CT is a conventional method in the respiratory system. Many diseases of the respiratory system can be diagnosed by plain CT. It routinely provides transverse section images from the apex of lung to the base without contrast enhancement. There are different observing windows, such as lung window which is used to observe the structure of lung and mediastinum window which is used to see other details.

(2) Enhanced CT

Enhanced CT scanning is often performed after finding lesion by plain CT. It is performed by intravenous injection of contrast medium. Foci may be clearly visualized after enhanced CT scanning. It can be usually used to determine the origin of masses, differentiate diagnosis of benign or malignant masses, and evaluate the relation between tumor and great vessels. Patients who are allergic with iodine agents can not undergo this examination.

(3) Post processing technique

Post processing technique can show the lesion's character, position and the relationship with adjacent tissues.

① ***HRCT***: HRCT uses thinner sections (0.3mm-2mm) and smaller FOV to show greater lung detail. It eliminates the partial volume effect and improves spatial resolution. It is useful to evaluate diffuse lung diseases and small lung nodules.

② ***Multiplanar reformation***: MPR uses volume data of MSCT to reformate the images in coronal, sagittal and oblique positions. It is useful in judging the lesion's origin and its relationship with other tissues.

③ ***Minimum intensity projection***: It uses minIP to show global images of trachea and arbor bronchialis. It is useful in detecting the lesion of trachea and bronchi, such as bronchi tumor and bronchiectasis.

④ ***CT virtual endoscopy***: CTVE is a method to imitate bronchoscopes by the volume data of MSCT. It is useful in observing intracavitary lesion of bronchi.

⑤ ***Lung nodule analysis***: Lung nodule analysis technique uses gray level histogram to judge the percentage of different CT values in the nodule. It can compute doubling time of the nodule by comparing different volumes of examinations. It is helpful in identifying the peculiarity of the lung nodule.

(4) Energy spectrum

CT is useful in identifying the peculiarity of lymph nodes by energy spectrum curve analysis.

4 MRI

(1) Plain MRI

Plain MRI is a conventional method to get the T1-and T2-weighted images of axial, coronal and sagittal sections. It is used not only to discover the lesion of mediastinum and thoracic wall, but also to diagnose cyst. It is very important for the diagnoses of bigger masses of mediastinum and lung, for example, DWI can provide useful information of the lesion.

(2) Enhanced MRI

Enhanced MRI can evaluate blood supply of the lesion, detect cyst and necrosis and show its relationship with great vessels.

Lesson 2 Normal imaging of chest

Section 1 Radiography

1 Compages of thorax

The normal chest radiography is a comprehensive projection of intrathoracic and extrathoracic tissues and organs, including soft tissues, bone, heart and great vessels, lung, pleura, and diaphragm (Fig 4-2-1).

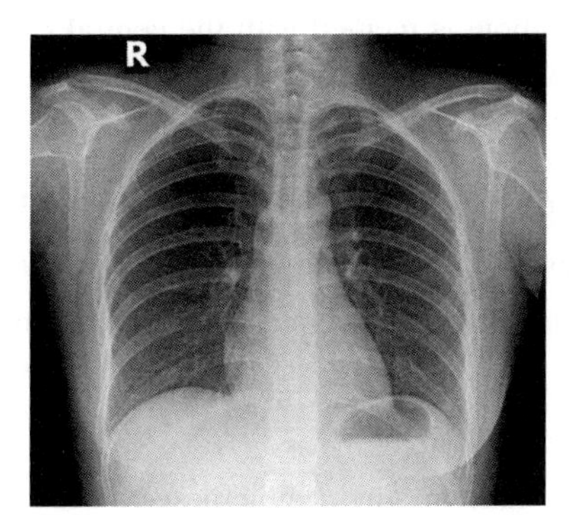

Fig 4-2-1 Normal chest radiography

(1) Soft tissues of chest wall

1) Sternocleidomastoid muscle and skin reflection over the clavicle

Sternocleidomastoid muscle in the neck may cause a homogeneous shadow in the apex of lung with a well-defined lateral margin. Skin reflection over the clavicle is on the upper border of the clavicle; there is a horizontal band-like shadow running parallel to the bone, which is produced by the fold of the skin and subcutaneous tissue.

2) Musculi pectoralis major

In young and strong males, it forms a fan-shaped shadow in the middle and outer bands of bilateral lungs with a well defined inferior margin, which is continuous with the skin fold of axilla.

3) Breast and nipple

The breast on each side of the thorax superimposes on lower lung field. It causes a hemispherical opacity with a smooth and clear inferior border.

The nipples sometimes appear as two small round shadows with intermediate density in the lower lung field, which are often found in elderly females.

(2) Bony thoracic cage

It is made up by thorax vertebra, ribs, sternum, clavicle, and scapula.

1) Thorax vertebra

Usually the upper four thoracic vertebral bodies can be seen, but the rest part of the thoracic vertebrae is merged with the central cardio-vascular shadow in the routine P-A view.

2) Ribs

The first to tenth ribs are connected to the sternum by costal cartilages that are invisible before calcified. Variations in the size or shape of one or more ribs are also common, which include cervical rib, bifurcation of rib and fusion of rib etc.

3) Sternum

In the P-A view, sternum almost superposes on the mediastinal shadows.

4) Clavicle

The medial ends of the clavicles should be equidistant from the midline.

5) Scapula

In the P-A view, the medial margin of scapula should not be misinterpreted as the thicken pleura and the secondary ossification center of the inferior angle should not be misinterpreted as fracture.

(3) Pleura

The pleura around the periphery of the lung is only visible in certain regions. On the right side, the horizontal fissure which separates the right upper and middle lobes can be seen on chest radiography. It appears as a thin and dense line. In the P-A view, it extends from the level of the sixth rib in the axilla to within 1cm of the hilum. In the lateral view, the horizontal fissure runs from the hilum straight to the anterior chest wall. The oblique fissures separate the lower lobe from the rest of the lung and are often visible on the lateral film. They begin at the level of the fourth or fifth thorax vertebra as a straight or convex line and extend to the diaphragm.

An azygos fissure is a common variation. It encloses the azygos vein and separates an azygos lobe from the rest of the right upper lobe.

2 Lung

(1) Lung field

Both lungs appear as translucent fields on chest film. Lung fields are divided into three equal parts longitudinally named inner, middle and outer zones. People also imagine drawing two transverse lines under the second and fourth anterior ribs respectively, and the lung field is divided into upper, middle and lower fields.

(2) Hilum

The hilar shadows consist of pulmonary arteries, veins and major bronchi. In the P-A view, hilar shadows are in the middle field and inner zone, and the left hilum is 1 ~ 2cm higher than the right. The hilum is divided into the upper part and lower part. The intersectant obtuse angle of right hilum is called hilar angle. The hilar angle is formed by the inner section of the superior pulmonary vein and the descending pulmonary artery. In the lateral view, the left and right hilar shadows overlap, and the right hilum is just anterior to the left; the hilar shadows appear as a long-tail comma.

(3) Lung markings

Lung markings are chiefly composed of pulmonary arteries, and pulmonary veins. Bronchi, lymphatic vessels and some interstitial tissues also participate in it. The normal markings always extend from the hilum toward the lung periphery in all directions.

(4) Lung lobes and segments

1) Lobes

The lungs are divided into lobes. The right lung has three lobes (upper, middle and lower lobes) and the left lung has two lobes (upper and lower lobes).

2) Segments

Each lobe consists of 2 ~ 5 bronchopulmonary segments anatomically. Bronchopulmonary segments are wedge shaped, with base lying peripherally and apex lying towards the hilum. Each segment has its own segmental bronchus.

(5) Trachea and bronchi

The trachea is divided into the left and right main bronchi at the level of the fifth or sixth thoracic vertebrae. At the bifurcation, the internal ridge that separates the two main bronchi is the carina. The bifurcation angle is normally 60°~85°. The main bronchi are divided into lobar bronchi, which in turn are divided into segmental bronchi. The segmental bronchi are subdivided into bronchiole, respiratory bronchiole and alveoli.

3 Mediastinum

The mediastinum is situated between the pleural cavities. It is behind the sternum and located before the vertebral column. The upper border is the thoracic inlet and the lower border is the diaphragm. Mediastinum contains heart, great vessels, trachea, main bronchi, esophagus, lymph tissue, thymus, neural tissue, fat tissue and other tissues. An imaginary plane extending from the sternal angle to the lower border of T4 vertebra divides the mediastinum into the superior and inferior mediastinum. They are subdivided into three parts: anterior, middle and posterior areas.

4 Diaphragm

The diaphragm consists of a peripheral muscular part and a central tendon. It separates the thoracic and abdominal cavities. The diaphragm attaches to the costal margin, sternum and the lumbar vertebrae. The diaphragm has three main hiatus: aortic hiatus, esophageal hiatus and vena caval foramen.

As viewed from the front, the diaphragm is divided into two domes. The level of the right hemidiaphragm is usually near the anterior end of the fifth or sixth rib, and the right dome is 1~2cm higher than the left. The diaphragm joins the thoracic wall to form acute angles, which are termed as costophrenic angles. The costophrenic angles are sharp in the P-A view. The posterior costophrenic angles are the deepest in the lateral view.

Movement of both domes is usually symmetrical. Eventration always involves the right dome of the diaphragm. It is due to deficiency of muscle or unevenness of tension. Eventration presents as unilateral elevation of the diaphragm. Changes of the shape and location of diaphragm may occur due to the pressure changes of thoracic cavity or abdomen cavity.

Section 2 CT

The tissues of thorax are very complex, such as lung, fat, muscle and bone. Their density and CT values are different. They have to be viewed by at least two window levels and window widths (Fig 4-2-2-A/B). The CT images of thorax are usually composed of different transverse sections, and they will be reformed by coronal or sagittal planes as necessary.

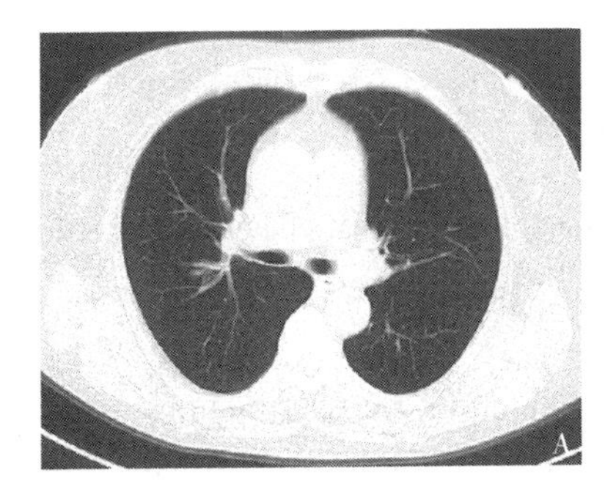

Fig 4-2-2-A Normal chest CT lung window

1 Chest wall

(1) Muscles of chest wall

The mediastinum window can identify pectoralis major, pectoralis minor, breast, latissimus dorsi, teres minor, subscapularis, and the fat of axillary cavity.

(2) Skeleton of chest

The bone window can show manubrium, body of sternum, xiphoid process, thoracic vertebrae, ribs, and scapula. Three-dimensional reformation technique can display the skeleton of chest spatially.

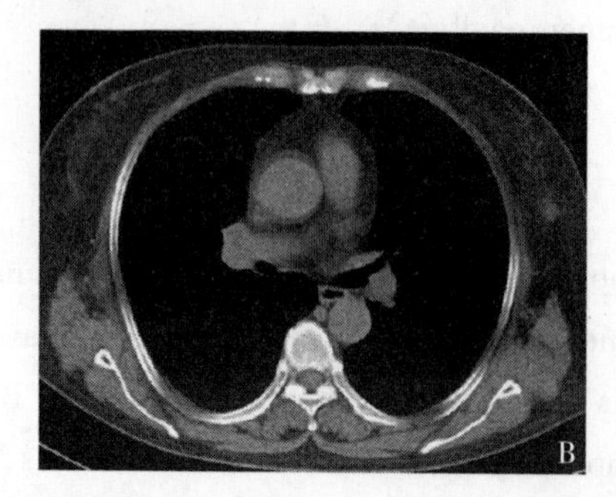

Fig 4-2-2-B Normal chest CT mediastinum window

2 Mediastinum

(1) Anterior mediastinum is located between sternum and heart. It mainly has thymus gland and lymph nodes. Thymus gland's density depends on its content of fat.

(2) Middle mediastinum has many structures such as trachea, main bronchi, great vessels, phrenic nerve, recurrent laryngeal nerve, pneumogastric nerve, lymph nodes and heart. The lymph nodes are mainly distributed along trachea and main bronchi.

(3) Posterior mediastinum is located between esophagus and thoracic vertebrae. It has esophagus, descending aorta, thoracic duct, azygos vein, hemiazygos vein and lymph nodes.

The lymph nodes of mediastinum are present as round or arch tissues, and its short diameter is not more than 10mm normally. It is abnormal if the short diameter is longer than 15mm.

3 Lung

(1) Lung field

The conventional CT can just detect lung field only or hilum by the image of one section. The vessels of the lung become thinner from center to periphery, and they are presented as round shadow on one section. The concomitant relationship, relative position, and lumen's size of bronchi and its vessels are constant. The size of bronchi is close to its concomitant pulmonary artery.

(2) Hilum

CT can show the hilum better than radiography. Enhanced CT is the best way to show the structure of hilum.

1) Right hilum

Right pulmonary artery is divided into two vessels: upper and lower pulmonary arteries.

2) Left hilum

Left pulmonary artery continues to left lower pulmonary artery across the left main bronchi. Left upper pulmonary artery is divided into two vessels to supply the corresponding lung segment.

(3) Fissura

Fissura is actually the margin of two adjacent lobes. It can be seen as a transparent zone in lung window. The fissura can be shown clearly as line shadow by HRCT.

(4) Lobe, segment and secondary pulmonary lobule

1) Lobe

Fissura is the marker to identify the lobe.

2) Segment

Bronchopulmonary segments are cone-shaped, with the apex lying towards the hilum.

3) Secondary pulmonary lobule

Secondary pulmonary lobule is often referred to as lung lobule, which is considered the anatomy unit of the lung. From HRCT, each lobule can be seen separated from an adjacent lobule by an interlobular septum. The center of lung lobules is composed of lobule arteries and bronchioles. The parenchyma of lung lobule is made up of acini which are surrounded by areolar tissues.

4 Diaphragm

The diaphragm is a dome-shaped muscle. Most part of diaphragm is close to the organs such as heart, liver and spleen. The density of diaphragm is hard to identify because it is very similar to other organs. The lower part of diaphragm forms diaphragm angle.

Section 3 MRI

The MRI performances of normal thorax depend on the signal intensity of different tissues. The lung, fat, muscle and bone tissues show different black and white gradation in MRI images because of their different signal intensities in MRI.

1 Chest wall

The muscle, tendon, ligament, compact bone and fascia of chest wall show black or gray on T1WI and T2WI because they have shorter T1 and T2 relaxation time. On the contrary, fat and spongy bone show white on T1WI and gray on T2WI.

2 Mediastinum

Lumens of trachea and main bronchi have no signal on MRI. Great vessels can be seen because they are surrounded by fat, and the fat has high signal on MRI. The esophagus can be shown better because it has the similar signal with muscle. Lymph nodes present as round middle signal on T1WI and T2WI, and their diameters are the same as on CT images.

3 Lung

The lung markings on MRI can not be shown as well as in CT scan, because they have no signal.

4 Diaphragm

The diaphragm can be seen clearly in images of MRI's transverse section. It presents as a thin and curved low signal. The height and modality of diaphragm can be shown in images of MRI's coronal and sagittal views. The diaphragm has lower signal than liver and spleen.

Lesson 3 Imaging Signs of Chest Diseases

The diseases of chest can present different abnormalities such as appearance, size, number, density and signal. These abnormalities on images are pathological reflections of the diseases. It is helpful to know the imaging signs of chest diseases for diagnosis.

Section 1 Pulmonary diseases

1 Obstruction of bronchi

Obstruction of bronchi is caused by intracavitary or extrinsic compression. There are mainly three obstruction types, namely obstructive emphysema, obstructive pneumonia, and obstructive atelectasis, according to different etiological factors, degrees, and duration.

(1) Obstructive emphysema

Emphysema is a permanent enlargement of the air spaces distal to the terminal bronchiole accompanied by inconvertible destruction of their walls. Emphysema can be classified into two kinds: i. e., localized and diffused.

1) Radiography

①***Localized obstructive emphysema***: It presents that increased translucency can be seen in local part of the lung. The scale of it depends on the position of obstruction. One side of lung's emphysema can be shown as that the lung's translucency has been increased; lung markings are rare; mediastinum has moved to the unaffected side; and diaphragm of the affected side has moved down.

②***Diffused obstructive emphysema***: Both lung fields demonstrate hyperlucency on radiography, and bullous emphysema are usually seen. In advanced stage, the lung volume has been increased; the hemidiaphragm has been flattened; the retrosternal space has been enlarged; and the intercostal space has been widened. Changes of heart and great vessels include long and narrow heart shadow, enlargement of pulmonary artery, and attenuation of peripheral lung markings. Pulmonary hypertension can be seen in the worst case.

2) CT

CT can show the position and reason of obstructive emphysema (Fig 4-3-1). The presentation on image in CT is the same as in radiography.

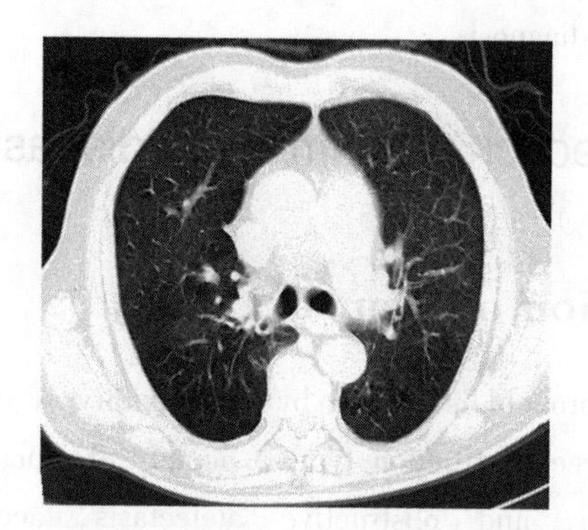

Fig 4-3-1 Emphysema, both lung fields demonstrate hyperlucency on CT

(2) Obstructive atelectasis

Obstructive atelectasis refers to a loss of lung parenchyma caused by the reduced influx. Reasons that may cause atelectasis include obstruction of bronchus, extrinsic compression from extra-pulmonary diseases, and contraction of intrapulmonary cicatrization. The most common reason is obstruction of bronchus. The lobe collapses because air in alveoli is absorbed during 18 ~ 24 hours after complete obstruction of the bronchus. The obstruction may occur in major bronchus, lobes, segments or bronchioles, resulting in one-side, lobe, segmental, or lobular atelectasis, respectively.

1) Radiography

①***One-side atelectasis***: The atelectatic lung shows homogeneous high density because it is devoid of air. The mediastinum has moved to the affected side. The intercostal space becomes narrow. The diaphragm gets higher and the unaffected side shows compensatory emphysema.

②***Lobe atelectasis***: The general demonstration includes atrophy of the obstructed lobe, increase of its density, and the compensatory emphysema of unobstructed lobe nearby, which is reflected by displacement of fissures and the movement of hilum towards the sick lobe (Fig 4-3-2-A).

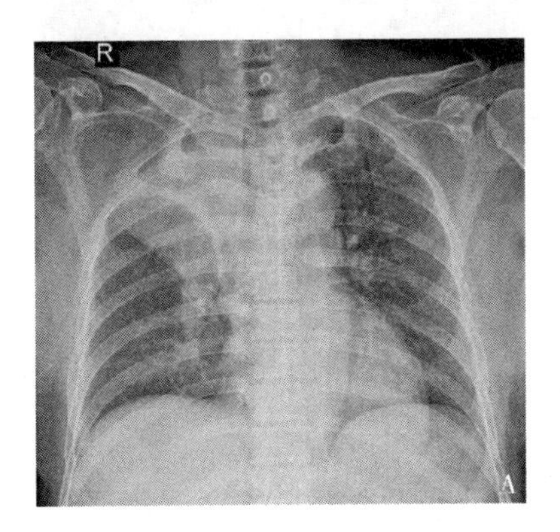

Fig 4-3-2-A Radiography: obstructive lobe atelectasis

③***Segmental atelectasis***: The simple segmental atelectasis is rare. It presents shadows like triangles with basement outwards and the apex towards the hilum in the P-A view.

④***Lobulus atelectasis***: It is often seen in lobular pneumonia, presenting as small patching shadows.

2) CT

①***One-side atelectasis***: The sick side presents soft tissue's density because of constriction. It becomes enrichment when given enhanced CT. The enhanced CT can show the position and reason for obstruction of main bronchi.

②***Lobe atelectasis***: Lobe atelectasis presents as a condensing shadow of triangle, with the apex towards the hilum in most cases (Fig 4-3-2-B).

③***Segmental atelectasis***: The segmental atelectasis is often seen as the internal or external segment of right middle lobe. The segment atelectasis presents

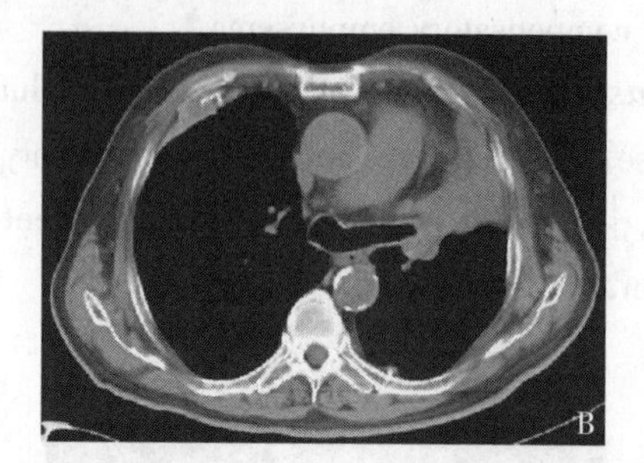

Fig 4-3-2-B CT: obstructive lobe atelectasis

as a condensing triangle shadow of soft tissue's density. That is often close to right side of the heart.

④*Lobulus atelectasis*: The performance of CT is similar to radiography.

3) MRI

The lobe or segmental atelectasis presents higher signal in T1WI images and high signal in T2WI images.

2 Consolidation

Consolidation means the replacement of air in the alveoli by pathological fluid, cells or tissues, which may be inflammatory exudation, edema fluid, blood, and granuloma or tumor tissues. The scale of consolidation can be acinus, lobule, segment or lobe. The causes of pulmonary consolidation include infection, pulmonary edema, pulmonary contusion, hemorrhage, infarction, pulmonary tuberculosis, alveolar carcinoma and mycoses.

(1) Radiography

The scale of consolidation varies. The inflammatory exudate within airspaces and interstitium of the affected lung causes the opacification and air-filled bronchioles outlined by adjacent fluid-filled alveoli in affected lung produce the air bronchogram.

The onset may be so acute that opacification is often at its maximum on the initial radiograph (Fig 4-3-3-A). Consolidation may not spread uniformly throughout the lobe. From the initial focus of infection inflammatory edema spreads via the air passages and the pores of Kohn, and as a result consolidation may conform to segmental boundaries. Resolution is accompanied by diminution of the density of the opacity as air returns to the lobe, and it is usually complete, with the lung architecture being restored to normal.

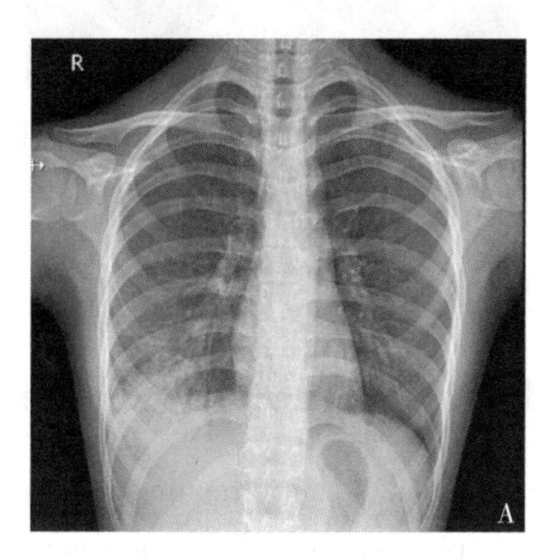

Fig 4-3-3-A Radiography: consolidation of right lung

(2) CT

The acute consolidation with effusion can present homogeneous high density shadow on lung window and soft tissue density shadow on mediastinum window. Air bronchogram can be seen in the bigger lesion (Fig 4-3-3-B).

The lesion of chronic consolidation can be seen higher density than acute one. The shadow looks like plum petals with limpid borders when the lesion occurs only in acinus.

(3) MRI

The consolidation with effusion presents ill-defined border lamellar high signal in T1WI images and higher signal in T2WI images. Sometimes, air bronchogram can be seen because the lesion has air-filled bronchus and vascular flow void. The signals' intensity differs because of the different content of protein in effusion.

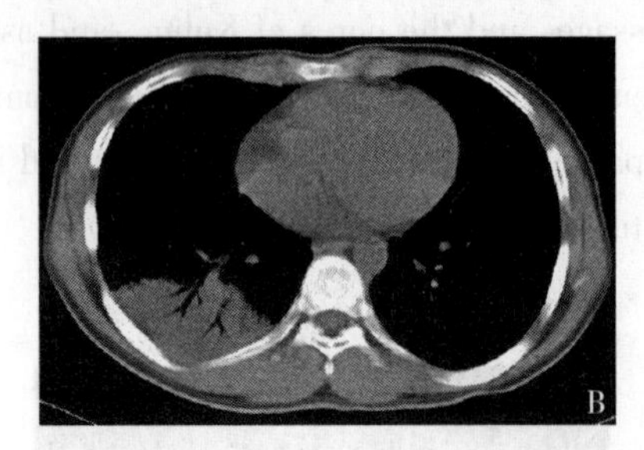

Fig 4-3-3-B CT: consolidation, air bronchogram of right lung

3 Cavity and intrapulmonary air containing space

Cavity: The central portion of the intrapulmonary diseases undergoes liquefaction and necrosis and is coughed up through the communication with bronchial tree and replaced by air. The process is called cavity. Cavity is often seen in tuberculosis, lung cancer or fungus.

The wall of thick cavity is more than 3mm in thickness, and that of thin cavity is less than 3mm. Intrapulmonary air containing space refers to abnormal enlargement of primary intrapulmonary interspaces, including bullae and bronchogenic cysts.

(1) Radiography

1) Thin cavity

The wall of cavity is composed of thin fibrous, granulation and caseous tissues. It presents as round or irregular shape. The margin of cavity is clear. There are spot-like lesions around the cavity. This kind of cavity is often seen in pulmonary tuberculosis or metastatic tumor.

2) Thick cavity

The wall of cavity is more than 5mm in thickness. There are high density lesions around the cavity. The inner wall of cavity is slick or unsmooth. This kind of cavity is often seen in pulmonary tuberculosis or peripheral lung cancer. The cavity of peripheral lung cancer has wall nodules.

3) The wall

The wall of intrapulmonary air containing space is thin and its depth is less than 1mm. There is no consolidation around the lesion and no liquid in the cavity.

(2) CT

CT is more sensitive than radiography and can show the details of cavity (Fig 4-3-4-A). CT can present the position, size, wall, thickness, and periphery lung of the cavity. The intrapulmonary air containing space mainly contains congenital lung cyst and bulla, and the former is bigger (Fig 4-3-4-B).

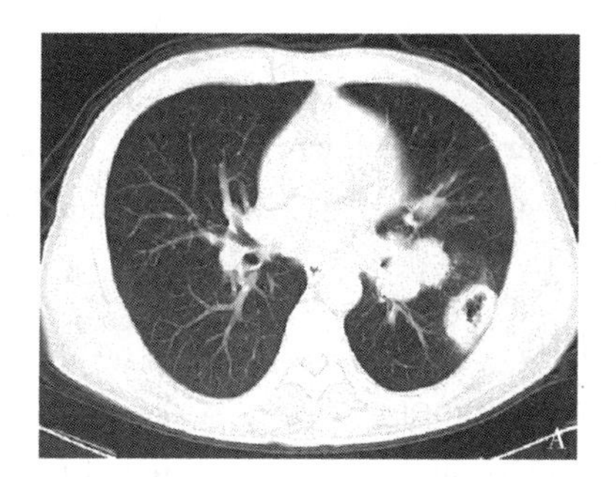

Fig 4-3-4-A CT: cavity with thick wall

(3) MRI

The cavity presents low signal shadow on T1WI or T2WI because of air. The wall of cavity presents middle signal shadow on MRI. MRI is not better than CT in showing details of the cavity's wall.

4 Nodule and mass

The lesion can be seen as nodule or mass when it shows modality of pathology. Radiographically, a nodule is defined as a lesion smaller than 3 cm in diameter. Those larger than 3 cm are termed as masses. Nodule or mass can be single or multiple. The usual causes of a solitary lesion are pulmonary carcinoma, tu-

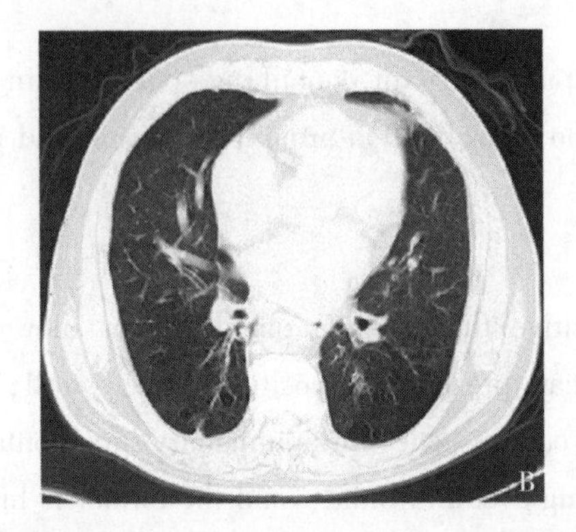

Fig 4-3-4-B CT: intrapulmonary air containing space

berculoma, and inflammatory pseudotumor when the lesion is single. The usual causes of multiple lesions are metastases, necrotic granuloma and multiple lung cysts.

(1) Radiography

1) Lung benign lung tumor

It always has an envelope and presents as a round mass with smooth margin. The hamartoma can have calcification that looks like popcorn.

2) Lung malignant lung tumor

It always grows up by invasive way and doesn't have a sharp margin. It shows a lobulated, notched, or infiltrating outline. Pleural retraction is also seen in pulmonary carcinoma.

Tuberculoma tends to be a smooth discrete nodule with spot calcifications and satellite lesions. The presence of fat and "popcorn" calcification will indicate a hamartoma, which is a benign neoplasm in the lung. Pulmonary metastases produce multiple well-defined shadows in the bilateral lung fields and vary in size.

(2) CT

CT can show more details of the nodule or mass (Fig 4-3-5-A/B/C/D). It can analyze signs, including modality, structure and margin, which are useful for diagnosing the disease.

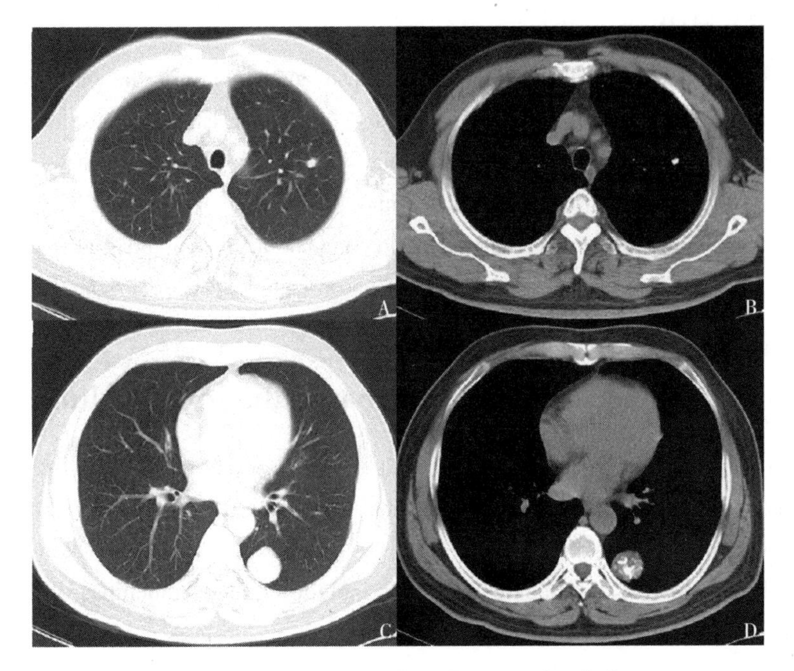

Fig 4-3-5-ABCD CT: nodule and mass with calcification

The CT can show signs of lobulation, vacuole signs, barb signs, and pleural indentation signs, and all of these signs can be seen in peripheral lung carcinoma frequently. It is helpful in identifying hamartoma if fat density can be found in lesion. Tuberculoma tend to have draining bronchi with thick wall. It is always surrounded by many satellite lesions of different sizes.

The enhanced CT is also useful in diagnosing the diseases. Tuberculoma tend to be circular periphery enhanced slightly. Benign lung tumor can show no enhancement or mild homogeneous enhancement. Malignant lung tumor can be enhanced evidently. Inflammatory pseudotumor can show circular or mild enhancement.

Acinus nodules are defined as consolidation within acini, which appear as plum petals, no more than 1cm in diameter (always less than 4mm). It can be seen in inflammation or acute miliary pulmonary tuberculosis. Miliary nodules are usually widespread in distribution and approximately equal in size.

(3) MRI

The signals in MRI are different because components of the mass include vessels, fibrous connective tissues, muscles, and fats. Chronic granuloma, caseating pulmonary tuberculosis, and hamartoma can be seen as lower signal on T2WI. Lung cancer or metastatic tumor may present higher signal on T2WI. The necrosis of lesion and cyst can present low signal on T1WI and high signal on T2WI. The lesion full of vessels cannot show signal because of the flow void effect.

5 Reticular, linear, and band shadows of lung

Reticular, linear, and band shadows of lung are due to interstitial diseases. Common etiological factors include effusion, phlogocyte, fibrous connective tissue, or granulation tissue.

The common interstitial lung diseases include chronic bronchitis, idiopathic pulmonary fibrosis, carcinomatous lymphangitis, asbestosis, and connective-tissue disorders.

The images vary because the interstitial lung diseases have different pathological peculiarities, scales or durations.

(1) Radiography

Extensive interstitial diseases present as mottling, honeycomb, reticular or nodular shadows (Fig 4-3-6-A). A honeycomb pattern indicates extensive destruction of lung tissues, with lung parenchyma replaced by thin-walled cysts.

Localized fibrosis may present as a few or numerous irregular parallel or radiating linear shadows of bands with varying thickness, which show high density on chest film. It is often seen after the recovery of pulmonary tuberculosis.

Interlobular proliferation or liquid accumulation may form septal lines on chest film, which is most commonly encountered in venous pulmonary hypertension and interstitial pulmonary edema. There is a common type of septal line: Kerley's B lines, which are short, thin horizontal lines at the periphery of the lung near the costophrenic angles, about 2cm in length and 1mm-2mm in width.

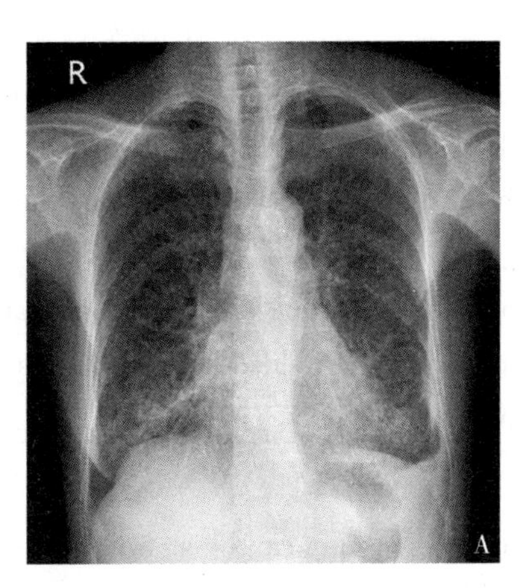

Fig 4-3-6-A Radiography: reticular, linear and band shadows of lung

(2) CT

CT, especially HRCT, is of great value in detecting early slight fibrosis and displaying subtle changes of interlobular septa thickness (Fig 4-3-6-B).

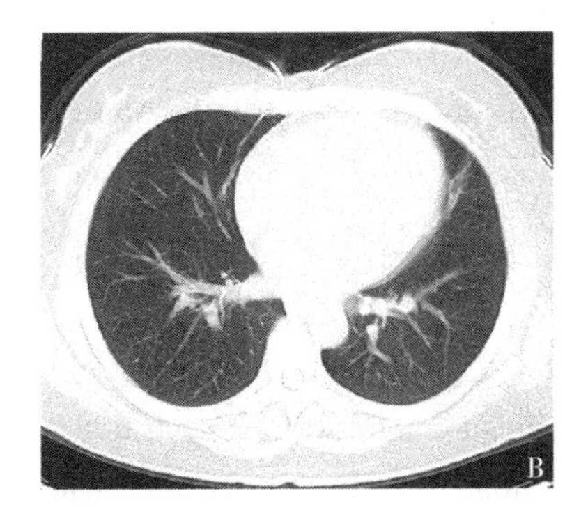

Fig 4-3-6-B CT: band shadows of both lungs

At the early stage of interstitial lung diseases, there are line shadows connecting with pleura, which are 1cm-2cm in length. They become polygon mesh shadows.

In the middle stage of interstitial lung diseases, there are adjacent thick interlobular septa that link together in extensive pulmonary fibrosis. They are 2cm~5cm in length, presenting as arc lines parallel to chest wall within 1cm to pleura, and are called subpleural lines.

At the late stage of interstitial lung diseases, there are shadows like honeycomb near the pleura in lower lung fields. They will expand to whole lung fields at later stage of pulmonary fibrosis.

(3) MRI

The bigger band shadows of lung can be shown in MRI images. They present as middle signals on T1WI or T2WI.

6 Calcification

Calcification usually occurs in areas of necrosis or degeneration. Pulmonary calcification may be a common finding in tuberculosis, hamartomas, silicosis, metastasis of osteosarcoma, and pulmonary microlithiasis.

(1) Radiography

The radiographic appearance may be tiny flecks, miliary spots or nodular shadows of very high density. The edge is very well defined and the size varies. Tuberculosis calcification is always located in the upper parts of lung and it presents as spots. The calcification of silicosis can be seen multiple, nodular shadows, and be full of two sides of lung. Calcification of eggshell type is often seen in lymph nodes.

(2) CT

The density of calcification is higher than soft tissue on mediastinum window and its CT value is more than 100HU. The lamellar calcification is always a benign lesion and it is common to occur in granuloma. The calcification of hamartomas has a typical popcorn pattern. The calcification of peripheral lung cancer is complex. It can be a single spot or multiple patches. The calcification of eggshell type in hilum lymph nodes can be seen in silicosis. Generally, the larger proportion of calcification accounts for, the more possibility of a benign lesion is. The small suffused nodular calcification is always seen in pulmonary microlithiasis or silicosis.

(3) MRI

MRI shows calcification poorly because it presents no signal on image.

Section 2 Pleura diseases

1 Pleural effusion

Many diseases can cause pleural effusion. The etiological factors include infection, tumor or allergic reaction etc. The pleural fluids may be blood, pus, lipid or chyle, transudates or exudates.

(1) Radiography

Pleural effusion is defined as an abnormal accumulation of fluid in the pleural cavity. The radiological appearance of pleural effusion is due to the amount and location, regardless of its nature and cause.

1) Free pleural effusion

The most common radiological appearance is blunting of the costophrenic angle. The posterior costophrenic angle is the first place to accumulate pleural effusion. Therefore, small effusions (up to 250ml) become apparent in the P-A view. With increasing fluid, a homogeneous opacity extends upward and covers the diaphragm and lung fields. The small amount of pleural effusion means that upper edge is up to the fourth rib, the middle amount of it is between the second and the fourth ribs, and the large amount of it is over the second rib (Fig 4-3-7-A). A massive effusion may cause complete opacification of the hemithorax with contralateral displacement of the mediastinum.

2) Localized effusion

Encapsulated effusion: It refers to the pleural fluid that has become loculated or encysted between layers of visceral pleura. It usually appears as oval opacity, its margin partially well defined and will convex to lung fields. The edge of effusion connects the chest wall with obtuse angle.

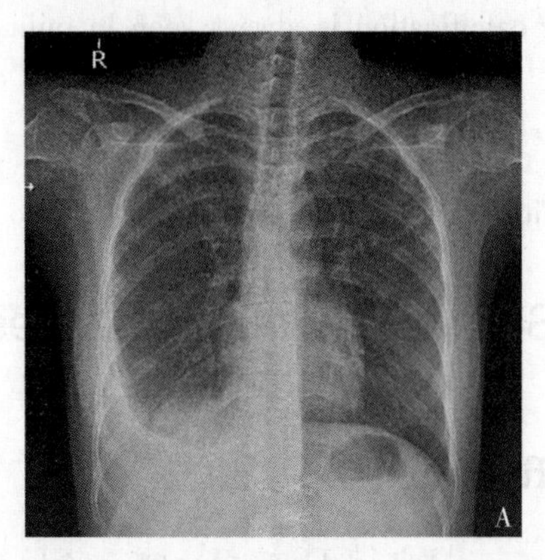

Fig 4-3-7-A Radiography: free pleural effusion of right pleural cavity

Interlobar effusion: It refers to a collection of pleural fluid between lobes, such as within the major and minor fissures. The typical radiographic appearance is opacity with a lentiform shape and sharply defined margins on the lateral radiograph.

Subpulmonary effusion: It is caused by fluid accumulating between the inferior surface of the lung and the diaphragm. It can always be seen in the right side. It may simulate elevation of the hemidiaphragm due to its well-defined superior margin. In fact, the costophrenic angle may appear deep and sharp and fluid may be seen in the fissures on supine position.

(2) CT

All effusion can be identified as liquid density on the section image. It presents as belt or crescent shadow with clear margin (Fig 4-3-7-B/C).

(3) MRI

In general, the effusion always presents low signal on T1WI and high signal on T2WI.

(4) Ultrasonography

There is abnormal liquid dark area between the two layers of pleura.

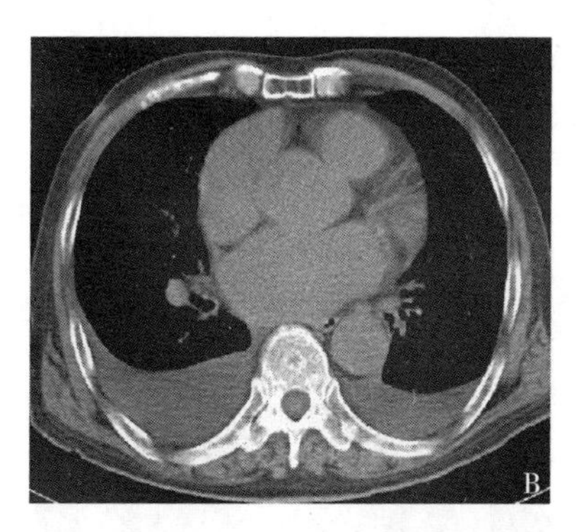

Fig 4-3-7-B CT: free pleural effusion of both pleural cavities

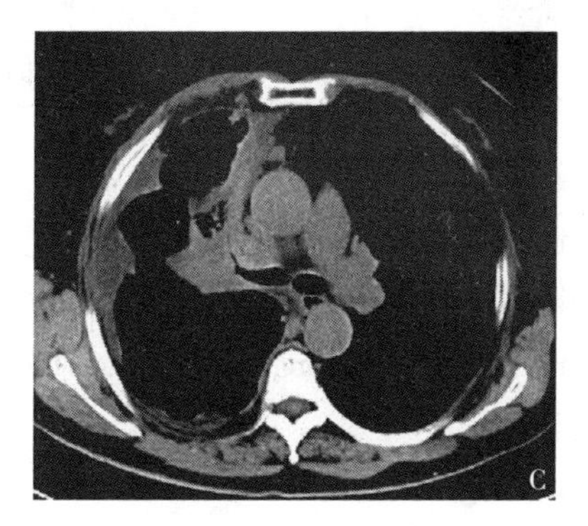

Fig 4-3-7-C CT: encapsulated effusion of right pleural cavity

2 Pneumothorax and hydropneumothorax

Pneumothorax is defined as the presence of air in the pleural space. Pneumothorax means that the pleural tear permits air to enter the pleural space. Hydropneumothorax is defined as the presence of both air and fluid within the pleural space.

(1) Radiography

On chest radiography, pneumothorax presents no lung markings and as gas density (Fig 4-3-8-A).

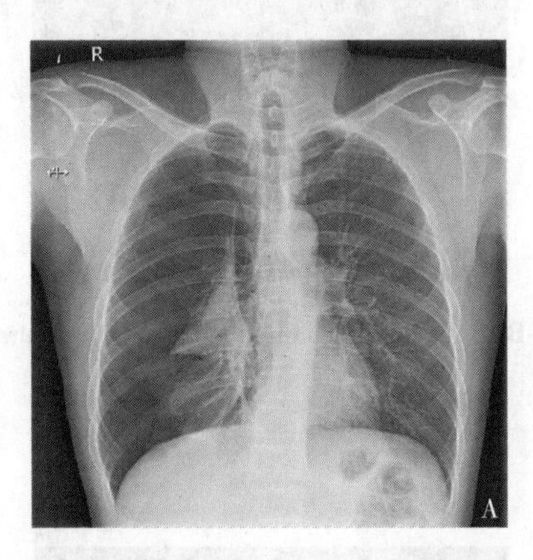

Fig 4-3-8-A Radiography: pneumothorax of right pleural cavity

1) Pneumothorax of small amount

A visible white line at the periphery of the lung and absence of lung markings beyond the line identify the pneumothorax. The pneumothorax is clear when the patient is expiring.

2) Pneumothorax of great amount

The area of pneumothorax occupies median or outer zone of lung fields. The inner zone of lung fields is lung that is compressed, and the lung presents as homogeneous soft tissue density. The intercostal space of the same side widens. The mediastinum shifts toward the normal lung and the diaphragm moves down.

3) Hydropneumothorax

Air fluid level can be shown at the erect position when there is hydropneumothorax. Transversal air fluid level can be seen when hydropneumothorax becomes serious.

4) Localized or multilocular pneumothorax and hydropneumothorax will form when there are pleura adhesions.

(2) CT

Pneumothorax may be shown as a low density zone with belt shape at lateral zone of lung fields (Fig 4-3-8-B). The inside bracket-shaped pleura can be seen as soft tissue density line shadow which is in parallel with chest wall. The lung has been compressed with different degrees and can move towards the hilum as a ball. The mediastinum shifts toward the normal side and the diaphragm moves down.

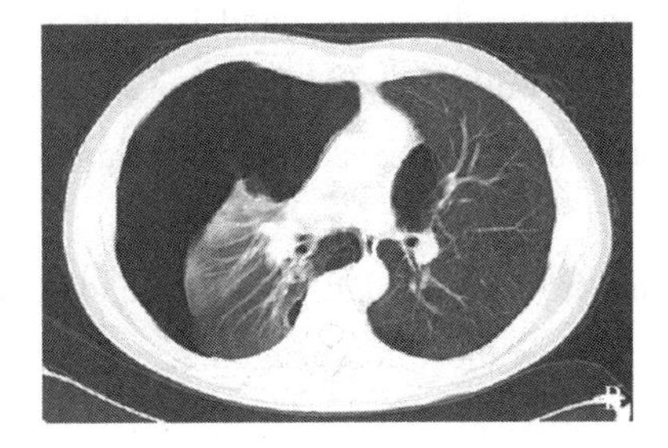

Fig 4-3-8-B CT: pneumothorax of right pleural cavity

The liquid is distributed at the dorsal side because of gravity and air is at the abdominal side when hydropneumothorax happens. The well-defined air-fluid level and margin of lung that has been compressed can be shown clearly.

(3) MRI

MRI can not present pneumothorax, but it can show the liquid signal of hydropneumothorax.

3 Pleural thickening, adhesion, and calcification

Pleural thickening may follow a variety of inflammatory processes that involve the pleura. The pleural thickening often exists with adhesion, and they are always at costophrenic angle. The pleural calcification is often caused by tuberculosis, hemorrhage and pneumoconiosis.

(1) Radiography

Localized pleural thickening and adhesion changes predominantly affect the dependent areas with blunting of the costophrenic angle.

Extensive pleural thickening and adhesion cause collapse of chest wall, narrowing of intercostal space, increase of lung field's density, exaltation of diaphragm, and movement of mediastinum.

Pleural calcification can be seen as lamellar, irregular or strip shadow, which is close to the margin of lung. The pleural calcification of encapsulated effusion can be shown as camber or irregular ring form.

(2) CT

Pleural thickening can be shown as band shadow with soft tissue density, which is located along chest wall. Its surface is not slick and its thickness is not homogeneous. The pleural thickening can be malignant if its thickness is more than 2cm.

Pleural calcification is always high density shadow which presents spot, band or block. Its CT value is close to skeleton.

(3) MRI

It can not display pleural thickening, adhesion and calcification as clearly as radiography and CT.

(4) Ultrasonography

Pleural thickening can be shown as middle echo of different thickness and scale between chest wall and lung on US. Pleural calcification can be shown as strong plaque echo with posterior acoustic shadow.

4 Pleural mass

Pleural mass is often seen in primary or metastatic tumor. The commonest primary tumor is mesothelioma. Others are fibroma, leiomyoma, and neurofibroma. Pleural tumor may be localized or diffuse. Lesions of diffuse pleural tumors are all malignant, often along with pleural effusion. The pleural mass can also be seen in pleural plaque of empyema or asbestosis.

(1) Radiography

Features of chest radiograph are well-defined, irregular, homogeneous, hemispheroid opacities, accompanied with pleural effusion in diffuse mesothelio-

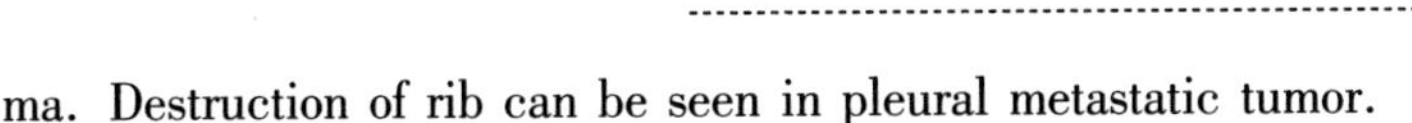

ma. Destruction of rib can be seen in pleural metastatic tumor.

(2) CT

Pleural mass can be presented as soft tissue density mass which is widely connected with chest wall. Pleura tail sign can be revealed on CT scan appearing as regional thickening of adjacent pleura. Obvious enhancement of masses can be seen on enhanced CT scan. Diffuse pleural mass can be shown as thickness of pleural with many uneven nodules. Pleural plaque of empyema or asbestosis is companied with calcification.

(3) MRI

Pleural mass can be shown as middle signal on T1WI and different high signals on T2WI.

(4) Ultrasonography

Pleural mass can be shown as round, middle echo mass which is connected with chest wall on US image. The benign pleural mass' echo is homogeneous, but the malignant one is heterogeneous and nonencapsulated.

Section 3 Mediastinal diseases

Radiography, CT and MRI can all show mediastinal diseases. Radiography can only present emphysema and air containing abscess of mediastinum. CT and MRI can identify the etiological factors of mediastinal diseases.

1 Radiography

Mediastinal and pulmonary lesions can both cause the mediastinal changes in shape and position. Change in shape probably means the widening of mediastinum (Fig 4-3-9). It can be caused by tumor, inflammation, hemorrhage, enlargement of lymph nodes, fat and abnormal vessels, among which tumor is the commonest cause. Mediastinum may shift to the affected side by atelectasis and diffuse pleural thickening, and may also shift to the normal side by the massive pleural effusion, huge pulmonary tumor, and hemilateral mediastinum tumor.

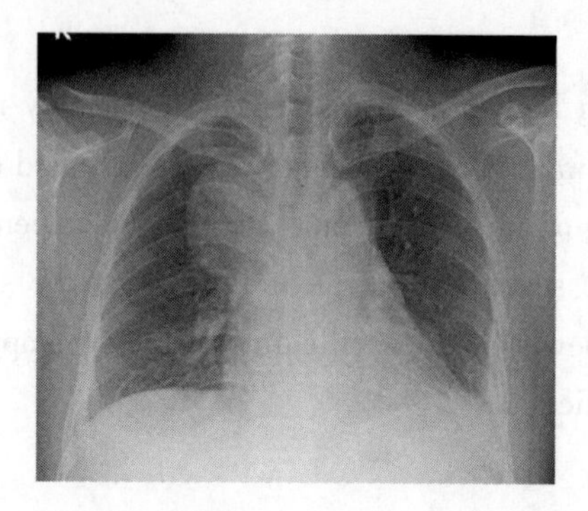

Fig 4-3-9 Radiography: widening of right mediastinum

2 CT

According to the CT value, mediastinal diseases can be classified into four kinds, which are fat, solid, cyst, and vessel. The fatty type of mediastinum disease is often located at right cardiophrenic angle. The solid disease can be seen in benign or malignant tumors, enlargement of lymph nodes. The cystic disease can be presented as round, liquid density shadow at different positions. The aortic aneurysm has camber calcification in its wall.

Enhanced CT is useful in identifying vascular or nonvascular and benign or malignant masses. The vascular disease shows apparent enhancement. The benign mass shows homogeneous, lower grade enhancement. The malignant mass is often presented as heterogeneous, apparent enhancement. The cystic disease can only present lower enhancement of its wall. The vessel in disease with fat density can be enhanced.

3 MRI

The solid tumor presents higher signal than muscle on T1WI and high signal on T2WI. The simple cystic disease is often presented low signal on T1WI and apparent high signal on T2WI. The fatty mass has high signal on both T1WI and

T2WI. The high signal of fat can be depressed by the technique of fat-suppression. The disease with abnormal vessels has heterogeneous signal because of turbulent flow.

Lesson 4 Diagnosis of Diseases

Section 1 Bronchiectasis

Irreversible abnormal dilatation of bronchioles on imaging confirms the diagnosis of bronchiectasis. The incidence of bronchiectasis has no difference between males and females. It often occurs in children and young adults.

[**Pathology and clinical manifestations**]

Acquired bronchiectasis is often caused by chronic infection. Inflammation can damage the muscle, elastic tissue and cartilage of bronchial wall. Involved bronchi are dilated, inflamed, and easily collapsible, resulting in airflow obstruction. Additionally, severe cough and deposition of secretions may result in high pressure of bronchi. The wall of bronchi can be dragged by atelectasis and diffuse lung fibrosis.

The classification of bronchiectasis is based on anatomic and morphologic patterns of airway dilation. It can be classified as three types: cylindrical bronchiectasis; varicose bronchiectasis; and cystic or saccular bronchiectasis. One or all three types can occur in the same patient. The lower lobes are most commonly affected and it can exist in both sides of the lung.

The three main symptoms of bronchiectasis are chronic cough, copious purulent or mucopurulent sputum, and hemoptysis.

[**Imaging appearances**]

1 Radiography

The chest radiographic findings can be normal. Sometimes the lung markings can increase, and radiolucent shadow-like rings can be seen.

2 CT

CT, especially HRCT, has become the most reliable method in the evaluation and noninvasive diagnosis of bronchiectasis.

(1) Cylindrical bronchiectasis

It is confirmed by the presence of "Tram-track" sign due to dilated bronchioles with its accompanying vessels. "Signet-ring" sign represents dilated bronchioles closely related to its adjacent vessels.

(2) Varicose bronchiectasis

It is identified by an irregular or beaded outline of the bronchi, with alternating areas of constriction and dilation.

(3) Cystic bronchiectasis

A cystic cluster of thin-walled cystic spaces looks like grapes, which often present air-fluid levels and bronchial wall thickening when infected (Fig 4-4-1).

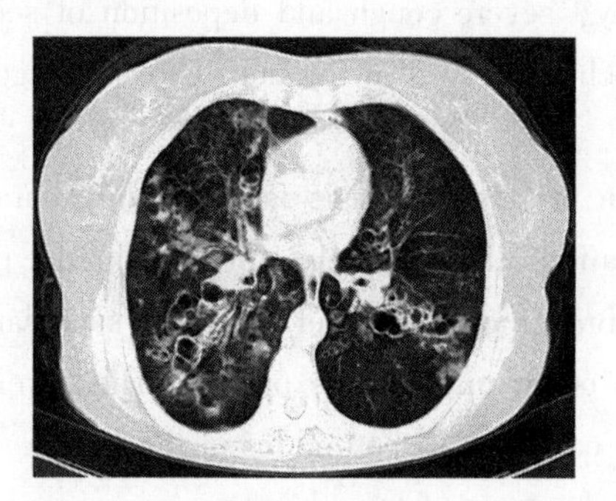

Fig 4-4-1 CT: cystic bronchiectasis

(4) Mucus plug of bronchi

The fluid-filled bronchi are revealed as sticks or nodules when they are perpendicular to the plane of the CT section, similar to the gloved finger shadows. The bronchi can be surrounded by plaque shadow of effusion or be presented as air fluid level when there is infection.

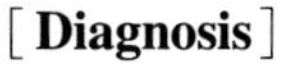

[**Diagnosis**]

Radiography can give a clue for bronchiectasis. HRCT can demonstrate the type and extent of bronchiectasis and can also help in evaluating the status of the surrounding lung tissues. All types of bronchiectasis have their characteristics. It is easy to diagnose bronchiectasis by its performance together with its clinical data.

Section 2 Pneumonia

Pneumonia is a common disease of lung. It can be classified on the basis of anatomy and etiological factors. In clinical practice the most useful classification is according to the etiology, and infection is the commonest cause of disease. Unfortunately, it is not possible to diagnose the organism by radiology alone. Pneumonia can be divided into three kinds according to anatomy, namely lobar, lobular and interstitial pneumonia.

1 Lobar pneumonia

[**Pathology and clinical manifestations**]

Lobar pneumonia is the most common bacterial pneumonia, often infected by pneumococcus. The process spreads rapidly leading to consolidation of an entire lobe or segment. Patient may have symptoms such as shivering, hyperpyrexia, chest pain and rusty expectoration. Laboratory examination can show the increase of total white blood cells and neutrophilic granulocyte.

Lobar pneumonia can be divided into four stages, i. e., congestion, red liver consolidation, gray liver consolidation, and dispersion according to pathology. The different stages of pathology can be shown by medical imaging.

[**Imaging appearances**]

(1) Radiography

1) Stage of congestion

The chest radiograph can be normal. Sometimes the lung markings can increase and the transparency of lung decreases.

2) Stages of red and gray liver consolidation

It presents as a homogeneous well-demarcated density of a segment, a lobe or the entire lung. Sometimes the "air bronchogram" can be seen (Fig 4-4-2-A).

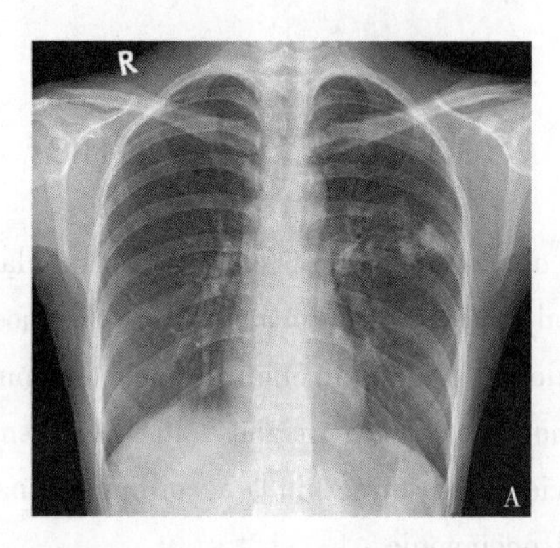

Fig 4-4-2-A Radiography: pneumonia of left lung

3) Stage of dispersion

The involved segment shows irregular and plaque shadow. The infection can disappear or become organized pneumonia.

(2) CT

In the stage of congestion, the affected area shows ground-grass opacity with ill-defined margin. Vessels loom in the area.

In the stages of red and gray liver consolidation, lobar or segmental dense shadows can be seen with a sharp border. When the bronchi remain aerated, they are seen as "air bronchogram" sign (Fig 4-4-2-B). In the stage of dispersion, there are patching shadows left due to the absorption. The shadow can disappear eventually.

[**Diagnosis**]

Acute lobar pneumonia can be confirmed by typical clinical appearance combined with chest radiography. The CT examination can be used for detection of early pneumonia.

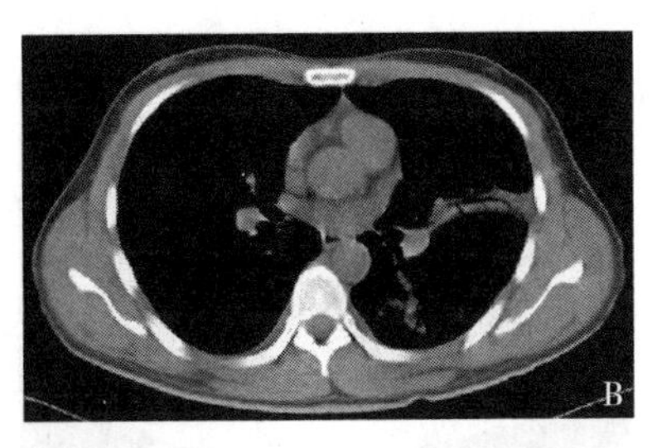

Fig 4-4-2-B CT: pneumonia, air bronchogram of left lung, free pleural effusion of both pleural cavities

2 Bronchopneumonia

Bronchopneumonia, also called lobular pneumonia, commonly occurs in old age and infancy or patients with concurrent disease.

[**Pathology and clinical manifestations**]

Microorganisms colonize the bronchioles and extend into the surrounding alveoli. In patients with acute bronchiolitis, the peribronchial alveoli are filled by inflammatory exudates, which lead to numerous discrete foci of consolidation. Lobular emphysema or atelectasis can be formed eventually.

Fever, bubble-like phlegm, chest pain, dyspnea, and cyanosis usually can be seen in these patients.

[**Imaging appearances**]

(1) Radiography

Shadows like patch and poorly defined opacities can be seen at the inner or middle zone of the lung fields. These patching opacities may produce segmental or large areas of consolidation that can become lobar pneumonia.

(2) CT

Scattered, nodular or patching opacities can be seen in the lower parts of both lung fields, together with small cavities, lobular hyperinflation, or atelectasis (Fig 4-4-3). The lesions can be cured after clinical treatment.

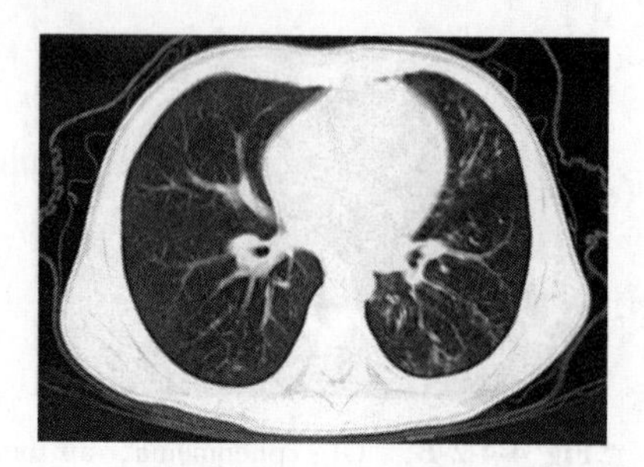

Fig 4-4-3 CT: bronchopneumonia of both lungs

[**Diagnosis**]

Typical cases can be diagnosed by apparent clinical symptoms and medical imaging. CT aims to acknowledge whether bronchiectasis develops in those patients who are deferred or recurrent.

3 Interstitial pneumonia

Interstitial pneumonia is defined as inflammation of the lung interstitium. Children are often affected, secondary to measles, pertussis or influenza.

[**Pathology and clinical manifestations**]

Infiltration by inflammatory cells of bronchial wall and lung interstitium is common. Consolidation occurs because of hyperaemia, edema of the bronchial. Inflammation can extend along the lymphatic, leading to lymphangitis and lymphadenitis.

Patients can have symptoms such as fever, cough, breathlessness, and cyanosis.

[**Imaging appearances**]

(1) Radiography

Interstitial pneumonia often affects both lungs, especially in the lower field. Radiography may demonstrate blur and exaggerated lung markings to form diffuse reticulations together with spot opacities. Interstitial inflammation around the hilum may result in the density of hilum increasing with hazy outline. Acute interstitial pneumonia often demonstrates diffuse emphysema due to obstruction of bronchiole.

(2) CT

In the early stage or non-serious cases, bronchovascular bundle enlargement can be seen and the lung field demonstrates patch shadow. Lymphaden enlargement can be seen in hilum and mediastinum. Slight pleural effusion sometimes can be shown in patients.

[**Diagnosis**]

Typical cases are easy to be diagnosed by medical imaging.

Section 3 Lung abscess

Lung abscess is a localized inflammatory disease, with central necrosis surrounded by pneumonitis. There are three kinds of paths of infection: inhale, blood and direct extension.

[**Pathology and clinical manifestations**]

The course of lung abscess is some degree of bronchial obstruction, inflammatory embolism of small vessels and tissue necrosis. The air-fluid level within the lesion is due to accumulation of pus in the dependent part and air in the non-dependent part. The thick walls are due to inflammatory reaction due to the inciting organism and adjacent air space opacification reflects pneumonic changes in the lung.

Complications include empyema, bronchopleural fistula formation, etc. Most lung abscesses are resolved with medical management consisting of antibiotics and postural drainage. Some lung abscesses become chronic lung abscesses with protracted course of disease.

Acute symptoms include shivering, fever, and chest pain. Copious foul-smelling sputum and increase of leukocyte number are present. Chronic symptoms include chronic cough, purulent sputum, hemoptysis, anaemia and clubbing.

[**Imaging appearances**]

1 Radiography

Lung abscess can be single or multiple. The lesion can be presented as compact mass shadow in the lung at the early stage. Lung abscess appears as cavitary lesions containing an air-fluid level at the later stage. The inner wall of the cavity tends to be smooth and sharp. The outer wall of cavity is ill-defined because of the surrounding pneumonia. Chronic abscess is indicated by progressive decrease in the size of the cavity and of the surrounding pneumonia.

2 CT

On CT film, lung abscess presents as a cavitary lesion with a relatively thick wall and ill-defined margin. It is easy for CT to demonstrate the position of abscess, the presence of pleural effusion and empyema (Fig 4-4-4). The enhanced CT can show apparent enhancement of the wall of lung abscess.

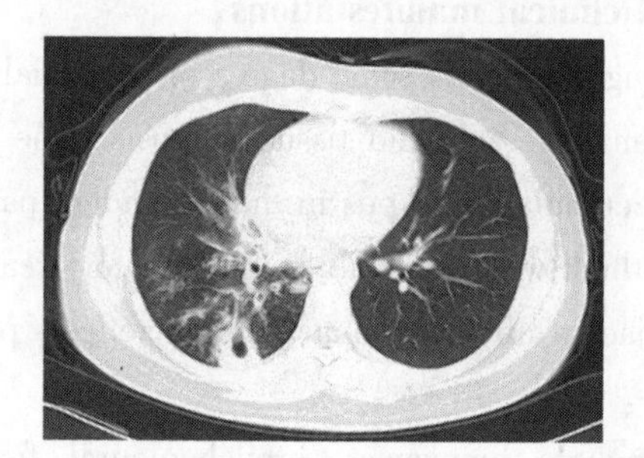

Fig 4-4-4 CT: lung abscess with cavity of right lung

[**Diagnosis**]

Thick-walled cavitary lung lesion with air-fluid level is the radiological feature of lung abscess.

Section 4 Pulmonary tuberculosis

Tuberculosis is a pulmonary and systemic disease caused by the mycobacterium tuberculosis. Infection is usually caused by inhalation of organisms from open cases of the disease. The incidence of tuberculosis has been increasing recently.

[**Pathology and clinical manifestations**]

The major determinants of the type and extent of the disease are the patient's age and immune status, the virulence of organism, and the mycobacterial load. The basic pathological changes are exudation, proliferation, and degeneration. All pathological changes can be coexistent. When the immune status is improved and proper medicine therapy adopted, tuberculous inflammation can be healed by resorption, fibrosis and calcification. Degenerative lesions are developed from exudative and proliferative lesions. These lesions may expand, dissolve and be liquefied, therefore cavity comes into being. Degenerative lesions may hematogenously spread into lung and systemic organs. Bronchogenic spread also may occur.

Primary tuberculosis is usually asymptomatic. Gradual onset of symptoms occurs over weeks or months. Symptoms range from tiredness, anorexia, low-grade fever, cough, chest pain and hemoptysis.

Diagnosis of tuberculosis is based on the comprehensive consideration of clinical findings, medical imaging and sputum culture.

The clinic classification of pulmonary tuberculosis in 2004:

①***Primary pulmonary tuberculosis***: including primary complex and intrathoracic lymph node tuberculosis;

② ***Hemo-disseminated pulmonary tuberculosis***: including acute, subacute and chronic hemo-disseminated tuberculosis;

③ ***Secondary pulmonary tuberculosis***: including infiltrative and chronic fibro-cavitary tuberculosis;

④***Tuberculous pleuritis***: including dry or exudative pleurisy and tubercular empyema;

⑤***Extra-pulmonary tuberculosis***: named according to the organ and its position.

[**Imaging appearances**]

1 Primary pulmonary tuberculosis

(1) Radiography

Primary tuberculosis usually occurs in childhood. The typical primary complex looks like dumbbell in shape.

It mainly consists of primary lesion, which is most commonly in a subpleural site in the well ventilated lower lobes. The lesion can present as round patching shadow. There is an area of peripheral consolidation and spread of infection from this along the draining lymphatic vessel may lead to enlargement of regional lymph nodes. This combination is referred to as a primary complex.

In the recovery stage of primary lesion, enlarged hilar or mediastinal lymph nodes are still present. Calcified densities can be seen in the nodes.

(2) CT

CT scan can show the size, number, contour and density of hilar and mediastinal lymph nodes. At the same time, enhanced CT can demonstrate early caseous necrosis inside the primary lesion, which appears as a relative low-density area.

2 Hemo-disseminated pulmonary tuberculosis

Disseminated pulmonary tuberculosis results from hematogenous spread of tubercle bacilli and consists of small tubercles widely disseminated in the lung. According to the virulence, amount of tubercle bacilli spreading into blood and the immunoreaction of body, it can be classified as acute, subacute and chronic disseminated tuberculosis.

(1) Acute miliary pulmonary tuberculosis

1) Radiography

Its typical appearances on chest radiograph are three kinds of uniform presentations that are widespread homogeneous millet-like nodules, uniformly distributed throughout the lungs and with similar density and size (1~3mm).

2) CT

CT can show the millet-like nodules earlier than radiography.

(2) Subacute and chronic miliary pulmonary tuberculosis

This kind of miliary pulmonary tuberculosis is due to a minority of tubercle bacillus spread into the lung in a long period recurrently.

1) Radiography

The miliary nodules are not uniform in size, density and distribution, mainly in the upper and middle fields. The lesions may be confluent, calcified and fibrotic (Fig 4-4-5-A).

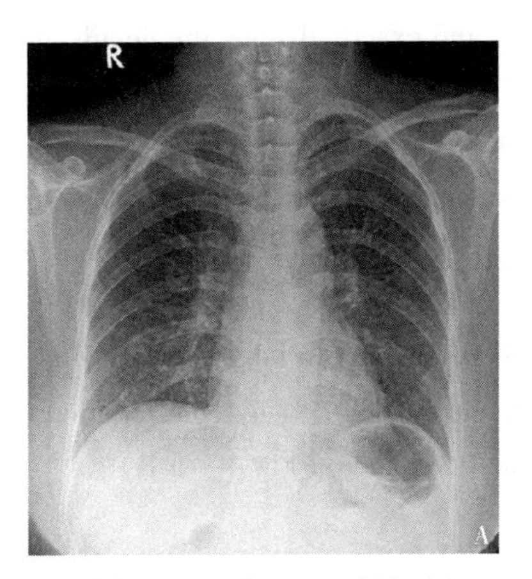

Fig 4-4-5-A Radiography: subacute and chronic miliary pulmonary tuberculosis

2) CT

The CT performance is similar to radiography. CT can show the details of lesion better.

3 Secondary pulmonary tuberculosis

It is the most common kind of pulmonary tuberculosis in adults.

(1) Infiltrative pulmonary tuberculosis

The lesion is always local because the body has specific immunity to tubercle bacillus. This follows the primary infection after a latent interval, however short or long, and is due to either reactivation or reinfection. It is now generally accepted that almost all post-primary tuberculosis is due to reinfection. The lesions usually start in the subapical parts of the upper lobes or in the apical segment of the lower lobes as small areas of exudative inflammation.

1) Radiography and CT

The appearance of infiltrative pulmonary tuberculosis tends to be various, which may give priority to one kind of sign or there may be a coexistence of several signs. CT can clearly and exactly display the details and surrounding structures of a lesion. Thereby, it is easier to use CT to diagnose and estimate the evolvement, compared to X-ray.

①Common findings are patchy shadows with ill-defined margin in the apical and posterior segments of the upper lobes or in the apical segment of the lower lobes.

②Caseous necrosis occurs within lobar or segmental exudation, called caseous pneumonia, which shows high-density consolidation on chest radiograph with multiple worm-eaten cavities inside (Fig 4-4-5-B).

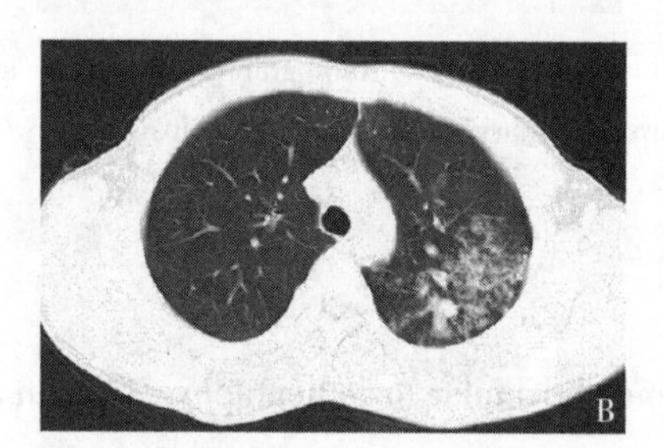

Fig 4-4-5-B CT: pulmonary tuberculosis, caseous pneumonia

③Lesions with proliferation which have spot shadows with sharp outline arrange in the form of "tree-bud" or "plum blossom".

④Tuberculoma appears as a sharply defined round or oval opacity, usually 2～3cm in diameter and with spotty, layered or annular calcification. Usually, there are discrete fibro-proliferations around the tuberculoma which are called "satellite lesions". Tuberculoma always has no or mild circular enhancement on enhanced CT.

⑤Cavitary diseases of tuberculosis are areas of increased radiolucency with a thin or thick wall and a smooth exterior margin. There are different kinds of "satellite lesions" around the cavitary diseases (Fig 4-4-5-C).

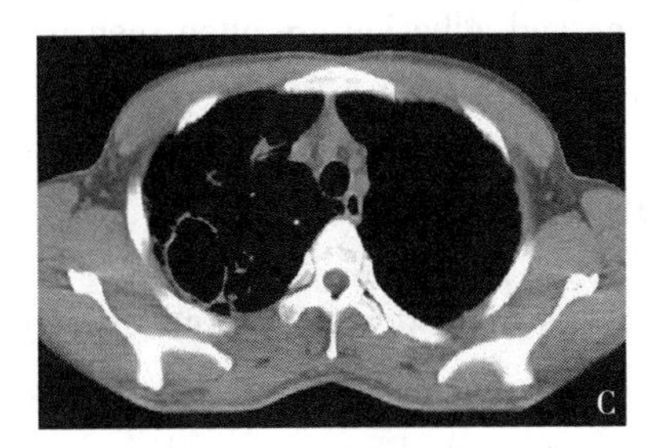

Fig 4-4-5-C CT: cavitary disease of infiltrative pulmonary tuberculosis

⑥Broncho-disseminated lesions are secondary to caseous necrosis within the opacity. Bronchogenic spread of the infection may occur by inhalation into uninfected areas when the necrotic, bacillus-laden contents of a cavity continue to drain into the bronchial tree. The lesion appears as patchy or lobular consolidation which is distributing along the bronchus.

⑦Interstitial tissue changes of lung may occur in some patients. HRCT can show reticular opacities, tiny nodules, ground-glass shadow, thick interlobular septum, and thickness of airway.

⑧Calcification or stripe shadow presents when proliferation lesion is healing.

(2) Fibro-cavitary pulmonary tuberculosis

It is the late period of secondary pulmonary tuberculosis. It leads to protracted course of pulmonary tuberculosis and bad destruction of lung tissues, and eventually forms fibrotic cavities.

Radiography and CT

①Fibrotic cavities that are thick-wall cavities can be found in the upper lung fields.

②Surroundings with cavities are patchy exudations, caseous consolidations, different degrees of calcification or many fibrotic lesions.

③The shrinkage of upper lobes, elevation of hilar and abnormality of lung markings form the "weeping willow sign".

④Signs of compensatory emphysema also can be found in the uninfected lung.

⑤Pleural thickening and adhesion are often seen in both lungs.

⑥Mediastinum moves to the infected lung.

4 Tuberculous pleuritis

Tuberculosis pleurisy is divided into dry and exudative pleurisy. It may be alone or coexist with intrapulmonary lesion, often presenting as a unilateral pleural effusion. Patients can feel chest pain or dyspnea.

Radiography and CT

It can present as different degrees of pleural effusion. Pleural thickening and calcification can be seen in chronic cases. CT can show pleural effusion in pulmonary lobule, base of lung or encapsulated effusion better.

[**Diagnosis**]

Radiological manifestations are different for each type of pulmonary tuberculosis. It is easy to diagnose pulmonary tuberculosis by a combination of medical history, medical imaging, and laboratory examination.

Section 5 Diffuse pulmonary diseases

There are many causes of diffuse lung disease in addition to infection, neoplasia or a primary abnormality of the airways. The chest radiograph remains the basic radiological tool in diagnosing these patients.

1 Idiopathic pulmonary fibrosis

It is the commonest kind of idiopathic interstitial pneumonia.

[**Pathology and clinical manifestations**]

Idiopathic pulmonary fibrosis can be different degrees of fibrosis in pathology. The severe case can change the structure of lung, honeycomb appearance of lung, and bronchiectasis of traction.

The disease is often seen at middle age and more in males than females. Typically the patient develops aggravated cough and progressive dyspnoea, accompanied with clubbed fingers and pulmonary heart disease.

[**Imaging appearances**]

Radiography and CT

The radiography appearances are normal in the early stage of the disease. CT can show "ground-glass" haze. Both lungs can present reticular nodular shadow and bronchiectasis of traction in the aggressive stage. Finally, severe contraction of the upper and middle zones with "honeycombing", cyst formation with 3～15mm in diameter may occur (Fig 4-4-6).

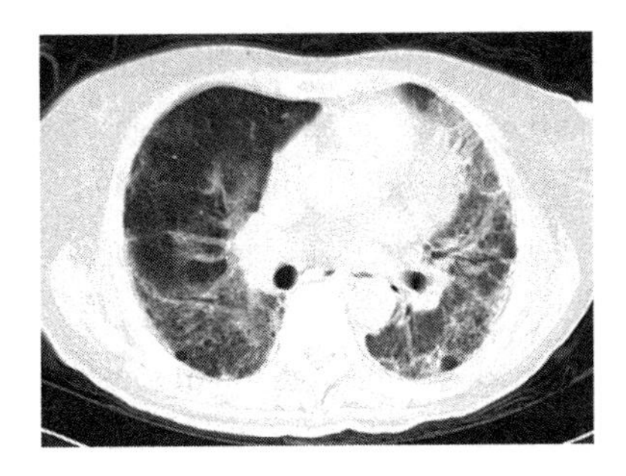

Fig 4-4-6 CT: idiopathic pulmonary fibrosis

[**Diagnosis**]

In the early stage, the chest radiograph may he normal. The performance of aggressive stage has characteristics which can be combined with clinical manifestation. Those are helpful to diagnose idiopathic pulmonary fibrosis.

2 Pulmonary alveolar proteinosis

This is a rare disease of unknown aetiology in which pneumocytes overproduce a proteinaceous lipid-rich material to a degree that overwhelms the capacity of the lung to remove it. This is probably the result of a response by the lungs to an irritant.

[**Pathology and clinical manifestations**]

The disease is more common in men than in women and can occur at middle age. The patient can feel short breath, expectoration and respiratory failure eventually. Most of the lung becomes consolidation in pathology.

[**Imaging appearances**]

(1) Radiography

The radiographic appearance resembles diffuse ground-glass shadow in both lungs. These opacities may become confluent. There can be "air bronchogram" sign in the consolidation. There may be apparent changes around hilum which can present as "butterfly-shaped". The performance is very similar to cardiac pulmonary edema.

(2) CT

The lesion can present as "map-like" with definite delimitation on HRCT. Thickening of the interlobular septa in addition to ground-glass shadow and consolidation produces the "crazy-paving" appearance, which is typical of this condition.

[**Diagnosis**]

Diagnosis is made by medical imaging which must be combined with clinical manifestation, lung biopsy, or bronchoalveolar lavage.

Section 6 Pulmonary tumors

A wide variety of neoplasms may arise in the lungs. While many lung tumors are overtly malignant and others are definitely benign, some fall histologically as well as in their clinical behavior between these two extremes. Pulmonary tumors may he classified histologically or according to their presumed tissue of origin.

Carcinoma of the bronchus is by far the most common and most important primary tumor of the lung.

1 Primary bronchogenic carcinoma

Approximately 98% of lung cancers arise centrally, i. e. in or proximal to segmental bronchi. The tumor arises in the bronchial mucosa and invades the bronchial wall. Tumor may grow around the bronchus and also into the bronchial lumen. The incidence and mortality of bronchogenic carcinoma has been rising in recent years. The most important and single aetiological factor is cigarette smoking. Air pollution and industrial carcinogen are also important etiological factors.

[**Pathology and clinical manifestations**]

Most carcinomas of the lung fall into one of′ two types, i. e., small cell lung cancer and non-small cell lung cancer. The latter includes squamous carcinoma, adenocarcinoma, adenosquamous carcinoma and large cell carcinoma, etc.

There are three types according to the origin positions: central pulmonary carcinoma, peripheral pulmonary carcinoma, and bronchioalveolar carcinoma. The central pulmonary carcinoma arises in the larger bronchi at or close to the hilum. The bronchioalveolar carcinoma arises in the bronchioles or alveoli and the remainder arises peripherally.

The early stage of lung cancer has no symptom. The common symptoms of late stage of lung cancer include persistent cough, expectoration, hemoptysis, chest pain and fever. Patients with lung cancer show a variety of symptoms depending on the lesion's position, size, invasion of surrounding structure, and paraneoplastic syndrome, etc.

[**Imaging appearances**]

(1) Central pulmonary carcinoma

1) The early stage of central pulmonary carcinoma is that the tumor grows in the lumen of bronchi, which does not involve the surrounding structures and has no metastasis.

①***Radiography***: It is normal, or sometimes local pulmonary emphysema and obstructive pneumonia can be seen in radiography.

②***CT***: It can clearly show the thickness of bronchi wall, stenosis of bronchi lumen and nodule in the bronchi lumen.

2) The late stage of central pulmonary carcinoma can be seen in radiography and CT definitely.

①***Radiography***: It can present hilar mass, which is the direct sign of central carcinoma, and which may be shown as lobulated or irregular shape. The tumors can be accompanied with obstructive pneumonia or atelectasis (Fig 4-4-7-A).

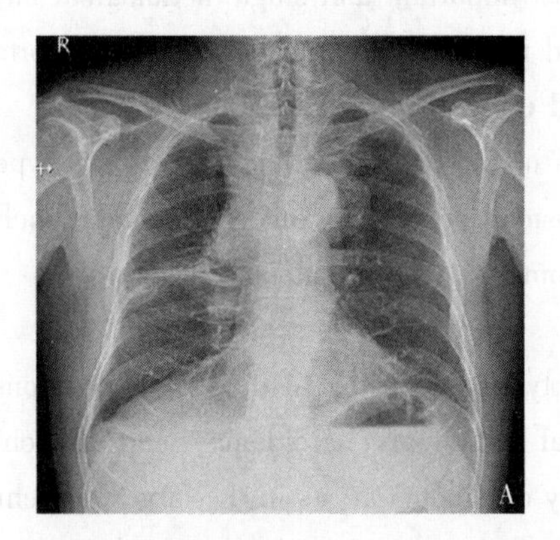

Fig 4-4-7-A X-ray: central pulmonary carcinoma with right hilar mass

②***CT***: It can present the wall of bronchi thickened irregularly, and circular or irregular bronchial lumen stenosis. Obstruction of the lumen leads to collapse, and often infection, in the lung distal to the tumor. Signs of atelectasis are: collapse or consolidation of the affected lung may occur. CT can show hilar or mediastinal lymph nodes and vessels that are associated with the central lung tumor (Fig 4-4-7-B).

③***MRI***: MRI is equally good for assessing tumors. MRI has been proved to be more accurate than CT in evaluating mediastinal and vascular tumor invasion. T1-weighted image shows the tumor as intermediate signal in contrast with the high signal from surrounding fat, enabling better delineation of chest wall inva-

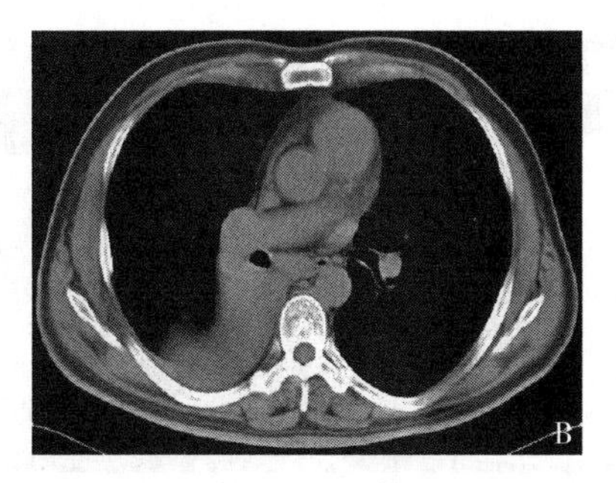

Fig 4-4-7-B CT: central pulmonary carcinoma with right hilar mass, obstructive atelectasis and enlarged mediastinal lymph nodes

sion, adjacent vessels, brachial plexus and spinal structures. The tumor can be shown as high signal in T2-weighted and DWI images, which can be helpful in demonstrating the extent of the tumor.

(2) Peripheral pulmonary carcinoma

1) The early stage of peripheral pulmonary carcinoma is that the tumor grows less than 2cm in diameter and has no metastasis.

①***Radiography***: It can present a nodular shadow in lung which has irregular shapes like lobulation, glitch and pleural indentation.

②***CT***: It can show characteristics, margin and surrounding structures of the tumor. Ground glass nodule (GGN) can be seen clearly in CT and GGN always has negative CT value (Fig 4-4-7-C/D).

1) The late stage of peripheral pulmonary carcinoma is that the tumor can be seen as big mass in the lung.

① ***Radiography***: With the tumor growing, the lesion becomes a lobulated mass with spiculated margin and pleural indentation. Cavitation occurs in those rapidly growing masses, always showing as eccentric thick-walled cavities with irregular and nodular inner surface. Calcification is rarely seen in the tumor (Fig 4-4-7-E).

② ***CT***: HRCT can show the details of tumor. It can present the

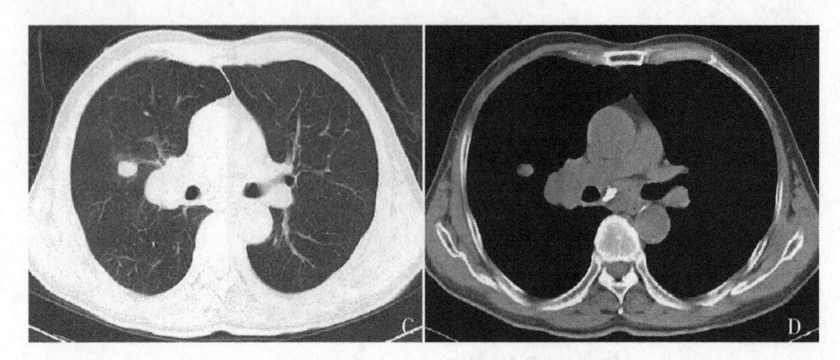

Fig 4-4-7-C/D CT: the early stage of peripheral pulmonary carcinoma with mass of right lung, enlarged hilar and mediastinal lymph nodes

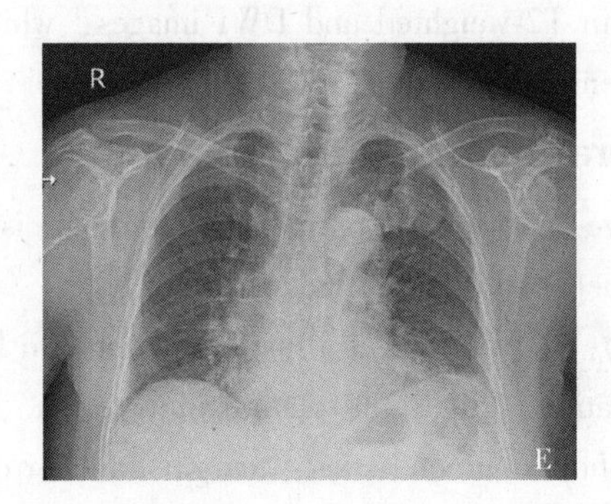

Fig 4-4-7-E Radiography: the late stage of peripheral pulmonary carcinoma with mass of left upper lobe

appearance, margin, internal structure and surrounding structures of the tumor. The tumor can be seen as short, apparent and homogeneous enhancement in multi-phase enhanced CT (Fig 4-4-7-F/G/H/I).

③***MRI***: T1-weighted image shows the tumor as intermediate homogeneous signal. The tumor can be shown as high signal in T2-weighted and DWI images.

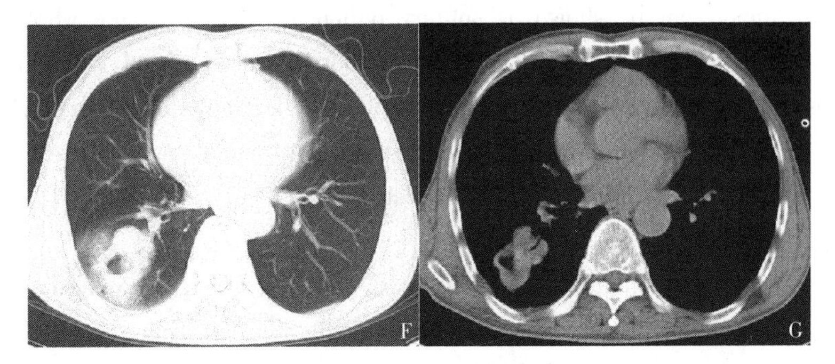

Fig 4-4-7-F/G CT: the late stage of peripheral pulmonary carcinoma with thick wall cavity

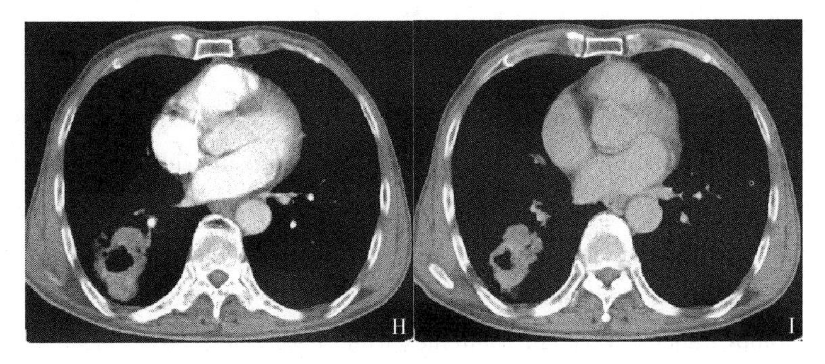

Fig 4-4-7-H/I Enhanced CT: the late stage of peripheral pulmonary carcinoma

The tumor can show heterogeneous signal when it has necrosis.

(3) Bronchioalveolar carcinoma

1) Radiography

Bronchoalveolar carcinoma may appear in a variety of ways, including a solitary pulmonary nodule, multiple nodules, and consolidation. The lesion has the tendency of fusion and becomes the consolidation of whole lobe of lung with the sign of "air bronchogram".

2) CT

The tumor can be shown as solitary pulmonary nodule in the whole lung which can be accompanied with extensive hilar and mediastinal lymph nodes. The lesion can be shown as a large patch of consolidation with the sign of "air bronchogram". The ground glass opacities in consolidated areas and the loom vessels inside are the important characteristics.

[**Diagnosis**]

Presence of speculated lung mass on CXR in an elderly chronic smoker is highly suspicious of primary lung carcinoma. Radiological features which help differentiate benign and malignant masses should be borne in mind. Bronchoscopy imaging-guided is used for final diagnosis.

2 Pulmonary metastasis

Many malignant tumors can spread via blood and lymphatics into lungs or directly invade the lungs.

[**Pathology and clinical manifestations**]

Metastases most commonly reach the lung hematogenously via the systemic veins and pulmonary arteries. They most frequently occur with tumors that have rich systemic venous drainage. Carcinoma of stomach, pancreas, and breast can involve the mediastinal lymph glands and spread along lymphatics of both lungs. Malignant tumors of mediastinum and chest wall may directly invade the lungs. Clinical appearances vary in patients with lung metastases. The common symptoms of pulmonary metastasis include cough, expectoration, hemoptysis and chest pain. The majority of these patients present with primary tumorous symptoms, along with severe debility. Some patients may be asymptomatic.

[**Imaging appearances**]

(1) Radiography

Metastases are more likely to be multiple than solitary. Most hematogenous metastases are sharply circumscribed with smooth edges. Metastases to the lung are usually bilateral, affecting both lungs equally, with a basal predominance. They are often peripheral and may be subpleural. Pulmonary metastases vary in size from millimetre to centimetre in diameter (Fig 4-4-7-J). The lymphatic metastasis can be shown as enlargement of hilar/mediastinal lymph nodes or radiated streak shadows that come from hilar. Also nodules look like string-of-beads can be seen.

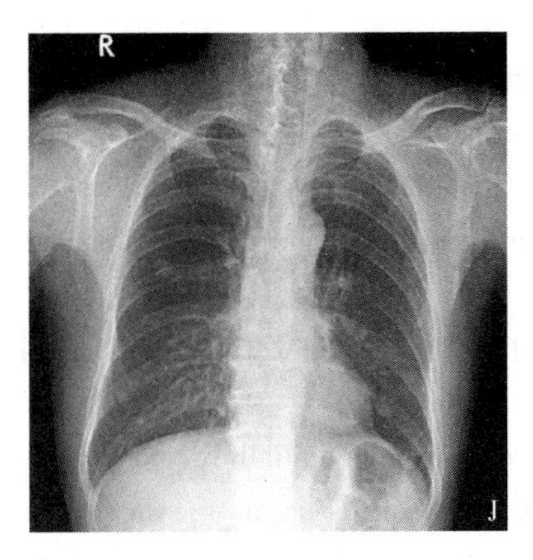

Fig 4-4-7-J Radiography: pulmonary metastasis of both lungs

(2) CT

CT is more sensitive than plain film in detecting metastases, showing subpleural location of multiple spheric nodules (Fig 4-4-7-K). Signs of cavitation, cyst and calcification are unusual in metastatic lesions. HRCT has particular ad-

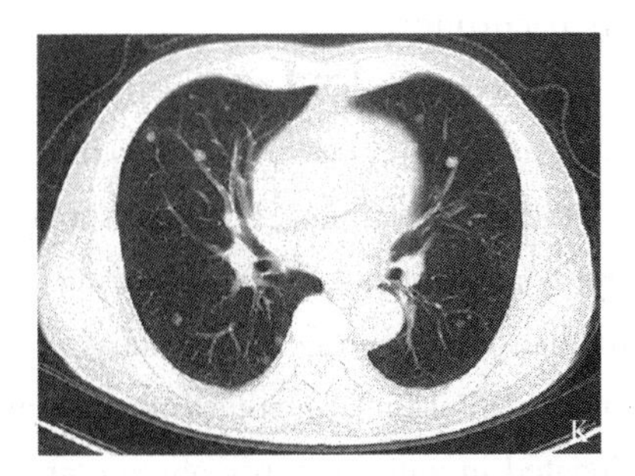

Fig 4-4-7-K CT: pulmonary metastasis of both lungs

vantages in displaying the lymphangitis carcinomatosa. In these cases a high-resolution CT scan may be undertaken to establish the diagnosis, when the typical appearances are nodular thickening of the interlobular septa and many tiny nodules along the bronchial and vascular bundles.

[**Diagnosis**]

Multiple round lung lesions in a patient with known malignancy most likely represent pulmonary metastases. CT thorax is more sensitive in detecting small pulmonary metastases. Sometimes medical imaging has to be combined with medical history, tumor marker in blood and puncture biopsy.

Section 7 Primary mediastinal tumor

Mediastinal disease is usually initially demonstrated on a chest radiograph and appears as a mediastinal soft-tissue mass, widening of the mediastinum or a pneumomediastinum.

However, the chest radiograph may appear normal in presenting mediastinal disease, which is subsequently clearly demonstrated by CT or MRI. The most common mediastinal abnormalities seen on a chest radiograph in adults are undoubtedly lymph node enlargement, vascular abnormalities and a hiatus hernia, but in infants and children the most common abnormality is seen in the thymus gland. Mediastinal tumors, cysts and lymph node masses tend to predominate in surgically treated patients mainly with thymic tumors, neurogenic tumors, benign foregut cysts, lymphoma, germ cell tumors, thyroid masses and mesenchymal and other tumors occurring.

The typical sites of the common and rare mediastinal masses are shown in the next part and it is helpful in locating a mediastinal mass into one of the anatomical compartments of the mediastinum. It is also important to remember that they can involve adjacent compartments. Mass occurring in the thoracic inlet with shift and distortion of trachea is frequently thyroid mass in adults and lymphangioma in children. The anterior division of mediastinum mainly consists of thymoma and teratoma. Masses located in anterior cardiophrenic angle are often lipoma and pericardiac cysts. The middle division of mediastinum mainly consists of lymphoma, and the following one is bronchogenic cyst. The posterior division of mediastinum mainly consists of neurogenic tumor.

[**Pathology and clinical manifestations**]

Benign mediastinal tumors can make the neighboring organs compressed, thus symptoms appear. When the superior vena cava is compressed by the tumor, there may be symptoms including dyspnea, and swelling of the face, neck, upper trunk and extremities, which form a complex syndrome named SVC syndrome. Compression of trachea may result in irritative dry cough or dyspnea. Compression of phrenic nerve may induce phrenic paralysis and hiccup. Lesions compressing the sympathetic nerves may result in Horner syndrome. Compression of esophagus may result in dysphagia. Malignant mediastinal tumors can present symptoms when they are very small and often invade the mediastinal structures. Some of the mediastinal tumors have the typical symptoms, for example, myasthenia gravis may present in about 1/3 patients with thymoma, and few patients with retrosternal goiters may manifest symptoms of hyperthyroidism.

[**Imaging appearances**]

1 Intrathoracic goiter

Thyroid disease is common and enlargement of the thyroid gland can be due to a number of causes including a non-toxic multinodular enlargement of the gland, thyrotoxicosis, thyroid adenoma, thyroid carcinoma, lymphoma and Hashimoto's thyroiditis. The enlarged thyroid glands in the neck extend into the mediastinum to produce retrosternal goitre. A mass developing within a heterotopic thyroid gland in the mediastinum is rare.

Retrosternal goitre is usually seen as an incidental mediastinal mass on a chest radiograph in an adult female patient. The goiter is often asymptomatic but can produce dysphagia, dyspnoea and stridor.

Retrosternal goitre on CT appears as an oval soft tissue mass in the superior part of the anterior or middle mediastinum, which fades off into the neck. The soft-tissue mass often contains central nodular or linear patterns of calcification and produces lateral displacement and compression of the trachea in the thoracic inlet. Rapid increase in the site of the mass indicates internal haemorrhage into a cyst.

The diagnosis is confirmed by CT (or MRI), which shows a mass of mixed soft-tissue attenuation which is enhanced after intravenous contrast medium and extends into the mediastinum from the tower pole of one of the lobes of the thyroid gland in the neck down towards the aortic arch. The mass may have a higher attenuation than muscle due to its iodine content and may contain foci of calcification or lesions of low attenuation due to cystic degeneration. MRI shows a mass of intermediate signal intensity in T1-weighted images and high signal intensity in T2-weighted images.

2 Thymoma

The normal thymus gland is seen as a triangular arrowhead or bilobed structure in children and young adult patients on CT, but undergoes fatty involution in elderly adult patients. Enlargement of the thymus gland can be due to a number of causes including thymoma, hyperplasia of the gland, thymic carcinoma, lymphoma, carcinoid and germ cell tumors, thymic cysts and thymolipoma. Thymomas are the commonest of the thymic tumors in adults and 10%~15% are invasive or malignant.

A thymoma is usually seen as an anterior mediastinal mass on a chest radiograph in an adult patient. The thymoma is often asymptomatic but can also present with myasthenia gravis, red cell aplasia or hypogammaglobulinaemia, as well as many other conditions.

A thymoma appears as a well-defined round or oval soft-tissue mass which projects to one side of the anterior mediastinum when it is large, but may be undetectable on the chest radiograph when it is small, indicating the need for CT. The soft-tissue mass may also contain curvilinear or nodular calcification. The presence of vascular encasement or pleural metastases indicates an invasive thymoma and a very large soft-tissue mass with less radiographic density than expected for its size, which alters in shape on respiration, indicating a thymolipoma.

The diagnosis of a thymoma is confirmed by CT (or MRI), which shows a mass of soft-tissue attenuation which may contain areas of low attenuation due to cystic degeneration. MRI shows a mass of intermediate signal intensity in T1-weighted images and high signal intensity in T2-weighted images. CT also demonstrates an enlarged but normal-shaped gland in thymic hyperplasia, a cystic mass containing fluid in a thymic cyst or a fat-containing mass in a thymolipoma. Thymoma can be enhanced uniformly after intravenous contrast medium.

3 Teratoma

The teratoma of the mediastinum is in the middle of anterior mediastinum. It includes the cystic and solid tumors, and the solid one is called dermoid cyst. The dermoid cyst contains tissues of ectoderm and mesoderm and is usually seen on CT as cyst density. The solid tumor contains tissues of three germ layers and is usually seen on CT as mixed density (Fig 4-4-8-A/B/C).

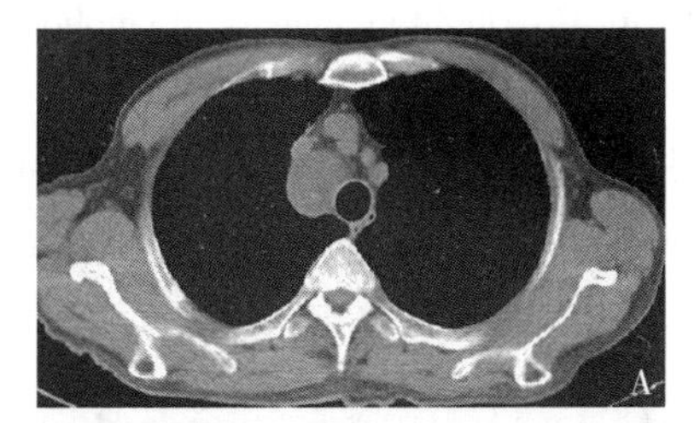

Fig 4-4-8-A CT: teratoma in the middle of anterior mediastinum

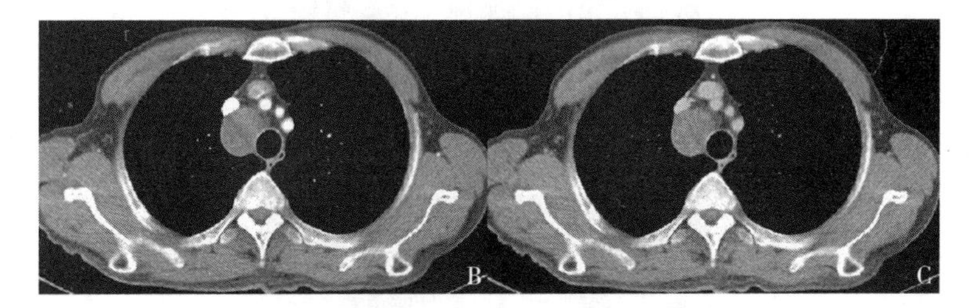

Fig 4-4-8-B/C Enhanced CT: teratoma

A fat-fluid level or even a rudimentary tooth is of course a diagnostic radiological sign. Rapid increase in the size of the mass indicates internal haemorrhage or the development of malignancy. The diagnosis is confirmed by CT (or MRI), which shows a cystic mass containing fluid, soft tissue, fat, calcification or hone. MRI shows a mass of variable high signal intensity in T1-weighted images if it contains fat, protein or blood.

4 Lymphoma

Lymphoma is often located in the anterior or middle of mediastinum. The enlargement and wavy margin of mediastinum can be seen on chest film. The hilar and mediastinal lymph nodes enlargement can be seen on CT and they are presented as homogeneous soft tissue density.

Lymphoma usually has intermediate signal intensity in T1-weighted images and appears high signal in T2-weighted images. Lymphoma can be enhanced on CT or MRI when contrast medium is injected. It usually grows with surrounding blood vessels (Fig 4-4-8-D/E/F). Diagnosis of lymphoma is mainly based on clinical presentation and histology of excised lymph node.

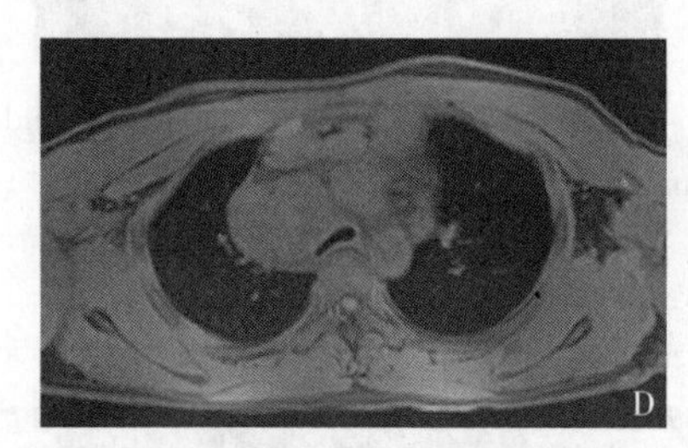

Fig 4-4-8-D MRI: lymphoma on T1-weighted image

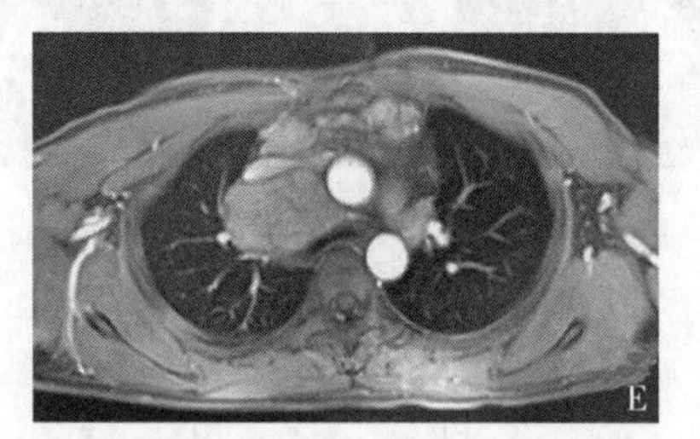

Fig 4-4-8-E Enhanced MRI: lymphoma

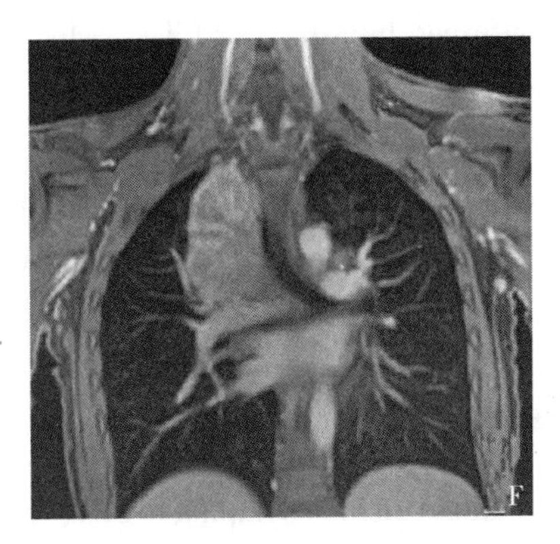

Fig 4-4-8-F Enhanced MRI on coronal view: lymphoma

5 Neurogenic tumors

The neurogenic tumors of the mediastinum develop from either the peripheral nerves or the thoracic sympathetic chain ganglia. They are known as the neurofibroma or neurilemmoma and ganglioneuroma. The majority of the neurogenic tumors are benign.

Neurogenic tumors are usually seen as an incidental posterior mediastinal mass on a chest radiograph in a child or young adult patient. The tumor is often asymptomatic, but can produce back pain or spinal cord compression. It extends through an intervertebral foramen into the spinal canal producing a "dumb-bell" tumor which is usually a neurofibroma. A neurogenic tumor appears as a well-defined round or oval soft-tissue mass in the paravertebral gutter, which usually projects to only one side of the posterior mediastinum. The nerve sheath tumors are usually circular in shape whereas the ganglion cell tumors are more elongated. The ganglion cell tumors may contain nodules of calcification, which is rare in the nerve sheath tumors. Neurogenic tumors may also involve adjacent bones to produce splaying of several thin posterior ribs, a localised pressure erosion defect of a vertebral body, enlargement of an intervertebral foramen and rib notching. Rapid increase in the site of the mass in association with bony destruction and a pleural effusion indicates the development of malignancy.

The diagnosis is confirmed by MRI (or CT), which shows a mass of intermediate signal intensity in T1-weighted images and high signal intensity in T2-weighted images with enhancement after gadolinium injection. MRI also demonstrates any intraspinal extension or cystic degeneration, but not tile presence of calcification. CT shows a mass of soft-tissue attenuation which is enhanced after intravenous contrast medium and may contain calcification.

6 Cystic masses

The cystic masses mainly include lymphatic cyst, bronchial cyst and pericardial cyst. The cyst has relationship with origin organ and can be localized easily. The cyst contains clear fluid density on CT and its CT value varies from 0 HU to 20 HU. The CT value can reach 30 HU or 40 HU if the cyst has protein or hemorrhage in it. The enhanced CT can distinguish the cyst and the solid tumor because the solid tumor can have apparent enhancement. MRI is better than CT to diagnose cyst. It can differentiate hemorrhage in the cyst sensitively.

[**Diagnosis**]

Diagnosis of mediastinum tumor is mainly based on medical image presentations such as the location of lesion, the density or signal of lesion, the margin of lesion and the changes of adjacent structures.

CT and MRI are the imaging modalities of choice to assess extent of intrathoracic involvement. They can also help in staging the disease and assessing response to treatment.

Section 8 Pleural diseases

The pleural diseases are originated or involved in plural. They can be divided into primary or secondary pleural diseases.

1 Pyothorax

Most of pyothorax is direct extension within an infected adjacent organ.

[**Pathology and clinical manifestations**]

The patients in acute phase can have symptoms such as hyperpyrexia, breathlessness and chest pain. The causation of pyothorax can be tuberculosis or other etiological factor.

[**Imaging appearances**]

(1) Radiography

It can present as pleural effusion or bronchopleural fistula in acute phase. And it can present pleural thickening, adhesion and calcification in chronic phase.

(2) CT

CT has the advantage of evaluating the underlying lung and mediastinal structures to identify the cause of the effusion. The wall of pyothorax is thick, smooth and homogeneous. And the wall of abscess cavity can be enhanced apparently on contrast enhanced CT.

[**Diagnosis**]

Lateral decubitus film, ultrasound or CT thorax helps to detect pyothorax. It is easy to diagnose by combination with typical clinical manifestation.

2 Tumor of pleura

The tumor of pleura can be divided into primary and secondary diseases.

(1) Primary tumor of pleura

Localized fibrous tumor and diffuse mesothelioma of pleura are two kinds of common pleural tumors.

[**Pathology and clinical manifestations**]

Patients with localized fibrous tumor can be asymptomatic. But patients with diffuse mesothelioma of pleura can have symptoms such as chest pain, dyspnea and cough.

Most of localized fibrous tumors are benign. But diffuse mesothelioma of pleura is always malignant. The tumor of pleura has unknown causation of disease.

[**Imaging appearances**]

1) Radiography

Sometimes pleural effusion is the only sign can be seen on radiography. The radiographic appearance is of a well-defined lobulated mass adjacent to the lung field when the tumor grows larger and the broad bottom of tumor is adhesive to chest wall.

2) CT

On CT localized fibrous tumor may show at any area of pleura. It presents as round, homogeneous density and sharp margin. It can be shown as homogeneous enhancement.

The usual appearance of diffuse mesothelioma of pleura is nodular pleural thickening which is accompanied with pleural effusion. Some patients with diffuse mesothelioma of pleura have signs such as enlargement of mediastinal lymph node and rib involvement.

3) MRI

The localized fibrous tumor is always shown as regular shape and homogeneous signal.

But the diffuse mesothelioma of pleura is usually shown as irregular shape and inhomogeneous signal. Its nematodes pleural effusion can be seen as short T1 signal and long T2 signal.

[**Diagnosis**]

The presence of pleural effusion with mass effect in a patient should raise the suspicion of primary tumor of pleura. Contrast enhanced CT thorax is the imaging modality of choice for assessing the extent of involvement and to provide supporting evidence of diagnosis. Aspiration of pleural fluid clinically or under imaging guidance confirms the diagnosis and helps to institute the appropriate treatment.

(2) Metastatic tumor of pleura

The metastatic tumor of pleura is secondary to the other tumor by blood or lymph.

It is common in lung cancer, breast cancer and tumor of gastrointestinal tract.

[**Pathology and clinical manifestations**]

The main symptoms of metastatic tumor of pleura are persistent chest pain and dyspnea due to pleural effusion. There are multiple sporadic nodules on pleura and pleural effusion.

[**Imaging appearances**]

1) Radiography

It is difficult to find small metastatic lesion on radiography. The effusion may obscure the pleural masses.

2) CT

Plain CT can show pleural effusion. Some patients with metastatic tumor of pleura can show sporadic nodules on pleura, irregular nodular thickness of pleura and enlargement of mediastinal lymph nodes (Fig 4-4-9). The nodules of pleura can be seen of apparent enhancement on enhanced CT.

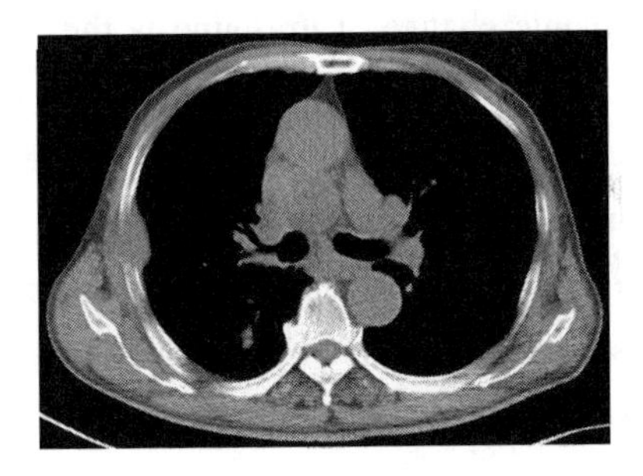

Fig 4-4-9 CT: metastatic tumor of right pleura

3) MRI

Plain MRI can show multiple sporadic nodules on pleura on T2-weighted image. The nodules of pleura can be seen of apparent enhancement on enhanced MRI and the signs are clearer than those on enhanced CT.

[**Diagnosis**]

In the presence of imaging appearances and primary tumor, the diagnosis is almost certain. But if necessary, percutaneous needle biopsy is probably the investigation of choice.

Chapter 5

Imaging of the Circulatory System

Medical imaging is very important in diagnosing diseases of the circulatory system. It can show the external contour and internal structure of the heart and great vessels. Radiography is the commonest examination of the circulatory system, though it cannot display the internal structure of the heart. Angiocardiography is the most precise method of visualization of intra-cardiovascular chambers and haemodynamic change. Ultrasound is the preferred examination in cardiological diagnosis, but it is also a very operator dependent technique. CT is an important method in the detection of calcification in the coronary arteries. It is often the first-line technique for diagnosing acute aortic diseases. MRI is progressing rapidly and there is a very considerable amount of potential for future development. The main strength of cardiac MRI techniques lies in their flexibility and the combination of anatomical and functional studies.

Lesson 1 Heart and Pericardium

Section 1 Imaging methods

1 Radiography

(1) Cardiac radiography

The commonest imaging examination of heart is radiography. Radiograpy is used for the thorax usually and the heart is examined meanwhile as one part of it. The conventional projection positions are: postero-anterior position, left anterior oblique position, right anterior oblique position and/or left lateral position.

(2) Cardiac angiography

Contrast medium is injected into the cardiac cavity through the catheter in the blood vessels. It is applied to study internal structure, motion and haemodynamics. It is divided into two types, the right/left heart angiography and coronary arteriography. The therapy is also achieved simultaneously.

2 Ultrasonography

Transthoracic echocardiography has become an important modality in assessing cardiac structure and function. The diagnostic work includes the combination of M-mode, 2-D (B-mode) with D-mode (PW, CW, and CDFI). Integrated application of these methods can improve the accuracy of heart diseases diagnosis. Heart lies inside the thoracic cavity and most part of it is covered by the lung tissue, which makes it hard for sound waves to penetrate bony tissues or air-containing lungs and specific acoustic windows are needed. The commonly used positions are gaps between ribs on the left chest, the apex area of heart, the area under the xiphoid process and the stermum nest.

(1) 2-D (B-mode) echocardiography

2-D (B-mode) is two-dimensional and real-time in showing different planes of heart clearly and directly. Therefore, it can show the structure of heart in detail, and display the spatial location and the connection of each part clearly. It has better spatial resolution and is the basic inspection method of ultrasonic echocardiography.

(2) M-mode echocardiography

It is one-dimensional time-motion curve. It often describes the movement of valves and the wall of the heart.

(3) D-mode echocardiography

It contains CDFI, PW, CW and tissue Doppler.

(4) Other methods and new technologies

The other methods and new technologies include the tissue tracking imaging, ultrasound contrast, stress echocardiography, transesophageal echocardiography and real-time three-dimensional echocardiography, etc.

3 CT

CT gives excellent quality images of intra-thoracic anatomy. The technique can be effective in the diagnosis of abnormalities of heart and great vessels.

Recent advances in high-speed multislice CT can have a great prognostic value in the detection of calcification in the coronary arteries that has practical utility and temporal resolution. But the multislice CT is radiational and cannot show directly in complex oblique planes. This is often the first-line technique for diagnosing acute aortic disease in combination with high-dose contrast injection, such as aortic dissection

4 MRI

MRI is an important examination which can show both the external and internal cardiac structures without contrast medium. MRI has become a particularly powerful tool for evaluating cardiac diseases. It can distinguish adjacent tissues from blood. MRI can use a lot of ranges of imaging planes, such as transverse, coronal, sagittal and complex obliques. In an examination plane of a cardiac cycle, a gradient-echo technique can be used to perform flow sequences.

MRI has a main strength in diagnosis of heart because of its flexibility and can combine the anatomical with functional studies. The more complete assessment of haemodynamic lesions can be diagnosed by MRI flow studies, such as valve abnormalities and congenital heart defects.

Section 2 Normal imaging findings of heart and pericardium

1 Radiography

(1) Chest radiography

The normal chest radiography can show a part of contour of heart and great vessels, while pericardium cannot be seen due to lack of contrast. Poster-anterior film can display two edges of heart (Fig 5-1-1).

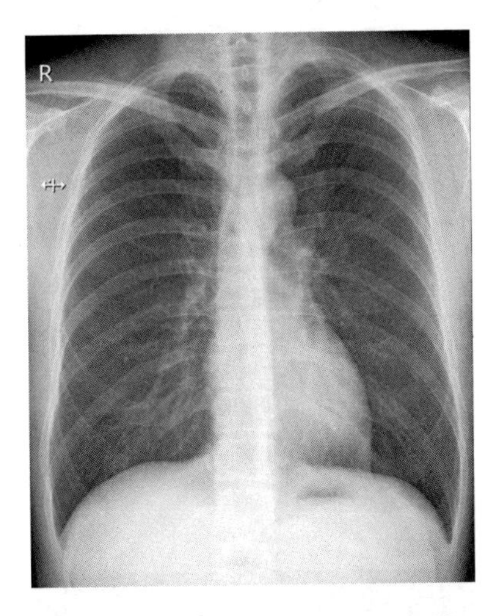

Fig 5-1-1 Normal poster-anterior film

(2) Heart contour

The shape of heart is divided into horizontal, oblique and vertical.

(3) Size

The cardiothoracic ratio is the most common method of describing heart size that is expressed as a percentage of the heart size with respect to internal thoracic diameter. The normal value is less than or equal to 0.5 (Fig 5-1-2).

2 Ultrasonography

(1) 2-D (B-mode) echocardiography

The common imaging planes are described as the following figures, such a parasternal long axis-left ventricle (Fig 5-1-3), parasternal short axis-mitral valve (Fig 5-1-4), four/five chambers (Fig 5-1-5) and so on.

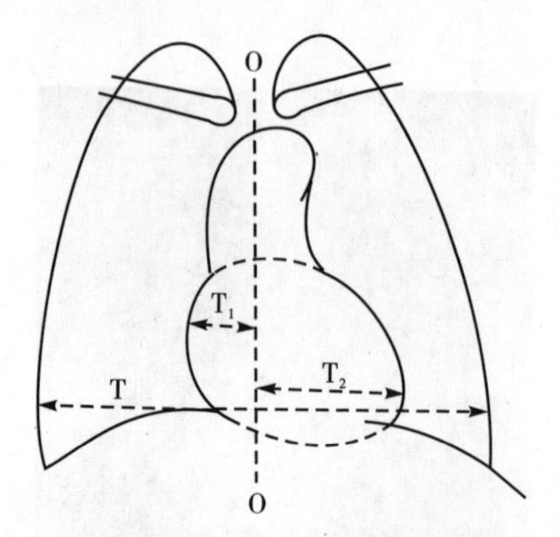

Fig 5-1-2 Cardiothoracic ratio

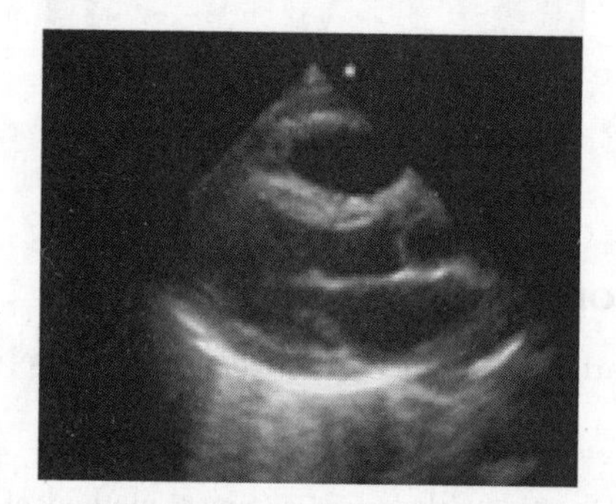

Fig 5-1-3 Parasternal long axis-left ventricle

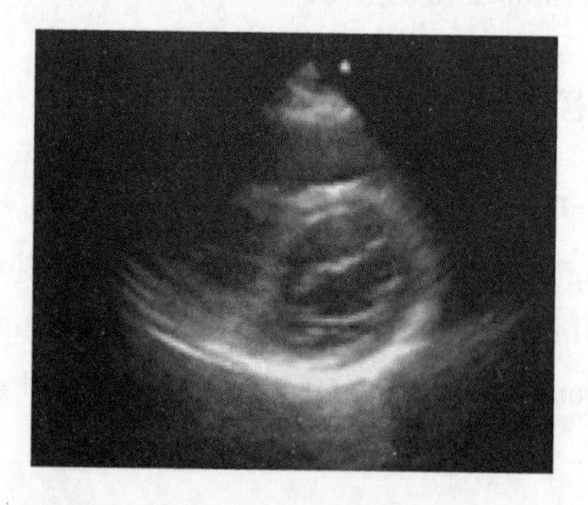

Fig 5-1-4 Parasternal short axis-mitral valve

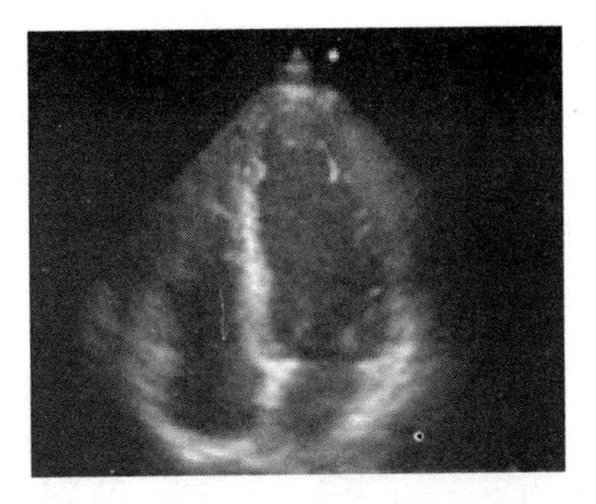

Fig 5-1-5 Apical-four chambers

(2) M-mode echocardiography

1) Normal M-mode of mitral valve

In diastole two peaks are formed which are called E and A peaks respectively. This is caused by the initial opening of valve in ventricular diastole and atrial contraction at the end of diastole. When diastole begins, the anterior mitral leaflet executes a rapid anterior motion, coming to a peak to form E peak. Then the ventricle is filled rapidly with blood from left atrium, and the valve drifts close. While the left atrium contracts, the mitral valve opens in a shorter anterior and terminates at peak A, which occurs just after P wave on ECG. In normal M-mode of mitral orifice, E peak is larger than A peak (E>A). C-D segment represents the closing of mitral valve in systole. The posterior mitral leaflet is approximate mirror of the anterior leaflet. We summarize M-mode features of mitral valve in a simple way: Double peaks, mirror image, opposite movement. (Fig 5-1-6)

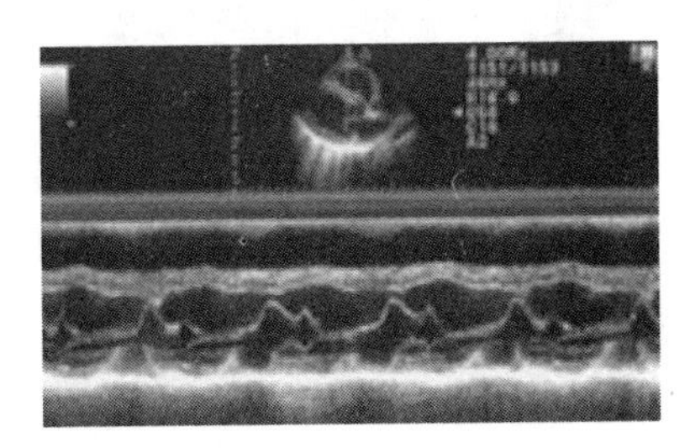

Fig 5-1-6 Normal M-mode of mitral valve

2) Normal M-mode of aortic valve

In diastole it opens a hexagon line. In systole it closes a straight line.

The superior curve represents the right coronary leaflet and the inferior curve represents the non-coronary leaflet. (Fig 5-1-7)

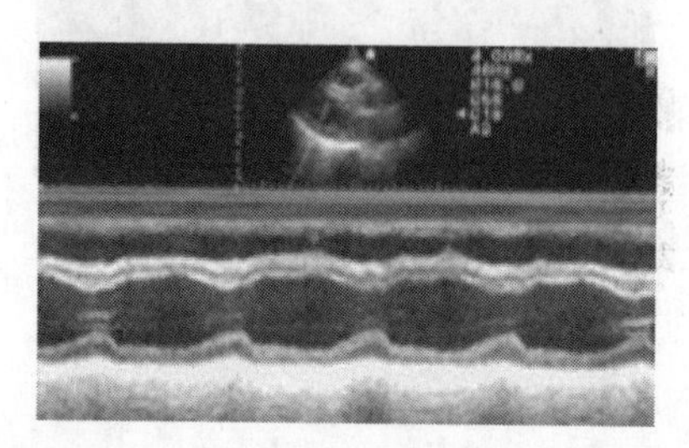

Fig 5-1-7 Normal M-mode of aortic valve

3 Normal M-mode of interventricular septum and posterior wall of left ventricle

In systole, interventricular septum moves forward and in diastole backward. Posterior wall of left ventricle moves in an opposite direction with interventricular septum in systole and diastole respectively. (Fig 5-1-8)

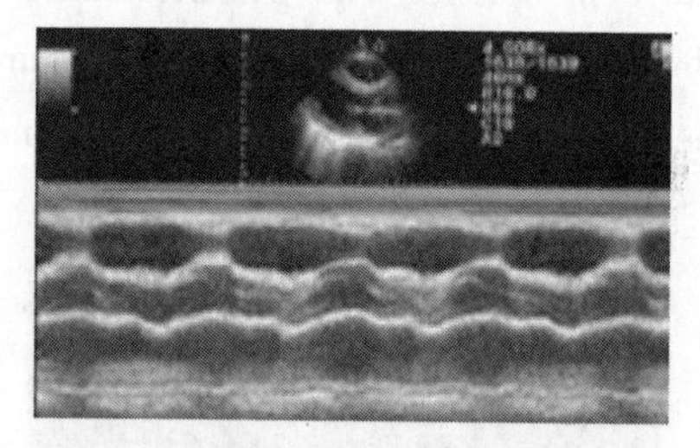

Fig 5-1-8 Normal M-mode of ⅣS and posterior wall of left ventricle

(3) CDFI

In the four chambers and parasternal long axis-left ventricle, normal mitral valve and tricuspid valve show as diastolic blood flow toward the probe of the red blood flow signals, and the left ventricular outflow tract and aortic valve show as systolic blood flow to the blue blood flow signals deviating from the probe. (Fig 5-1-9)

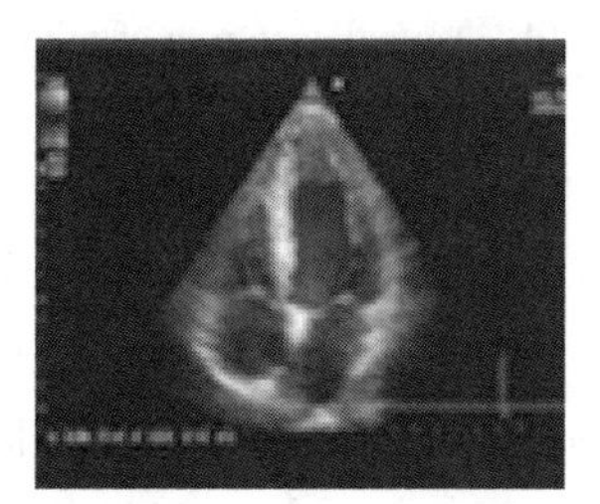

Fig 5-1-9 Four chambers Aortic valve shows blue blood flow

(4) D-mode echocardiography

We have discussed PW, CW and spectrum in detail in the preceding chapter.

1) Normal spectrum of mitral orifice

Apical-four chambers plane is often used. The sample volume is located under cusps of mitral valves of left ventricle. The blood flow in diastole is luminar flow. The spectrum shows positive direction (above baseline), narrow band with double peaks (E and A peaks). There is empty window between spectrum and borderline. In normal D-mode of mitral orifice, E peak is larger than A peak (E>A). The mechanism of formation of E and A peaks is the same as that of M-mode. CDFI shows a wide, red, bright blood flow from left atrium to left ventricle through mitral orifice in diastole when mitral valve opens. (Fig 5-1-10)

2) Normal spectrum of aortic orifice

Apical-five chambers plane is used. The sample volume is located near orifice of ascending aorta. The blood flow in systole is luminar flow. The spectrum

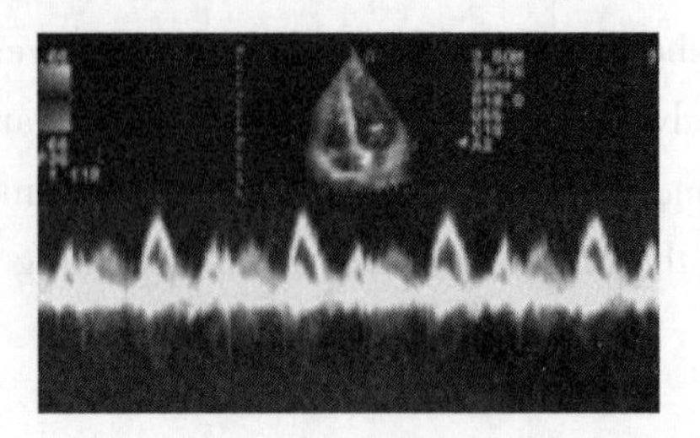

Fig 5-1-10 Normal spectrum of mitral orifice

shows negative direction (below baseline), narrow band with single peak. There is empty window between spectrum and borderline. The shape of spectrum is triangle with steep ascending branch and obtuse descending branch. The formation of single peak is caused by injection of blood flow from left ventricle to ascending aorta through aortic orifice. CDFI shows a blue blood flow from left ventricle to ascending aorta through aortic orifice in systole when aortic valve opens. (Fig 5-1-11)

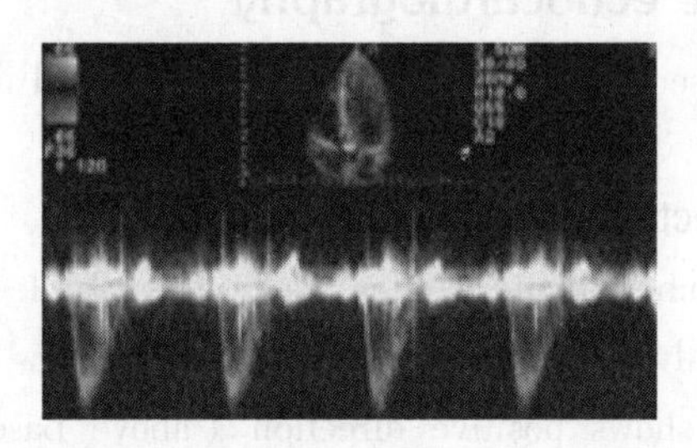

Fig 5-1-11 Normal spectrum of aortic orifice

3 CT

(1) Axial plane

It is the most common, and it can show cardiac structure and atrio-ventricular anatomy. The pericardium will be seen as 1 ~ 2mm thickened arching zones, like soft tissue density (Fig 5-1-12-A/B/C/D).

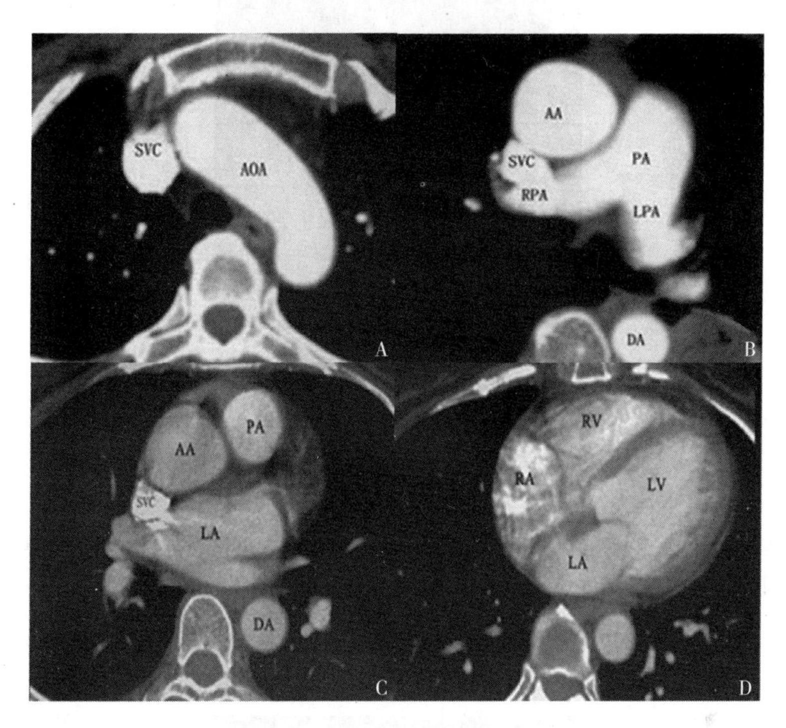

Fig 5-1-12-A/B/C/D

A: aortic arch level, B: tracheal carina level, C: aortic root level, D: left ventricle level

AOA: aortic arch; SVC: superior vena cava; AA: ascending aorta; DA: descending aorta; PA: pulmonary artery; RPA: right pulmonary artery; LPA: left pulmonary artery; RA: right atrium; LA: left atrium; RV: right ventricle; LV: left ventricle

(2) Short-axial

It is perpendicular to the long axis of heart. The level of left ventricular body will show ventricular wall and septa. The round filling defects refer to anterior and posterior papillary muscles (Fig 5-1-12-E).

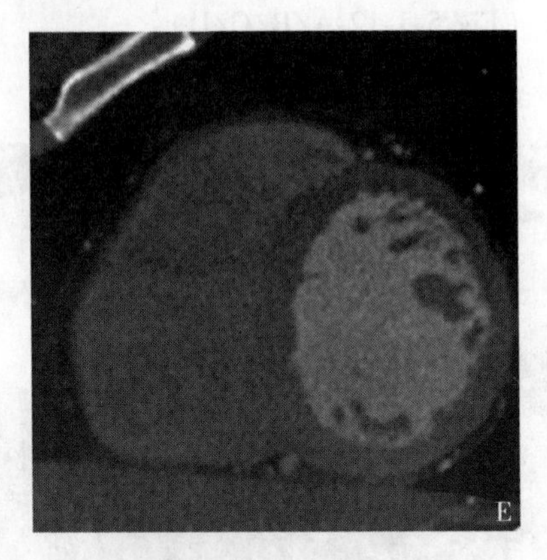

Fig 5-1-12-E　Short-axial

(3) Long-axial

It can show the valve, left ventricular outflow tract and apex. On the level of outflow tract, the outflow tract, aortic valve and ascending aortic root can be observed (Fig 5-1-12-F).

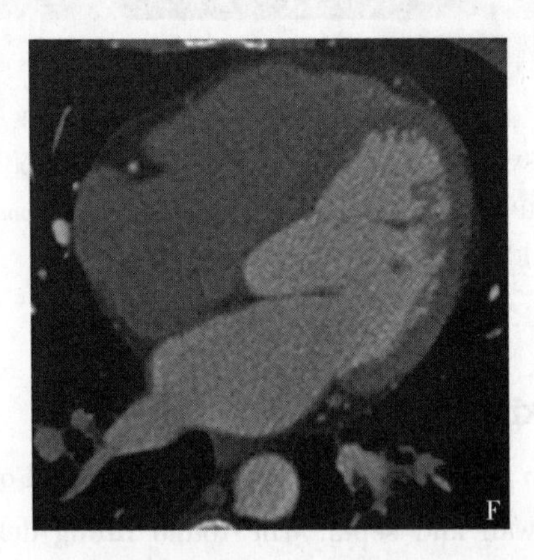

Fig 5-1-12-F　Long-axial view

4 MRI

MRI findings are consistent with CT at the position of axial, coronal, sagittal plane (Fig 5-1-13-A/B/C).

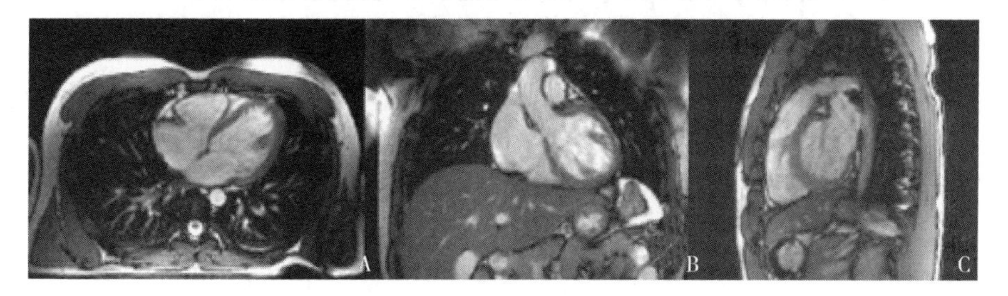

Fig 5-1-13-A/B/C MRI

(1) Myocardium

The myocardium shows moderate signal in T1-and T2-weighted images. The thickness of right ventricular wall is equivalent to a third of the left.

(2) Endocardium

The endocardium will present as thin linear signal, slightly higher than the myocardial signal.

(3) Valve

The valve shows intermediate intensity in MR, including mitral, tricuspid and aortic valves.

(4) Pericardium

It presents as a linear low signal. The thickness of pericardium is not more than 4mm.

(5) Coronary artery

The coronary artery can be seen instability and poor reproducibility in images of MRI because of interference of cardiac and respiratory motion.

Section 3 Imaging signs of heart and pericardium diseases

1 Position, shape, and size abnormalities

(1) Position abnormality

The diagnosis of position abnormality should depend on CT and MRI images or angiocardiography, but not radiography.

1) Overall position abnormality

①Heart displacement, which deviates from its normal position due to the lung disease or deformity.

②Heart translocation, which presents cardiac congenital dissociation, co-existing with thoraco-abdominal organ transposition and heart malformation.

2) Atrio-ventricular relative position abnormality

The left and right sides are reversed, for example, the right atrium or ventricle is on the left side.

3) Atrio-ventricular connection abnormality

The left atrium connects with the right ventricle, and the right atrium connects with the left ventricle.

4) Connection between cardiac ventricle and great vessels

The left ventricle should connect with aorta and the right one with pulmonary artery. When the great vessels fail to develop, the connection will be affected.

(2) Shape and size abnormality

1) The shape of heart

The shape of heart is divided into mitral, aortic and whole largamente type (Fig 5-1-14-A/B/C). Cardiac enlargement includes ventricular hypertrophy and chamber dilatation. Cardiothoracic ratio is the simplest method which defines cardiac enlargement, and the normal value is below 0. 5.

2) Internal structure abnormality

It mainly refers to the abnormal atrio-ventricular septa and valve.

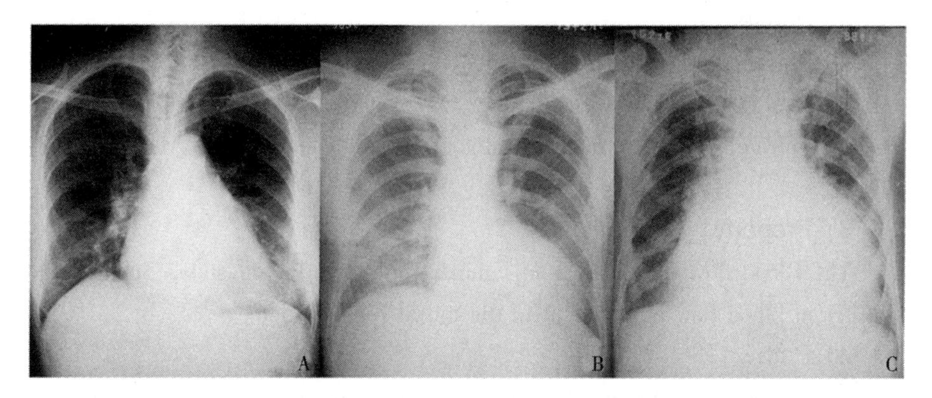

Fig 5-1-14-A/B/C Mitral, aortic and whole largamente type

A: mitral type: pear-shaped, bulging pulmonary artery segment, left ventricular enlargement, often seen in mitral valve disease and atrial septal defect. B: aortic type: the aortic arch is broadening, heart enlargement, often seen in aortic valve disease and hypertensive heart disease. C: Heart enlarges to both sides, often seen in heart failure and a large amount of pericardial effusion

2 Abnormal cardiac motion and blood flow

(1) Abnormal motion

We can make the evaluation on the abnormal cardiac motion by observing the ventricular motion. The evaluation method includes echocardiography, ventriculography, MSCT and MRI. The echocardiography can display the abnormal motion and blood flow in real-time, directively and sensitively. According to the heart contraction amplitude and coordination, the abnormalities can be divided into enhancement, weakness, disappearance and contradictory motion.

(2) Abnormal blood flow

It mainly depends on ultrasound.

1) Velocity

The velocity of blood flow is higher or lower than the normal. Most heart diseases can cause the abnormal blood flow. For example, in the Left Ventricular Diastole of MS, the blood flow velocity increases markedly around the mitral valve. The blood flow velocity decreases obviously around every heart valve.

2) Phase

The duration of blood flow is longer or shorter than normal, or the blood flow happens in the phase without flow. For example, there is no blood flow in the left ventricular outflow tract normally, but it happened in the Aortic regurgitation.

3) Property

The Blood flow translates from laminar flow to turbulent state. Such as the left atrium blood flow is turbulent in the mitral regurgitation

4) Path

Blood flow goes through the channel that does not exist in normal heart, such as a left to right shunt in atrial septal defect.

3 Coronary abnormalities

It can be classified as congenital and acquired.

(1) Coronary angiography

It is the most reliable method for the diagnosis of coronary artery disease, but it is an invasive examination (Fig 5-1-15).

(2) Ultrasonography

Initial segment of coronary arteric stenosis, atherosclerotic plaques, and arterial stenosis can be evaluated. The dilated wall of coronary arterial initial segment can be seen. Ultrasound can display coronary artery expansion such as coronary artery fistula. It can also observe the pathological changes of coronary artery origin, coronary arterial line and fistula.

(3) MSCT

As the most important noninvasive method, it can show arterial stenosis and occlusion or origin, morphology, abnormality of coronary artery (Fig 5-1-16-A/B).

(4) MRI

MRI can display the proximal and middle abnormalities of the coronary artery.

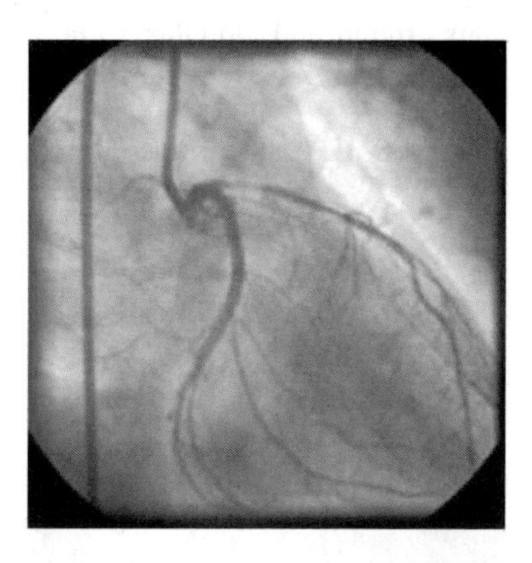

Fig 5-1-15 Coronary angiography

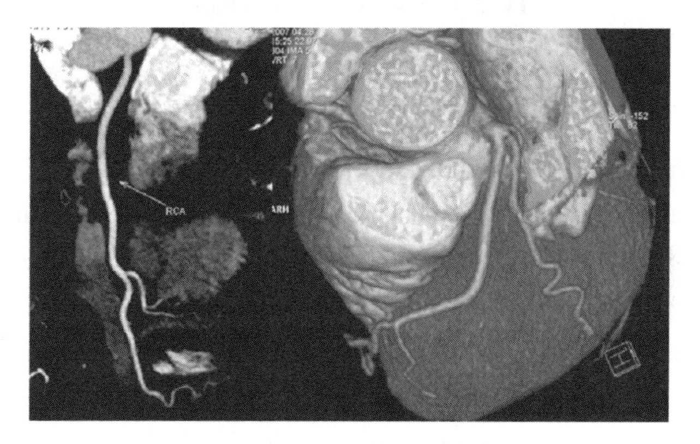

Fig 5-1-16-A/B MSCT

4 Pericardial lesions

(1) Pericardial effusion

1) Radiography

The appearances that can be identified on radiography depend on the amount of effusion. A large collection of effusion can cause massive enlargement of cardiac shadow, which looks round and globular (Fig 5-1-17-A).

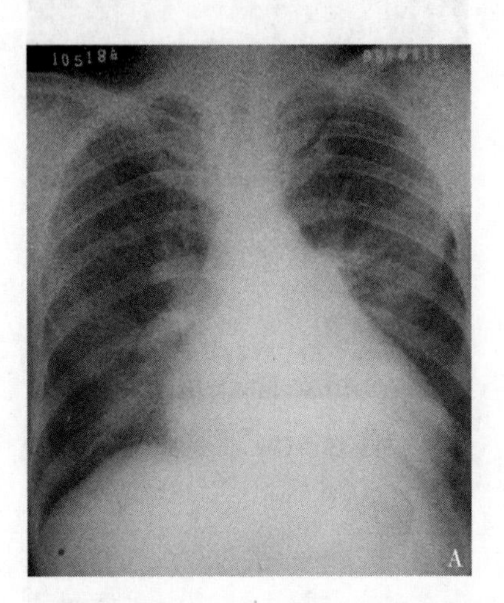

Fig 5-1-17-A Pericardial effusion
The heart enlarges to both sides.

2) Ultrasonography, CT, and MRI

①***Ultrasonography***: 2D echocardiography is the best imaging technique for detection of pericardical effusion. It can not only estimate the amount but guide tapping. Anechoic area is found in left ventricle border or left ventricle wall (in the pericardium).

②***CT***: CT can show broadening pericardial cavity with water-like density fluid, and evaluate the amount of effusion (Fig 5-1-17-B).

③***MRI***: Fluid can be seen as short T1 signal and long T2 signal on plain MRI (Fig 5-1-17-C).

(2) Pericardial thickening

1) Radiography

The appearances of abnormal heart morphology, broadening superior vena cava and pulmonary congestion can be shown.

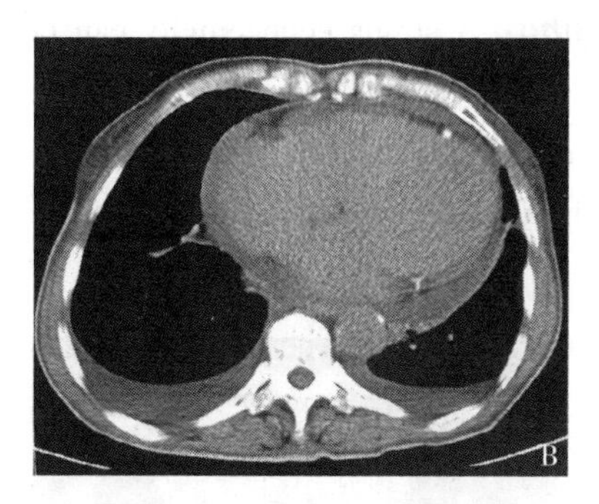

Fig 5-1-17-B Pericardial effusion

CT shows a large amount of liquid density in pericardium

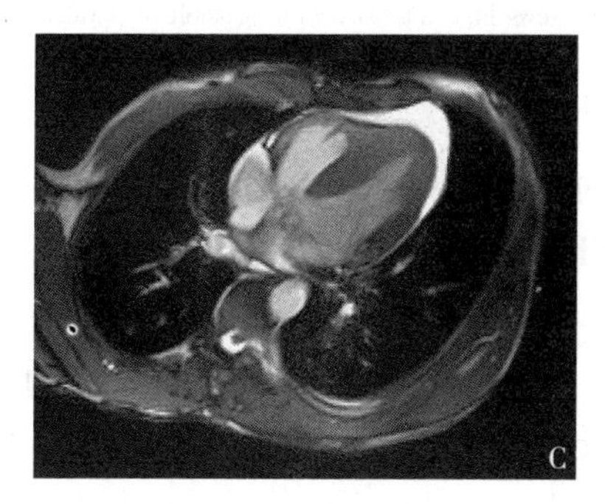

Fig 5-1-17-C Pericardial effusion

a large amount of liquid intensity with long T2 signal in pericardium on T2WI

2) Ultrasound, CT, and MRI

They can directly display the thickened pericardium that is above 4mm.

(3) Pericardial calcification

1) Radiography

The calcification presents as eggshell on radiography.

2) Ultrasonography, CT and MRI

①***Ultrasonography***: A strong echogenicity can be seen in calcified pericardium.

②***CT***: CT has high sensitivity and specificity to diagnosis calcification, which can show pericardial high intensity with linear or eggshell (Fig 5-1-18).

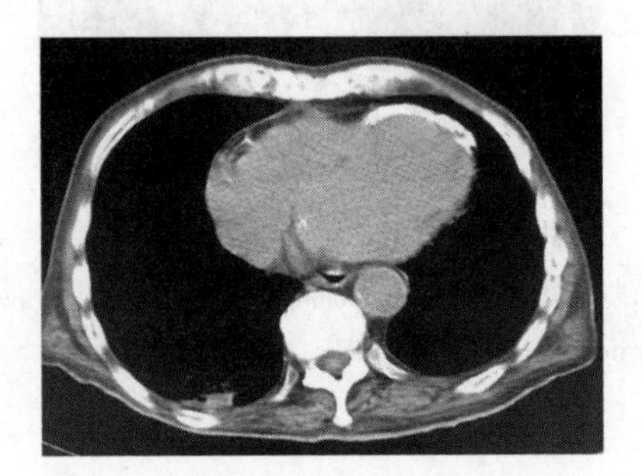

Fig 5-1-18 Pericardial thickening

CT shows high intensity with eggshell in pericardium

③***MRI***: It demonstrates no or low signal on MRI.

(4) Pericardial mass

1) Radiography

This is frequently noted in radiography as pericardial effusion.

2) Ultrasonography, CT, and MRI

①***Ultrasonography***: It appears as mass or irregular shape. The echo level is hyperechogenic.

②***CT***: CT shows the pericardium with the density which is similar to soft tissue.

③***MRI***: MRI can display shape, size and edge of mass combined with film sequence, and can observe the mass activity, too.

(5) Hilar and pulmonary vessels change

1) Hilum

The appearance of bilateral hilar enlargement can be seen in pulmonary congestion and pulmonary plethora. Pulmonary dilatation can be judged by the diameter of descending branch of the right pulmonary artery that exceeds 1. 5 centimeter in adults.

2) Abnormal artery

①***Pulmonary congestion***: It may occur as a result of increased blood flow with a left to right shunt. The arterial branches will broaden proportionally and extend toward the periphery.

②***Pulmonary arterial hypertension***: It often occurs in pulmonary heart diseases and pulmonary embolism. The proximal pulmonary arteries are enlarged and then taper toward the periphery, which is called hilar truncation (Fig 5-1-19).

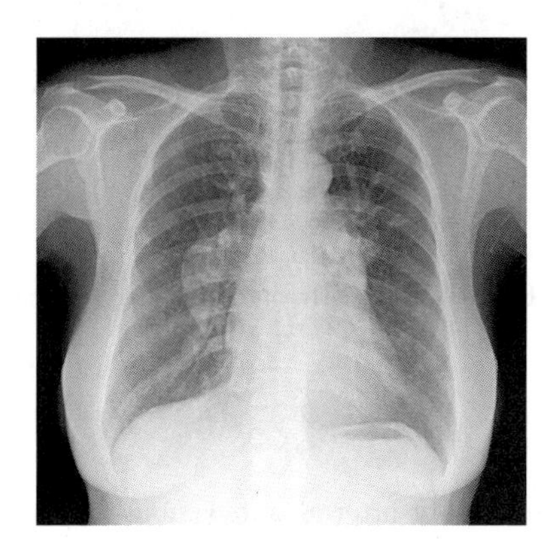

Fig 5-1-19 Pulmonary arterial hypertension

A dilatation of the pulmonary artery, pulmonary markings thickening, often seen in pulmonary heart disease and pulmonary embolism

③***Pulmonary oligaemia***: It is due to heart diseases of reducing cardiac output, such as tricuspid stenosis and pulmonary stenosis. The findings of thin arteries and hyperlucent lung fields can be seen on radiography.

3) Pulmonary venous hypertension

The causes are increase of left atrial pressure, left ventricular resistance and pulmonary venous pressure. The appearances of pulmonary congestion, pulmonary interstitial edema and alveolar pulmonary edema can be seen on radiography (Fig 5-1-20-A). Pulmonary interstitial edema are associated with Kerley B lines-horizontal subpleural lines, 1~3mm in thickness and 2~3cm in length, most frequently identified at the costophrenic angles (Fig 5-1-20-B).

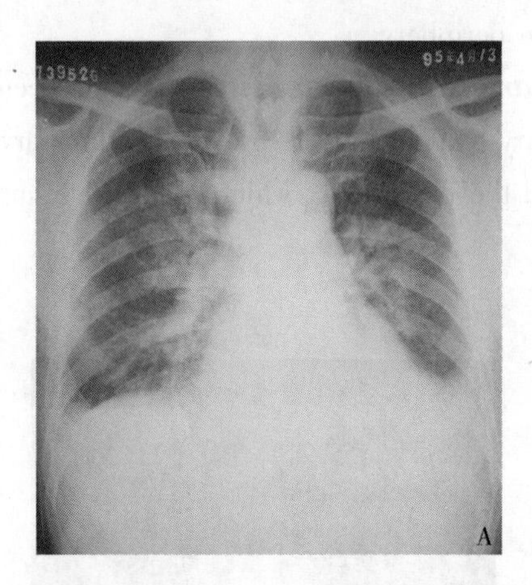

Fig 5-1-20-A Alveolar pulmonary edema

4) Mixed type

The findings of pulmonary arterial and venous hypertension can be seen on chest radiography.

Section 4 Diagnosis of diseases

1 Coronary atherosclerotic heart disease

Cardiac imaging techniques are very important in diagnosing this disease. It is a multifactorial and complex process of the development of coronary atheroma.

[**Pathology and clinical manifestations**]

The development of atheromatous plaques in the coronary artery is related to a variety of clinical syndromes. The conditions, such as stable angina or ischaemic cardiomyopathy, will occur because of chronic increase in the size and oc-

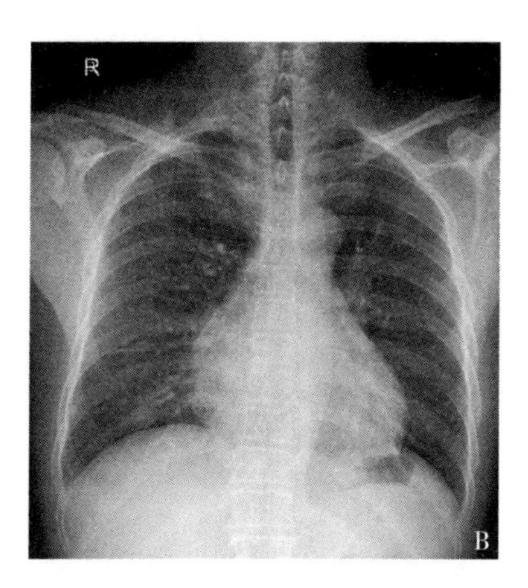

Fig 5-1-20-B Pulmonary interstitial edema

clusive nature of the plaques. A variety of acute coronary syndromes include unstable angina, myocardial infarction, heart failure and sudden death. The factors leading to these syndromes are acute changes, especially plaque rupture.

[**Imaging appearances**]

(1) Radiography

The chest radiograph is usually normal except for myocardial infarction. The chest radiographic features include progressive enlargement of the heart and the development of pulmonary edema. It can show perihilar and peripheral parenchymal clouding and the septal lines, and finally the formation of alveolar pulmonary edema. If the left heart failure aggravates, pleural effusions will increase (Fig 5-1-21-A).

Coronary angiography is the most accurate examination method in combination with the left ventricular angiography.

(2) Ultrasonography

Echocardiography can show initial segment change of coronary artery, myocardial ischaemia, myocardial infarction and its complications.

1) Initial segment change of coronary artery

The irregular thickness of coronary arterial wall, aortic stenosis, and some-

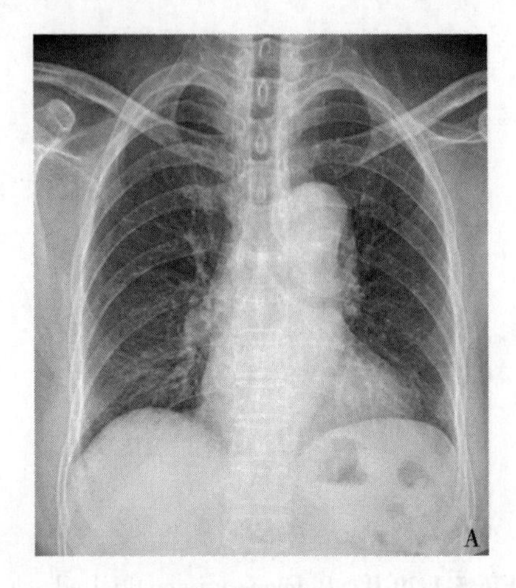

Fig 5-1-21-A

Coronary atherosclerotic heart disease enlarged cardiac shadow, prominent aortic nodes, and calcification in the aortic arch.

times the calcification can be seen.

2) Myocardial ischaemia

Regional wall movement abnormal appears in the corresponding wall segments when ischaemia occurs.

3) Myocardial infarction

①Regional wall movement abnormal appears in the corresponding wall segments. This is the most important diagnostic feature of myocardial infarction in echocardiography.

②The internal echo in myocardial infarction segments is abnormal. In acute myocardial infarction, it becomes hypoechogenic. In chronic myocardial infarction in which scar is formed, it becomes hyperechogenic and corresponding wall becomes thinned.

③In normal heart, the increase rate of wall thickness is more than 30%. But in myocardial infarction, it is less than 30%, zero or even negative. That means the wall thickness does not increase in systole but becomes thinned. This is the main difference between angina pectoris and myocardial infarction.

④***Impairment of left ventricle function***: EF, FS, CO, and SV are decreased. E peak velocity is decreased and A peak velocity is increased. E peak velocity is lower than A peak velocity.

⑤***Complications of myocardial infarction***: The common complications include ventricular aneurysm (Fig 5-1-21-B), formation of pseudo-aneurysm, ventricle thromboem-bolism, ventricular septal perforation, papillary muscle dys-function or rupture (Fig 5-1-21-C), and postinfarction syndrome. Ultrasound has high sensitivity and specificity in the diagnosis of them.

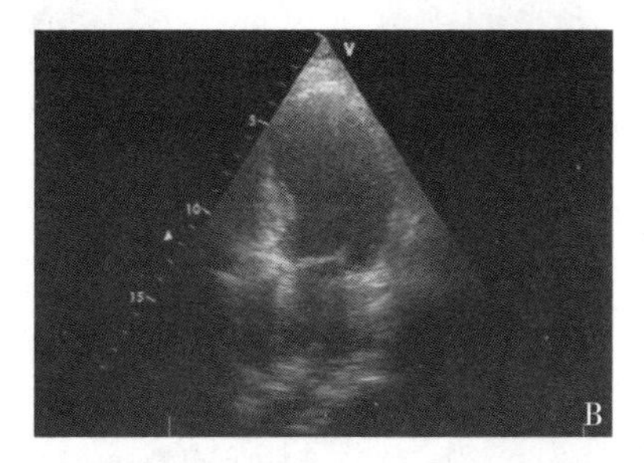

Fig 5-1-21-B Formation of real aneurysm

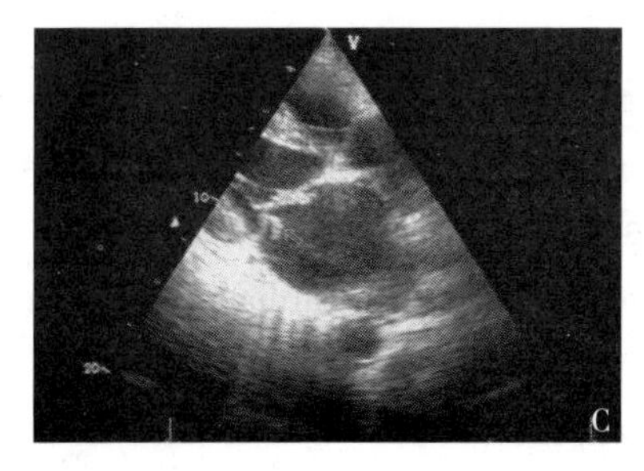

Fig 5-1-21-C Papillary muscle dysfunction or rupture

(3) CT

CT, especially CTA, has become the most reliable method in the evaluation and noninvasive diagnosis of coronary artery diseases. Fast CT scanning techniques have great advantages in the detection of calcification in the coronary arteries, because it is non-invasive and is performed quickly.

1) Anomalous coronary artery

CTA has been considered as great clinical potential for detecting or ruling out coronary artery stenosis. In addition, risk stratification can also utilize the imaging of coronary atherosclerotic plaque (Fig 5-1-21-D).

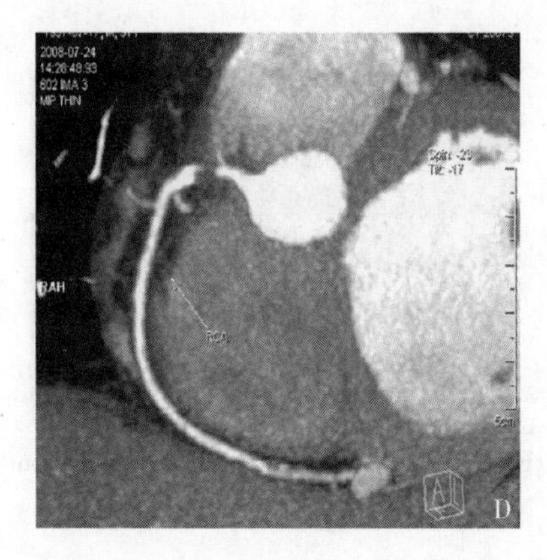

Fig 5-1-21-D Anomalous coronary artery

On coronary artery CTA examination, CPR shows low density of visible plaque formation within the arterial lumen, partial occlusion of the lumen.

2) Myocardial ischemia

Based on the different phases of cardiac cavity size, left ejection fraction can be calculated.

3) Myocardial infarction

CT shows that regional myocardial wall becomes thin. Myocardial wall will be not thickening in systolic phase. The segmental ventricular wall function abnormalities and reducing ejection fraction can also be seen.

(4) MRI

A modality to comprehensively visualize cardiovascular structures and functions can be achieved with technologic advances in cardiovascular magnetic resonance (CMR). The detection of calcification is not suitable in MRI. Before the high-resolution studies of coronary arteries are achieved on a routine basis, MRI cannot be used as a screening tool for coronary artery disease.

1) Angina

The decreasing of segmental cardiac motion on movie sequence and perfusion of ischemic myocardium can be shown.

2) Acute myocardial infarction

Myocardial infarction shows high signal on T2WI, but thickness of myocardial wall is often normal. The disappearance or decreasing of segmental cardiac motion on movie sequence and perfusion of ischemic myocardium can be shown. MRI can show delayed enhancement in myocardial infarction region.

3) Older myocardial infarction

Myocardial infarction shows low signal on T2WI, and thickness of myocardial wall becomes thinner. The appearances of segmental cardiac motion, perfusion of ischemic myocardium and delayed imaging is similar to the acute phase.

4) Complications after myocardial infarction

The complications mainly contain ventricular aneurysm, ventricular septal perforation and left ventricular papillary muscle rupture. Ventricular aneurysm displays dilated left ventricle toward the surface of heart. The walls of aneurysm show high signal in acute phase and then low signal in chronic phase. Ventricular septal perforation is revealed as discontinuity of ventricular septa and intraventricular left to right shunt. Left ventricular papillary muscle rupture can show mitral regurgitation due to mitral insufficiency.

[**Diagnosis**]

Coronary angiography is the golden standard for the identification of coronary heart disease. CTA can also help in evaluating the stability of plaque in coronary artery. Coronary heart diseases have its characteristics. It is easy to diagnose by its performance combined with clinical data.

2 Rheumatic heart diseases

Rheumatic heart diseases (RHD) include acute or subacute rheumatic carditis and chronic rheumatic valvular diseases. Myocardium and mitral valve are frequently involved.

[**Pathology and clinical manifestations**]

The basic pathological changes are swelling of the valve, valve stenosis and insufficiency.

There are no obvious clinical manifestations at the early stage. Patients with mitral stenosis can have symptoms such as dyspnea hemoptysis and cardiac diastolic murmur shivering, hyperpyrexia, chest pain and rusty expectoration. Patients with mitral insufficiency can have symptoms such as heart palpitation, shortness of breath, left heart failure and heart systolic murmur.

[**Imaging appearances**]

(1) Radiography

1) Mitral stenosis

The chest radiograph can show pulmonary congestion, pulmonary edema and enlargement of left atrium and right ventricle (Fig 5-1-22-A/B).

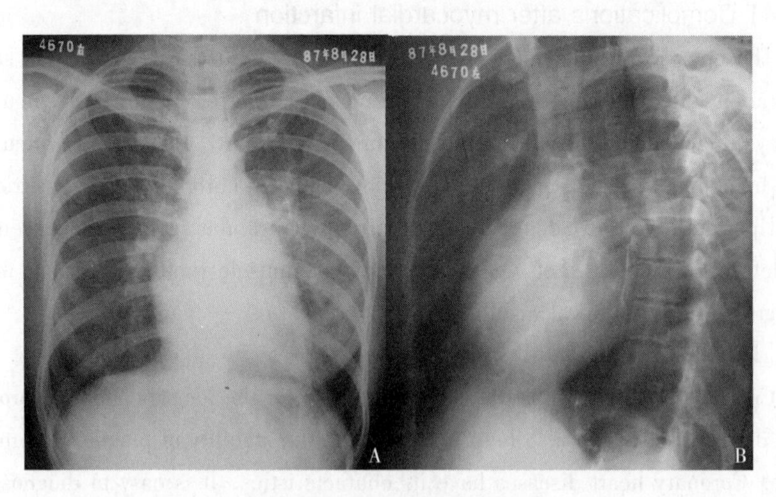

Fig 5-1-22-A/B Mitral stenosis

2) Mitral insufficiency

It presents as left ventricular enlargement due to moderate regurgitation.

3) Aortic stenosis

The enlargement of left atrium and ventricle can be shown, combined with limited expansion of ascending aorta.

4) Aortic insufficiency

The findings of left ventricular enlargement and expansion of ascending aorta or aortic arch can be seen in radiography.

(2) Ultrasonography

Echocardiography is the most important diagnostic examination for evaluation of valve disease.

1) Mitral stenosis (MS)

①***M-mode***: The M-mode diagnosis of mitral valve stenosis is based on an increase in echo production from the thickened, deformed, often calcified leaflets; a decrease in the opening amplitude of the valve; anterior motion of the posterior leaflet (city wall-like wave); and a decrease in the diastolic or EF slope.

②***Two-dimensional echocardiography***: MS alters the 2D appearance of the valve because it partially fuses the normally independent leaflets; an increase in echo production from the thickened, deformed mitral leaflets; a reduction in mitral orifice area; and it creates persistent gradient between the left ventricle (LV) and left atrium (LA). This gradient keeps the stenotic diastolic orifice opened to its maximum and causes the entire valve to dome or bulge into the ventricle throughout diastole. In the parasternal short axis plane, the opening of the valve can be imaged just above the tips of the papillary muscles. From this orientation, its maximum diastolic opening area can be measured by direct planimetry of the 2D image. This method is a reliable means of judging the considered severe, $<1.5cm^2$ as moderate, and $>1.5\ cm^2$ as mild mitral valve stenosis. Doppler echocardiography provides a constellation of measurements to estimate the severity of MS. These variables include the gradient across the valve, the inferred area by the pressure half-time, the continuity equation or the proximal flow convergence, and the pulmonary pressures at rest and during exercise from the tricuspid regurgitant jet velocity. Color flow mapping displays the acceleration field proximal to a stenotic mitral valve (arrow). Continuous wave Doppler recording shows that the peak and mean velocity are higher, indicating mitral valve stenosis (Fig 5-1-22-C).

③Indirect methods to identify the severity of MS include estimating the extent of leaflet calcification, the degree of LV underloading (i. e., volume decrease), the presence of RV and RA dilatation, and the degree of tricuspid regurgitation and pulmonary hypertension, as determined by Doppler of tricuspid reguritant jet.

④Transesophageal echocardiography shows the stenotic mitral valve and dilated left atrium with smoke.

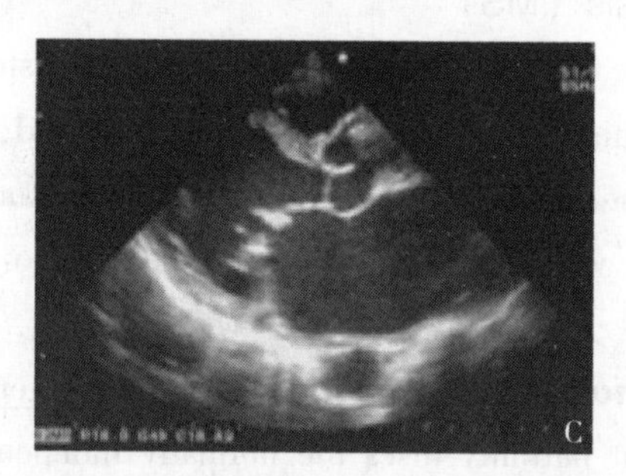

Fig 5-1-22-C Two-dimensional echocardiography

1) Mitral incompetence (MI)

①***Color flow Doppler***: The features of severe mitral regurgitation seen by color flow Doppler imaging arise from the high energy transfer of a volume of blood into LA, producing the characteristic "jet" in LA.

②***Two-dimensional echocardiography***: an increase in echo production from the thickened mitral leaflets; the mitral leaflets close at wrong place and fail to coapt; LA and LV enlargement.

2) Aortic stenosis (AS)

Aortic valvular stenosis caused by thickened and calcified trileaflet valve. The opening amplitude of leaflets is decreased. The varying degrees of concentric

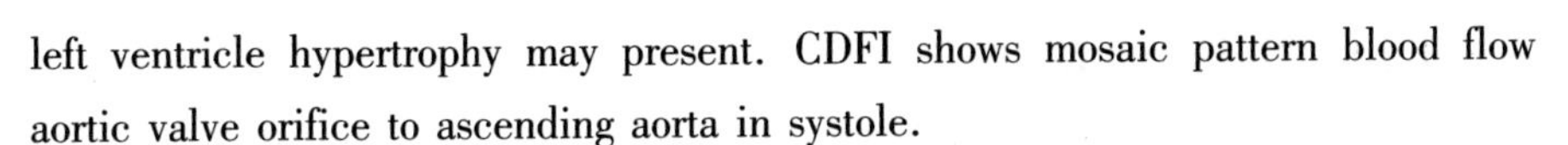

left ventricle hypertrophy may present. CDFI shows mosaic pattern blood flow aortic valve orifice to ascending aorta in systole.

3) Aortic incompetence (AI)

Aortic valve leaf closed line is double, anterior mitral diastolic rapid flapping wave. CDFI illustrates a holodiastolic flow reversal diastolic flow reversal in the abdominal aorta recorded with pulsed-wave Doppler.

4) Combined valvular disease

It has different combinations of the above signs. But because of the interaction, there are some differences in performance with single valve disease.

(3) CT

MSCT can display the calcification of valve and the thrombus on the posterior wall of the left atrium. Valvular insufficiency cannot be observed directly.

(4) MRI

The heart size, volume and thrombus can be seen on the SE sequence. Because of going through the valve lesions, abnormal blood flows will occur.

[**Diagnosis**]

Typical cases can be diagnosed by ultrasound. CT and MRI can not be the main method for diagnosis.

3 Cardiomyopathy

Primary cardiomyopathy includes dilated cardiomyopathy, hypertrophic and constrictive types, and the cardiomyopathy is common in clinical settings.

[**Pathology and clinical manifestations**]

The heart of patient with dilated cardiomyopathy is spherical. Left heart expands markedly. The surroundings of myocardial interstitum and blood vessels are fibrosis in different degrees. Myocardial cells assume hypertrophy, vacuolar degeneration or atrophy.

The most prominent symptoms include left ventricular failure, arrhythmia and systemic arterial embolism.

[**Imaging appearances**]

(1) Radiography

The abnormal cardiac enlargement of all four chambers or just the left ventricle can be seen usually. In the untreated patient the formation of engorgement of the pulmonary vasculature comes from the volume overload of the left atrium.

(2) Ultrasonography

The ventricles are dilated, especially for the left ventricle. The anteroposterior and lateral diameters of the left ventricle increase, and the shape of left ventricular turns from ellipse to ball. Endocardial motion is lower. Thrombus can be found which adheres to wall, mainly in the apex. Sometime pericardial effusion can be seen.

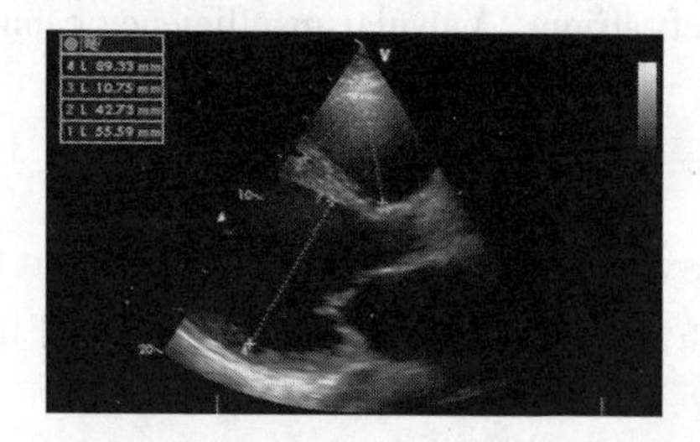

Fig 5-1-23 2D: Dilated cardiomyopathy

(3) CT

The thickness of ventricular wall is often normal or slightly thicker. Myocardial contraction function will decrease.

(4) MRI

The signal intensity of myocardium is moderate intensity, which is consistent and homogeneous in dilated cardiomyopathy. The shape and function are the same as those in CT scan.

[**Diagnosis**]

It can be confirmed by expanding heart chamber, excluding secondary factors.

4 Congenital heart diseases

(1) Atrial septal defect (ASD)

[**Pathology and clinical manifestations**]

ASDs are the second most common congenital lesions in adults (behind bicuspid aortic valves). These defects are often undetected until adulthood due to the lack of prominent clinical symptoms initially. If untreated, an ASD can eventually result in RV heart failure, pulmonary hypertension, atrial arrhythmias, or paradoxical embolization and ischemic cerebral events. There are five types of ASD based on the location of the defect in atrial septum: septum primum; septum secundum; sinus venosus ASD; coronary sinus ASD; and mixed ASD. The ostium primum atrial septal defect (ASD) and the ostium secundum ASD are the major types of this abnormality, and the latter is more common. The ostium secundum defect often lies in the level of the foramen ovale. The tissues of the septum primum or the atrioventricular valves cannot be involved.

There is a left to right shut with the appearance of ASD, and the right atrium and right ventricle will expand and the pulmonary blood flow increase, then leading to pulmonary arterial hypertension.

[**Imaging appearances**]

1) Radiography

If the pulmonary-to-systemic flow ratio is less than 2 : 1, it is usually normal in the chest X-ray, but if it exceeds this level, pulmonary plethora and cardiac enlargement will be seen. The right atria and right ventricular mainly expand with the increasing blood flow. The chest radiography will show centrally dilated pulmonary arteries and peripheral pulmonary vascular "pruning" in the patient with significant pulmonary arterial hypertension (Fig 5-1-24-A).

2) Ultrasonography

Both M-mode and 2D Ultrasound can show the abnormalities as follows:

The right atrium and ventricular are dilated, and the right ventricular outflow tract is widened; abnormal cardiac wall motions happen: the increased motion of right ventricular anterior wall and the decreased motion of ventricular septum. The continuity of the atrial septal upper and middle parts is interrupted

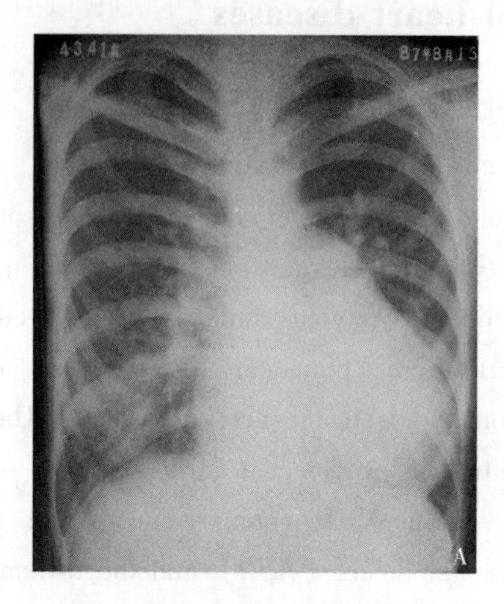

Fig 5-1-24-A ASD

Heart enlargement, combined with pulmonary arterial hypertension

(Fig 5-1-24-B/C).

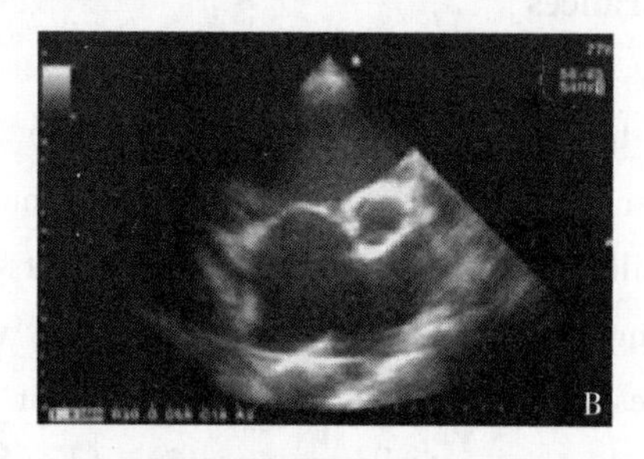

Fig 5-1-24-B 2D-ASD

3) CT

MSCT can show the diameter and location of septal defect.

4) MRI

The loss of septal signal and dynamic performance can be seen in movie se-

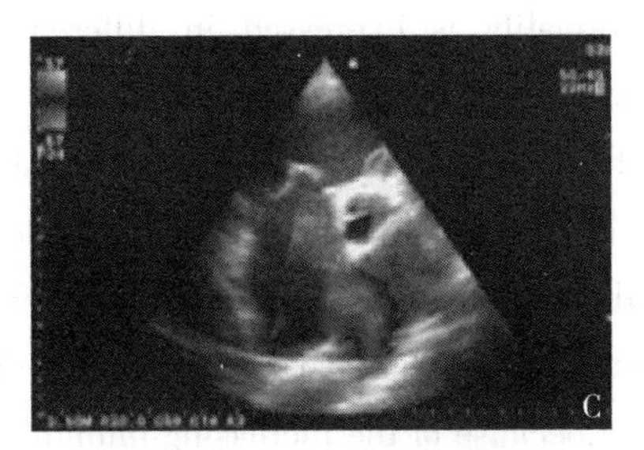

Fig 5-1-24-C CDFI-ASD

quence. Enhanced MRI can show abnormal communication between left and right atria (Fig 5-1-24-D).

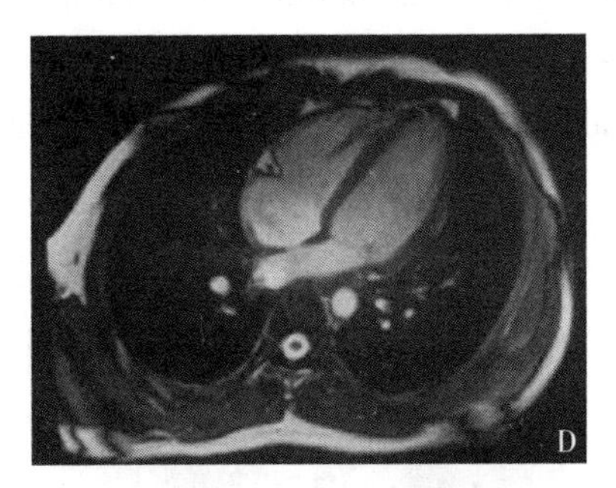

Fig 5-1-24-D ASD

Parts of atrial septal signal loss, abnormal blood flow from the left atrium to the right atrium

[**Diagnosis**]

The findings are usually normal in radiography. CT and MRI can be used in diagnoses.

(2) Tetralogy of Fallot

[**Pathology and clinical manifestations**]

It is a complex of four related abnormalities, containing pulmonary stenosis, ventricle septal defect (VSD), overriding aorta and right ventricular hypertrophy. This abnormality is expressed in different ways, which depend mainly on the severity of the pulmonary stenosis. In mild cases of pulmonary stenosis the abnormality behaves much like a simple ventricle septal defect, with possible defect caused by the reduced pulmonary blood flow.

More typically, the pulmonary stenosis will restrict pulmonary blood flow leading to cyanosis. Varying degrees of cyanosis and fainting spells on exertion will appear in childhood because of the increasing infundibular obstruction to lung blood flow with increasing heart work.

The characteristic systolic murmur by auscultation on the second and fourth intercostal spaces at the left sternal border can be heard.

[**Imaging appearances**]

1) Radiography

The chest radiography is often not classical, but in some cases the concavity in the left heart border can be seen. The distortion by the large right ventricle and pulmonary oligaemia can make cardiac apex prominently raised (Fig 5-1-25-A).

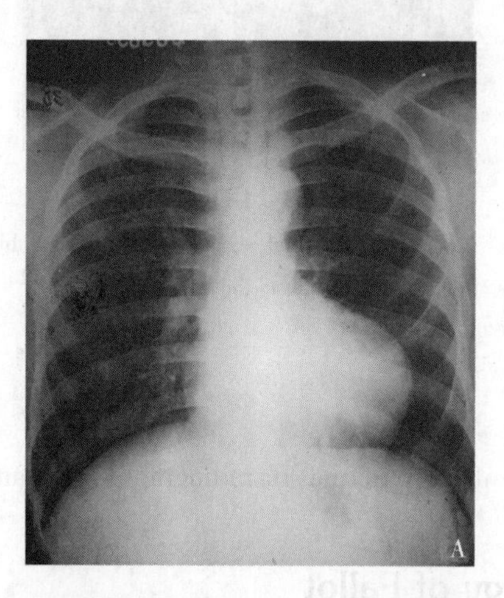

Fig 5-1-25-A Tetralogy of Fallot

Right ventricular is enlarged, apex is upturned, and heart shadow looks like shoe

2) Ultrasonography

Tetralogy of Fallot consists of four anatomic defects: ventricular septum defect, pulmonary stenosis, over-riding aorta and right ventricular hypertrophy. Parasternal long-axis view, parasternal short-axis view, right ventricular outflow tract long-axis view, Apical-four chambers and Apical-five chambers are commonly used.

Echocardiography: M-mode echocardiography shows right ventricular anterior wall thickening, stenosis of right ventricular outflow tract, dilated aorta shifted forward, right ventricular hypertrophy (RVH).

①***2D***: Parasternal long-axis view shows dilated aorta shifted forward, anterior wall and interventricular septum interruption, placement of the aorta shifted toward the right (over-riding of the ventricular septum by the large aorta), and aortic and mitral valves in continuous fiber.

More than one chamber shows that ventricular septal defect is typically located in perimembranous region with a left to right shunt (Fig 5-1-25-B).

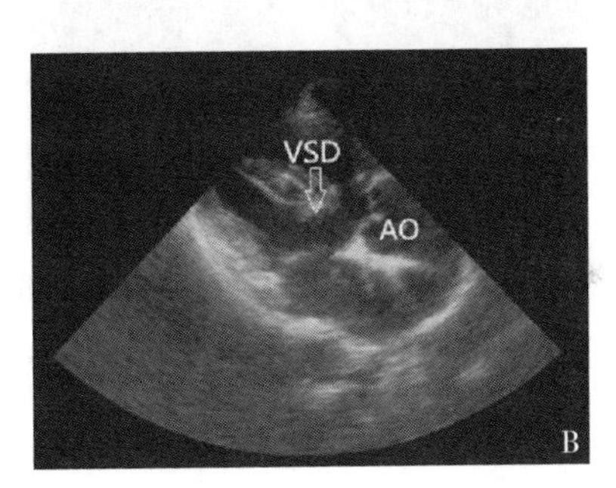

Fig 5-1-25-B Tetralogy of Fallot-VSD

Right ventricular hypertrophy (RVH), thickened RV wall, decreased left ventricular. (Fig 5-1-25-C).

Pulmonary artery infundibular stenosis is showed as (Fig 5-1-25-D).

②***CDFI***: In long axis-left ventricule section, the red blood flow from left ventricle to aorta and the blue blood flow from right ventricle to aorta can be seen. The mosaic pattern blood flow is shown in right ventricular tract and pulmonary

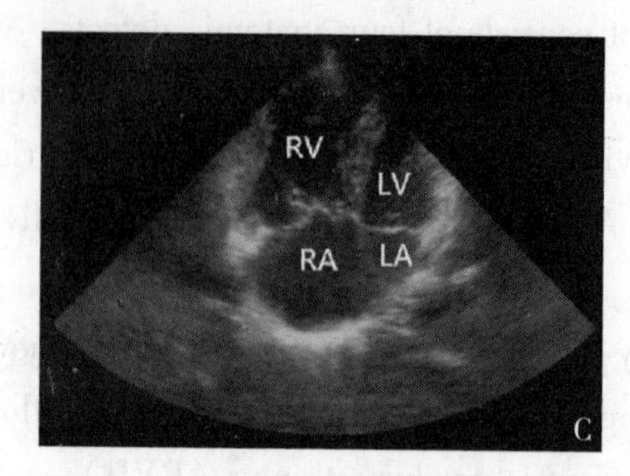

Fig 5-1-25-C Tetralogy of Fallot—thickened RV wall

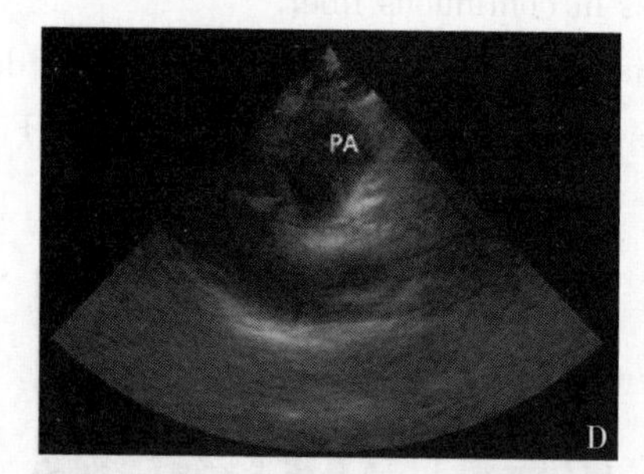

Fig 5-1-25-D Tetralogy of Fallot—pulmonary artery infundibular stenosis

artery (blood flow of pulmonary valves stenosis).

3) CT

CT shows the details of lesion better, such as pulmonary stenosis, right ventricular hypertrophy and the diameter of great blood vessels.

4) MRI

MRI can evaluate the morphological changes of heart. The pulmonary artery and its branches can be observed with enhanced MR.

[**Diagnosis**]

It is easy to make the diagnoses by the combination with clinical manifestation and classical findings in imaging. The abnormalities can be shown by CT and MR.

5 Pericarditis

[**Pathology and clinical manifestations**]

In healthy state, the pericardium normally contains a small amount of fluid (<25ml), which separates visceral layer from parietal layer. Pericardial effusion often results from tuberculosis, inflammation, tumors and trauma. Clinically, the pericarditis is divided into pericardial effusion and constrictive pericarditis.

Pericardial effusion: The commonest clinical abnormality of the pericardium is pericardial effusion. The rapidity with which the fluid collects can cause different degrees of symptoms. The clinic symptoms include fever, palpitation, dyspnea, hepatomegaly and hydroperitoneum.

Constrictive pericarditis: The inflammation of the pericardial sac will cause thickening and a reduction in compliance. The left ventricular filling will reduce.

[**Imaging appearances**]

(1) Pericardial effusion

1) Radiography

Pericardial effusion: The plain film appearances depend on the amount of fluid. A lot of effusion can cause massive enlargement of the cardiac shadow, which is round and globular in appearance. There is no particular chamber enlargement. A large globular heart on the plain film rather than congested lungs is the characteristic appearance (Fig 5-1-26-A).

2) Ultrasonography

Echocardiography is the best imaging technique for pericardial effusion. It can not only estimate the amount of the effusion but treat it by ultrasonography-guided puncture. The echocardiography findings are shown as Fig 5-1-26-B.

3) CT

CT can be used to visualize the pericardial diseases clearly. The pericardium is bordered by epicardial and mediastinal fat that can be clearly visualized.

Pericardial effusion: CT will demonstrate the presence of pleural effusions. The density of effusion is similar to water; the value is 10~40Hu (Fig 5-1-26-

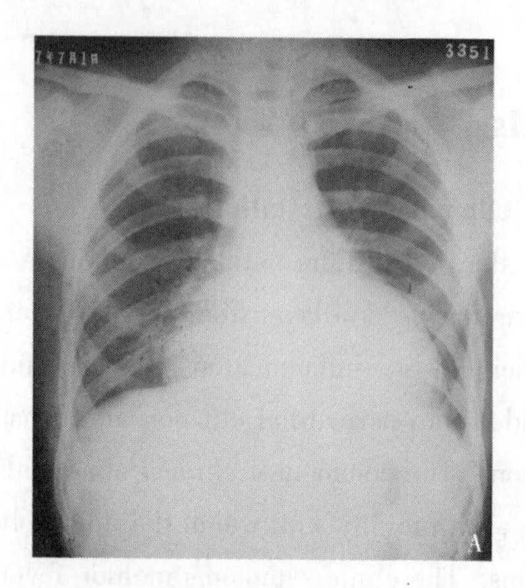

Fig 5-1-26-A Pericardial effusion

The heart enlarges to both sides.

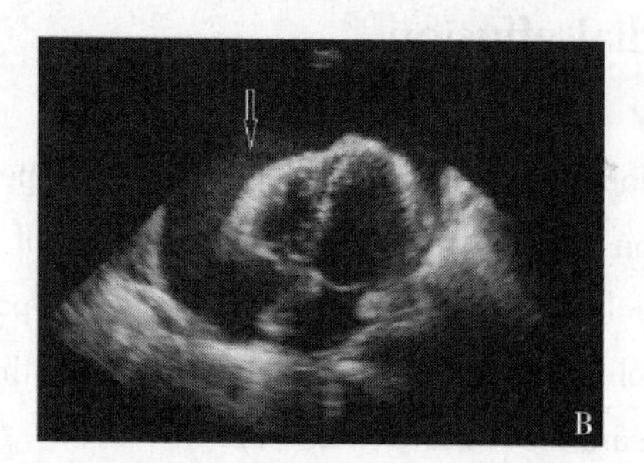

Fig 5-1-26-B Pericardial Effusion

C). If the fluid is bloody, the value of CT will be as high as 50Hu.

4) MRI

MRI is sensitive to show the signal of the pericardial effusion. The intensity of the signal on T1WI depends on the effusion's nature, and it is high signal on T2WI commonly (Fig 5-1-26-D).

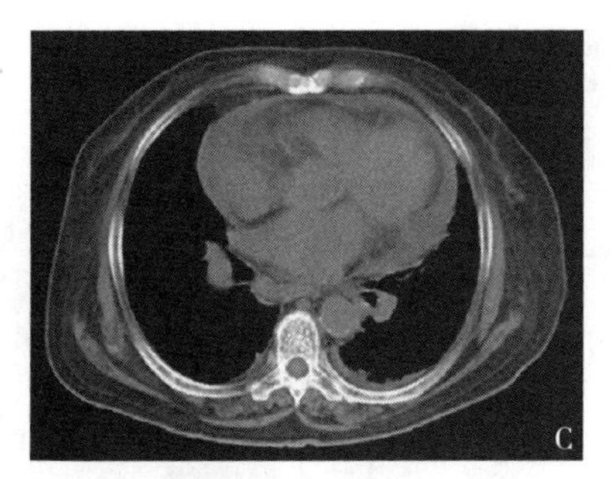

Fig 5-1-26-C Pericardial effusion

CT shows a large amount of liquid density in pericardium

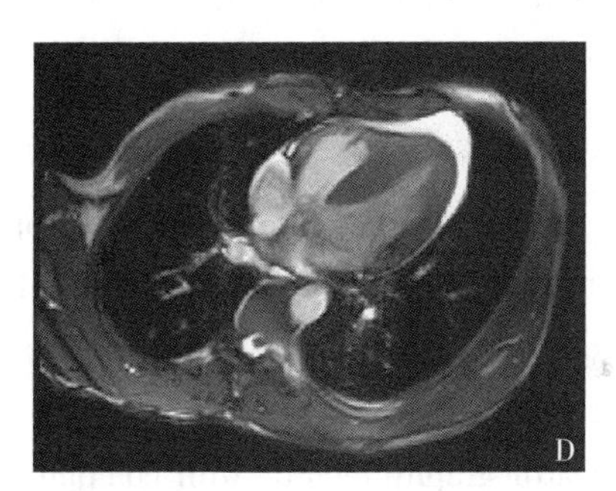

Fig 5-1-26-D Pericardial effusion

a large amount intensity with long T2 signal in pericardium on T2WI

(2) Constrictive pericarditis (CP)

1) Radiography

The heart is often normal on the plain film, but in some cases it can be shown nonspecifically enlarged. Pleuro-pericardial adhesions can cause the right border of the heart straightened and the cardiac outline roughened (Fig 5-1-27-A/B).

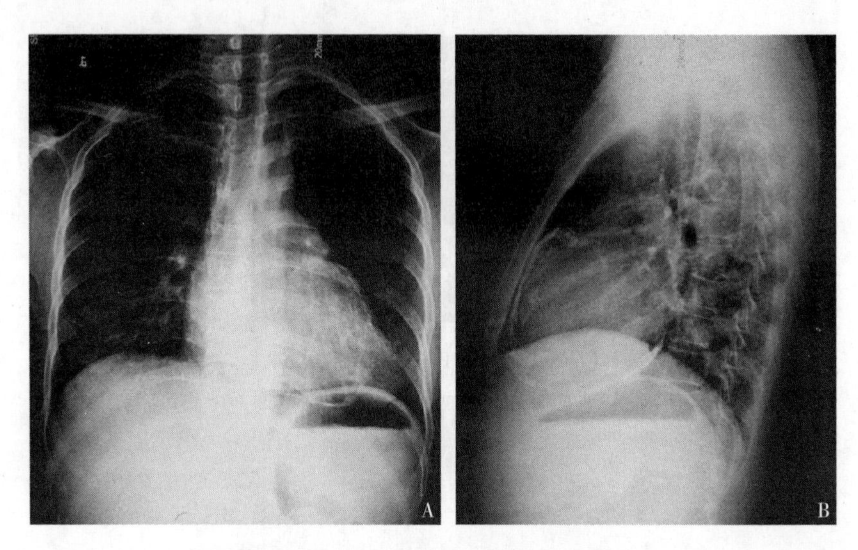

Fig 5-1-27-A/B Constrictive pericarditis

Eggshell calcification surrounds the entire heart

The obstruction of left atrial emptying and the development of pulmonary edema can be produced by the presence of the atrioventricular groove calcification. But calcification may not necessarily be associated with constriction.

2) Ultrasonography

Transthoracic echocardiography records with computer programs. The thickened and calcified pericardium can be shown clearly.

3) CT

Constrictive pericarditis: CT can show the extent and distribution of pericardial calcification. So it is the most accurate method. Pericardial calcification is described as a fine irregular linear. Approximately one third of cases of constrictive pericarditis can be seen with calcification (Fig 5-1-27-C).

[**Diagnosis**]

Pericardial effusion and constrictive pericarditis can be confirmed by typical clinical appearance combined with imaging examinations.

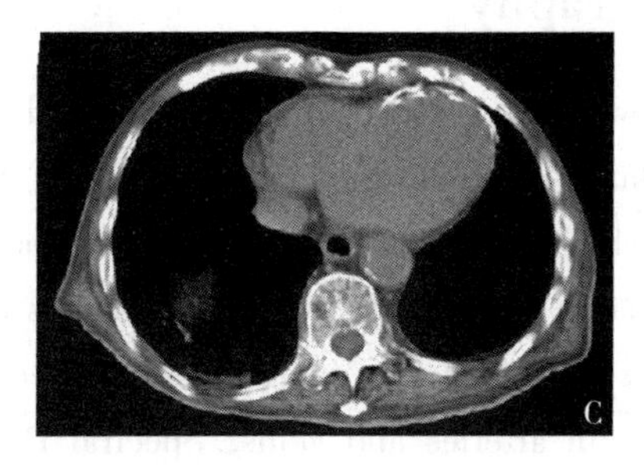

Fig 5-1-27-C Constrictive pericarditis
CT shows high intensity with eggshell in pericardium

Lesson 2 Great Vessels

Vascular diseases include arterial and venous diseases, such as atherosclerosis, arterial embolization, arterial dissection, aneurysm and venous thrombosis. CT is an important method for diagnosis of vascular diseases. MRI can also be used and it has the characteristic of no radiation.

Section 1 Imaging methods

1 Radiography

(1) Chest radiography

It is the preliminary method, and the projection position is the antero-posterior and lateral position.

(2) Angiography

Angiography is the golden standard in diagnosis of vascular diseases.

2 Ultrasonography

Ultrasonography is one of the main examinations and always be taken as the preferred one. Vascular B-mode ultrasonography relies on the use of ultrasound to produce a black and white anatomical image that can demonstrate the presence of disease along an arterial wall or the presence of thrombus in a vein. Doppler ultrasound can provide a functional map in the form of a color flow image, which displays the blood flow in arteries and veins. Spectral Doppler analysis enables Doppler waveforms to be recorded from vessels. It is then possible to visualize changes in flow patterns in vessels and calculate velocity measurements, enabling the sonographer to grade the severity of the vascular disease. A combination of B-mode imaging, color flow imaging and spectral Doppler recordings should be used throughout the examination.

Various transducers are available for vascular ultrasound examination of different parts. A 2.5 ~ 5 MHz sector scanning transducer is used for scanning the ascending aorta, aortic arch and pulmonary trunk. A 3 ~ 5 MHz curved array transducer is used for the aortoiliac segment. A 7 ~ 10 MHz linear array transducer is the most suitable probe for scanning the carotid artery, upper and lower extremity blood vessels.

3 CT

CTA is often taken as the first-line technique for the diagnosis of acute aortic diseases. It displays multiple vessel images in one examination.

4 MRI

MRI has no radiation and iodinated contrast side effect. Common or enhanced MRI shows findings similar to CTA or DSA after processing to obtain 3D reconstruction.

Section 2 Normal imaging findings of great vessels

1 Radiography

(1) Chest radiography can not show the vascular wall and intravascular structure.

(2) Angiography

The location, direction and diameter of vessels can be shown clearly.

2 Ultrasonography

(1) Normal findings of artery

The wall of every artery is composed of three layers: intima, media, and adventitia. All three layers can be visualized on B-mode images. The two transition zones between the lumen and the intima and between the media and the adventitia produce two parallel echogenic lines, with an intervening zone of low echoes that corresponds to the media. The thickness of the intima cannot be directly imaged from the ultrasound image since it typically measures 0. 2 mm or less. There is a close correlation between histology and ultrasound-based measurements of the intima-media thickness (IMT). IMT is a measure of early atherosclerosis and vascular remodelling that can be assessed quickly, non-invasively, and cheaply with high-resolution ultrasound. Normal arterial segments can be interrogated rapidly using color flow imaging. There should be color filling to the vessel walls. The color image normally demonstrates a pulsatile flow pattern, with the color alternating between red and blue due to flow reversal during the diastolic phase in normal lower limb arteries. Flow in normal carotid arteries is forward flow throughout the cardiac cycle. In arteries, each cycle of cardiac activity produces a distinct wave on the Doppler frequency spectrum that begins with systole and terminates at the end of diastole. (Fig 5-2-1-A/B)

(2) Normal findings of vein

The vein shape is often oval and its size will vary with respiration. The walls

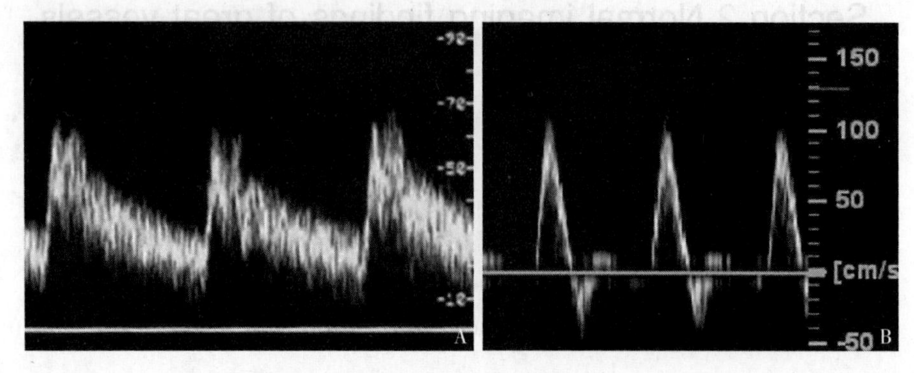

Fig 5-2-1-A/B Spectral Doppler waveforms of normal artery.
A: internal carotid artery; B: common formal artery.

of the normal veins are thin and smooth and will completely coapt, obliterating the vein lumen, with slight pressure from the transducer. The lumen of the vein should be anechoic, without internal echoes. Valves, if present, may be associated with slight dilatation in the vein lumen. They appear as delicate linear structures that move freely in the lumen. Color flow imaging should demonstrate spontaneous flow with no evidence of a color void. Venous flow back to the heart is influenced by respiration, the cardiac cycle and changes in posture. Compression of the local vein will produce augmentation and increased blood flow signals toward the heart in the proximal vein. Spectral Doppler interrogation should demonstrate these variations.

3 CT

Vessels can be shown as moderate density by strong comparison of peripheral fat and gas, round, oval or ribbon-like. Enhanced CT will show vessels that taper from the proximal to the distal. The image of CTA is similar to that of DSA.

4 MRI

Plain MRI shows flow signal relevant to the velocity and direction. The vessel demonstrates hyper-intensity on enhanced MRI.

Section 3 Imaging signs of great vessels diseases

1 Position abnormalities

They contain abnormal connection, abnormal relative location relationship between the aortic and pulmonary arteries, abnormal arterial origin and abnormal venous reflux, which chest radiography is hard to show.

2 Morphological abnormalities

They contain broadening, compression and stretching deformation of vessels. For example, aortic dilatation can be seen in arteriosclerosis.

3 Quantity abnormalities

The amount of blood vessels is more or less than normal.

4 Lumen abnormalities

(1) Dilatation

It often occurs in aneurysm. Aneurysmal dilatation is defined as a diameter of greater than 4 cm, with the dilatation involving all three layers of the aorta.

(2) Stenosis or occlusion

The thickening wall and intra-luminal mass and plaque can lead to arterial stenosis or occlusion.

5 Abnormal walls

(1) Thickening

It can be divided into congenital and acquired thickening, such as coarctation of the aorta and arteritis.

(2) Thinning

The main disease is aneurysm with a sudden increase of intravascular pressure.

(3) Shape abnormality

Ultrasonography, CT and MRI can evaluate the composition and type of plaque.

(4) Calcification

CT shows calcification clearly, mainly in atherosclerosis.

Section 4 Diagnosis of diseases

1 Pulmonary embolism

When the thrombosis or embolus blocks pulmonary arteries, the respiratory and circulatory system dysfunction will occur.

[**Pathology and clinical manifestations**]

When an organism thrombus, often from the lower limbs, embolises to the centra-pulmonary arteries, acute pulmonary embolism will occur. Seriously, it will lead to acute right heart failure, possible circulatory collapse and death with large embolism.

[**Imaging appearances**]

(1) Radiography

1) Plain film

It is relatively uncommon as a diagnostic technique. The typical appearance is triangular or wedge-shaped area of infarct.

2) Pulmonary angiogram

It can directly visualize the thrombus as the filling defect in the blood cavity.

(2) Nuclear medicine imaging

It has become an important method that can be used to diagnose pulmonary embolic disease with its high specificity of the positive test and the availability of the imaging technique.

(3) Ultrasonography

Echocardiography may show thrombus in proximal pulmonary arteries and, if normal, can exclude haemodynamically important PE. It cannot exclude smaller PEs. It may show signs of right ventricular (RV) strain or RV hypokinesis. McConnell sign, a specific pattern of RV dysfunction seen in patients with acute PE, is seen as mid-free wall akinesia or hypokinesis with normal apical motion on the apical four-chamber view. The ratio of RV end-diastolic area to LV end-diastolic area should be 0.6 or less. Values in excess of 0.6 indicate RV dilatation. Flattening or bowing of the ⅣS toward the LV often accompanies this finding and indicates significant RV volume overload. Due to ventricular interdependence, LV diastolic filling is impaired, leading to a reduction in cardiac output. Another indirect finding involves measuring the diameter of the inferior vena cava (ⅣC) during inspiration and expiration using a subcostal view. Lack of inspiratory collapse of the ⅣC by 50% suggests a right atrial pressure>10 mm Hg. This non-specific finding may lend further support to a suspicion of elevated right heart pressures. Deep venous thrombosis can be most frequently found in the deep veins of lower extremity.

(4) CT

CTA will show filling defect in the lumen of the vessel. The complete cut-off sign´ can be found in the more peripheral arteries because of the completely occlusion of thrombus. It can also show the presence of small unilateral or bilateral pleural effusions (Fig 5-2-2-A/B).

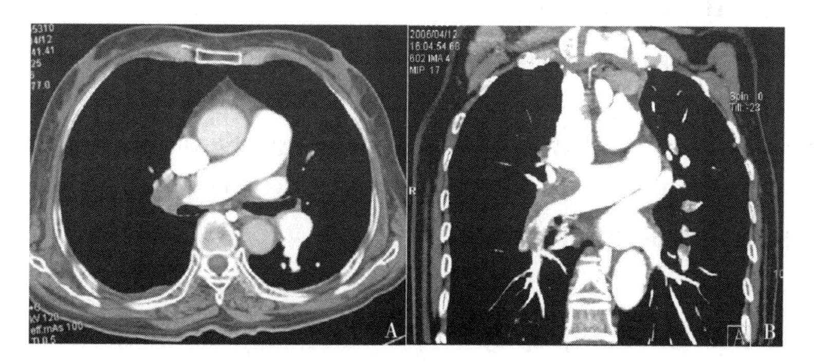

Fig 5-2-2-A/B Pulmonary embolism

Enhanced CT scanning, filling defect in the right main pulmonary artery lumen, lumen stenosis

(5) MRI

MRI has a potential of producing a 3D ventilation perfusion study. The segmental branches of the pulmonary circulation can be identified combined with the phased array body coils.

[**Diagnosis**]

Pulmonary angiography is the golden standard for the identification of pulmonary embolism. It is not difficult to diagnose by its performance combined with its imaging findings.

2 Aortic dissection (AD)

A devastating result of degeneration of the thoracic aorta is aortic dissection (AD). The major contributing factor is hypertension. It is often associated with aneurysmal dilatation of the aorta.

[**Pathology and clinical manifestations**]

The primary mechanism still remains unclear. The rupture of the intima with secondary extension into the media in aorta and a haemorrhagic change within the diseased media will lead to the occurrence of the dissection. The descending aortic dissection can extend down to the abdominal aorta. And the left renal arterial dissection can cause ischaemic change.

[**Imaging appearances**]

(1) Radiography

The widening of the mediastinum is the most common abnormality. The appearance of the dilatation of aortic knuckle and upper descending aorta leads to a prominent hump sign or unfolding of the arch. This radiological finding is more characteristic but less frequent. It can also show lateral displacement of each trachea.

(2) Aortic angiography

It can be seen true and false cavities and intimal rupture lesion.

(3) Ultrasonography

Sonographic characteristics of aortic dissection include a double-lumen artery with a visible intimal flap in aorta with gray scale imaging. The intimal flap may be seen fluttering within the vessel with each cardiac cycle. The echodense flap may separate the true and false lumens. Color flow imaging will further demonstrate two lumens. The false lumen may also thrombose. When there is a proximal and distal tear, blood flows on either side of the intima layer. Sometimes, however, there is antegrade flow in the true lumen and retrograde flow in the false lumen. When there is no distal tear, blood pools behind the detached intima layer, which leads to a reduction of the lumen and eventually an occlusion. The dissection weakens the wall of the aorta, which can lead to an aneurysmal dilatation and rupture.

(4) CT

Often periaortic haematoma in aortic dissection can be demonstrated on CT. Enhanced CT can show dissection flap in the aorta. But CT cannot produce particular information about the function of the aortic valve, and that is the major disadvantage. The development of aortic regurgitation can be seen occasionally when a dissection extends into the aortic root (Fig 5-2-3-A/B).

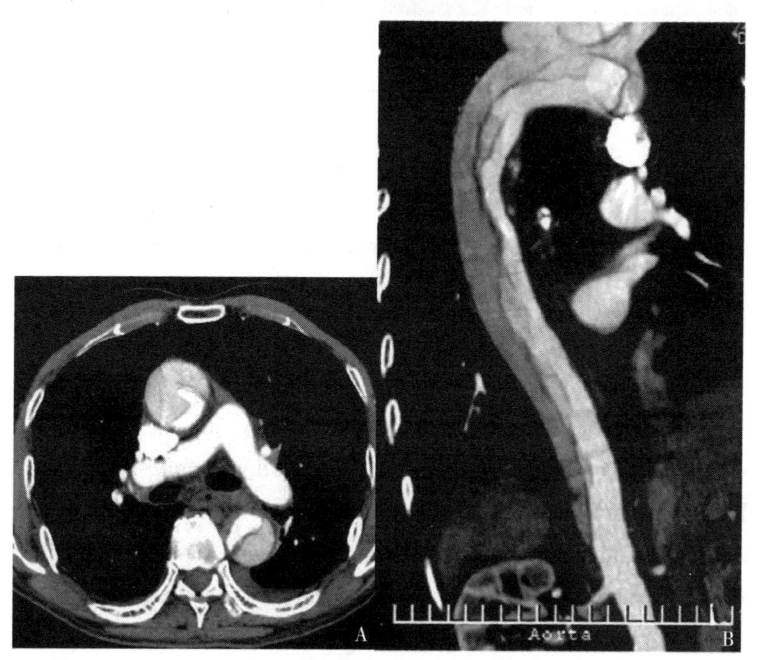

Fig 5-2-3-A/B Aortic dissection

Low density line in the thoracic aortic; the aorta is divided into two cavities of true and false; true lumen with high density

(5) MRI

The images of a tortuous aorta can be shown more easily using the multiplanar nature of MR. In addition, the important findings about the aortic valve and flow within the false lumen can be displayed clearly with the use of sequences on both the oblique and axial planes. The variable flow patterns in the true lumen and one or more false lumens can be often demonstrated (Fig 5-2-3-C/D).

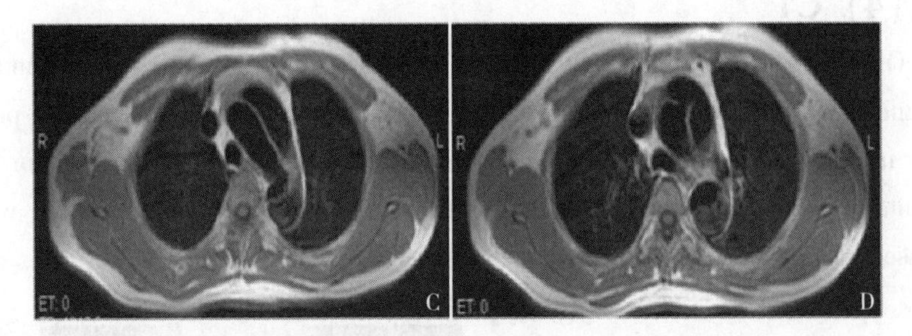

Fig 5-2-3-C/D Aortic dissection

Intimal flap shift inward the aortic arch; lumen is divided into two cavities of true and false

[**Diagnosis**]

Typical cases can be diagnosed by imaging of ultrasound, CT and MR, especially CTA.

3 Lower limb atherosclerosis

Lower limb atherosclerosis is lower extremity arterial wall thickening, stenosis and occlusion due to intravascular plaque deposition.

[**Pathology and clinical manifestations**]

The basic pathological changes are plaque deposition, calcification, and thrombosis formation. There are obvious clinical manifestations such as lower extremity arterial pulsation and lower limb skin temperature decrease.

[**Imaging appearances**]

(1) Radiography

1) Plain film

The chest radiograph can show calcifications in lower limb.

2) Lower limb angiography

Lower extremity arterial angiography can confirm the diagnosis, but it is invasive.

(2) Ultrasound

In the lower extremity, B-mode images are obtained initially, allowing a clear evaluation of anatomic structures and atheromatous plaques. Abnormal dilatations or arterial aneurysms should be measured using the B-mode image. The atheromatous plaques may be extensive and diffusely distributed. Calcification of the arterial wall, especially in diabetic patients, produces strong ultrasound reflections, and the walls of the calf arteries can appear particularly prominent. B-mode imaging in combination with color flow imaging is also useful for identifying acute occlusions where the lumen will appear clear or demonstrate minimal echoes on the image, because thrombus has a similar echogenicity to blood. When an arterial segment has been occluded for some time, the vessel may contract and appear as a small cord adjacent to the corresponding vein.

Arterial stenoses will be demonstrated as areas of color flow disturbance or aliasing. In addition, the color flow image of flow in a nondiseased artery distal to severe proximal disease or occlusion may demonstrate damped low-velocity flow, which will be seen as continuous flow in one direction. Color flow imaging reveals an absence of flow in the occluded segment of the vessel.

Spectral Doppler analysis should demonstrate flow velocity increased in the region where the lumen is narrowed. Conversely, vascular resistance is decreased as a result of collateral circulation and vasodilation in the distal part of the obstruction. As the disease progresses, the triphasic flow diminishes to a biphasic flow. This is due initially to the loss of elastic recoil caused by "hardening" of the arteries. If the disease progresses further, the flow loses its pulsatile nature to a monophasic signal. Any areas of color flow disturbance should be investigated with angle-corrected spectral Doppler to estimate the degree of narrowing. Velocity criteria for the assessment of lower limb stenoses are shown in Table 5-2-1.

Table5-2-1 Velocity Criteria for the Assessment of Lower Limb Stenoses

Percentage Stenosis	Peak Systolic Velocity (m/s)	Velocity Ratio
Normal	<1.5	<1.5 : 1
0~49	1.5~2.0	1.5~2 : 1
50~75	2.0~4.0	2~4 : 1
>75	>4.0	>4 : 1
Occlusion	–	–

(3) CT

Plain CT can show calcification. CTA can display intraluminal filling defects (Fig 5-2-4).

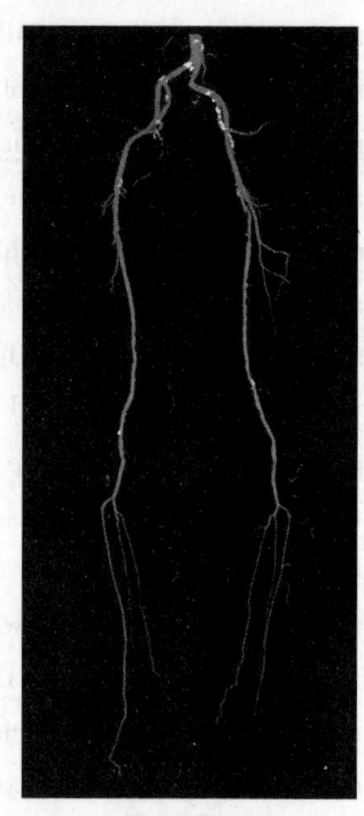

Fig 5-2-4

The left femoral artery with multiple low density plaque and calcified plaque; lumen shows irregular eccentric stenosis and occlusion

(4) MRI

The findings of MRA are similar to CTA.

[**Diagnosis**]

Typical cases can be diagnosed by imaging of ultrasound, MSCT and MRA.

4 Deep venous thromboses (DVT)

The origins of deep venous thrombosis (DVT) are multifactorial, such as slowing of the blood flow and increase of blood coagulation. Some conditions can cause DVT), such as malignant disease, age, obesity, trauma and surgery.

[**Pathology and clinical manifestations**]

If there is significant obstruction or inflammation produced by the thrombosis, clinical

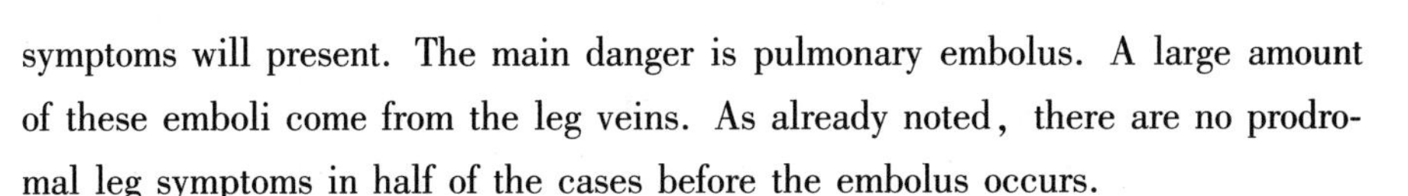

symptoms will present. The main danger is pulmonary embolus. A large amount of these emboli come from the leg veins. As already noted, there are no prodromal leg symptoms in half of the cases before the embolus occurs.

[**Imaging appearances**]

(1) Radiography

Phlebography shows venous thrombosis in deep veins of the calf. The clot shows as a central filling defect with marginal contrast. Wall thickening, luminal stenosis and formation of collateral circulation can also be seen.

(2) Ultrasonography

1) Acute thrombus (within 2 weeks)

Acute DVT presents as heterogeneous poorly echoes within the vein lumen and it frequently distends the vein diameter. Inability to completely obliterate the vein lumen with manual probe compression is the principal criterion for the diagnosis of DVT. The proximal edge may not be attached to the wall, instead it is surrounded by anechoic blood flow or color flow signals. This likely represents the most recently formed portion of the thrombus and may be seen sonographically as mobile or free floating with the lumen. Color Doppler imaging may demonstrate a filling defect within the thrombus involved segment. Spectral Doppler analysis will not detect flow from an occluded vessel or from within a thrombus. If incompletely obstructed, spectral Doppler will demonstrate spectral signals from the patent portion. If there is obstruction, there is a loss of phasicity distally. Loss of phasicity in the absence of thrombus implies a non-visualized central obstruction.

2) Sub-acute thrombus (more than two weeks)

Sub-acute thrombus becomes more echogenic. As a thrombus ages it may also resolve completely or partially. The vein diameter may become normal. The vein re-opening may occur and color Doppler imaging may show partial blood flow in the lumen.

3) Chronic thrombus (several months to years)

As a thrombus ages and reendothelializes, it retracts and recanalizes. Sonographically it becomes more irregular, stiff, and echogenic. Residual changes such as wall thickening, scarring, synechiae, or calcification are common. The vein may appear narrowed or of normal caliber. Wall thickening can prevent compression, which can mimic non-occlusive thrombus. Color Doppler imaging can aid in demonstrating a circumferentially thickened wall or flow signals in an irregular eccentric lumen. Respiratory phasicity (detected with spectral Doppler analysis) may normalize or remain decreased or absent. Valves may be damaged resulting in venous insufficiency. In some cases the thrombosed vein remains permanently occluded and collateral vessels may be found in the vicinity. A patent vein without an accompanying artery should raise suspicion that the main vein is thrombosed and a collateral vessel is being imaged.

(3) CT

MSCT can display wall thickening, luminal stenosis, and thrombosis or calcification formation. "Track sign" can be seen (Fig 5-2-5).

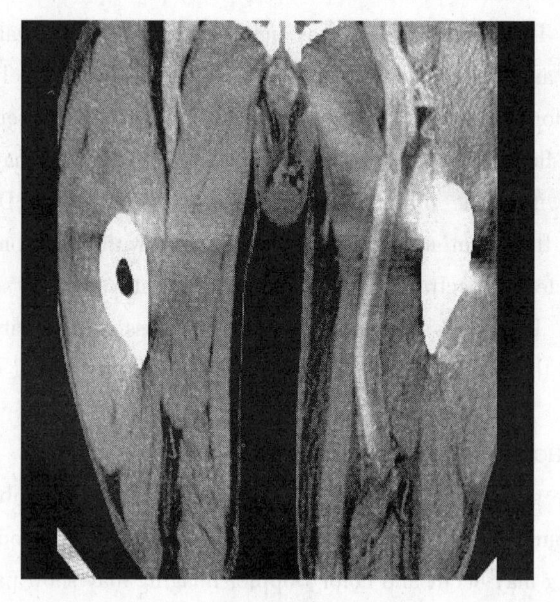

Fig 5-2-5

The left femoral vein with low density filling defect

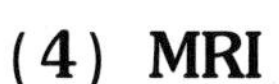

(4) MRI

Thrombus can be seen on the SE sequence. Acute thrombus signal is equal or high, while chronic thrombus signal is equal or low. Enhanced MRI can show filling defect, wall thickening, luminal stenosis and formation of collateral circulation.

[**Diagnosis**]

Typical cases can be diagnosed by ultrasound, CT, and MRI instead of phlebography.

Chapter 6

Imaging of the Digestive System

Lesson 1 Esophagus and Gastrointestinal Tract

Section 1 Imaging methods

1 Radiography

(1) Plain films

Plain radiography is only used for acute abdominal diseases related to esophageal and gastrointestinal diseases, including the metallic foreign body in esophagus and gastrointestinal tract, perforation and intestinal obstruction and so on.

(2) Barium meal examination

Esophagus and gastrointestinal tract belong to hollow visceras, and the initial imaging examination is always the barium examination.

The barium meal examination should be chosen according to the lesion's different suspect pathological change. Before the exam some preparations should be done. For example: the upper gastrointestinal barium meal examination needs fasting and water deprivation for at least 6 hours prior to the examination. The slow leak agent should be taken orally to clean the intestinal surface before the colon enema examination.

1) The radiography of esophagus, stomach, and duodenum

It is always called upper gastrointestinal radiography and used for the examination of the esophagus, stomach and duodenum diseases.

2) The small intestine radiography

The small intestine radiography includes oral contrast agent enterography examination and enteroclysis examination. The enterography can show the track of barium in small intestine until the barium reaches the ileocecus after the upper gastrointestinal examination. The enteroclysis uses the catheter which is inserted into the duodenojejunal flexure to inject barium and air to obtain the double contrast effect.

3) Colon barium enema examination

It is used in the examination of colon diseases, and always the double contrast barium enema exam is taken.

2 Ultrasonography

Ultrasonic examination is used less in the diagnoses of gastrointestinal tract diseases because of the gas in it. Endoscopic ultrasonography is sometimes used in the examination of stomach.

3 CT

The conventional CT includes plain CT scan and enhanced CT scan. Chest CT is always used to evaluate the thickness of esophageal wall, show the tumors and partial swelling lymph nodes. Abdomen CT has already been one of the main techniques for the diagnoses of gastrointestinal diseases. Before the examination, fasting and oral water are needed. CT can show the thickness of cavity wall, the tumors' location, the lesion's abnormal enhancement and the invasions outside the cavity walls clearly. At the same time, CT can observe the location of the intestinal tubes and whether stricture exists or not. Currently, CT is widely used for the examination of gastrointestinal tumors, inflammation, obstruction, ischemic diseases and so on.

Section 2 Normal imaging findings of esophagus and gastrointestinal tract

1 Esophagus

Radiography: the piriform fossa is bilateral symmetry and confluent in the central, then downwards to the esophagus. The upper esophagus is connected to the hypopharynx at the 6th cervical vertebra. The lower esophagus is connected to the cardia at the 10th ~ 11th thoracic vertebras. The esophageal contour is smooth and tidy. The esophageal wall is capable of expanding and contracting. The width of esophagus is 2 ~ 3 centimeters. The mucous membranes of esophagus show several longitudinal and parallel stripe images, which are slender and transparent. The dense lines located between the adjacent transparent stripes are the mucosal folds full of barium. The esophageal mucosal folds are downwards to the cardia and then to the gastric curvature mucosal folds. The esophageal anterior border has three impressions, which are aortic arch impression, left main bronchus impression and atria sinistrum impression.

2 Stomach and duodenum

The stomach can be divided into lesser gastric curvature, greater gastric curvature and three parts, namely gastric fundus, gastric corpus and gastric antrum. On the right side of the stomach contour is lesser gastric curvature, and on the right side of the stomach contour is greater gastric curvature (Fig 6-1-1).

(1) Shape of the stomach

The shape of stomach can be divided into four types according to the somatotype, tension and the condition of nerve function. a) steerhorn stomach: the stomach of steerhorn type shows transverse position and has high tension. Meanwhile, the gastric angle can not be shown obviously in this type. b) fishhook stomach: the gastric lower pole of this type is to the level of spina iliaca. The fishhook type stomach has medium tension and the gastric angle can be shown clearly. c) dolichogastry: it is also called asthenic type stomach. The position and tension of asthenic type stomach are all low. The upper side of the gastric cavity is narrow and the underside is wide in this type. The gastric lower pole of this type of stomach is usually lower than the level of spina iliaca. At the same time, this type of stomach is always seen among the asthenic people. d) cascade stomach: The gastric fundus of this type appears as sac and keeps retroverted. The gastric vacuole is big and the tension is high. The barium gets into the retroverted gastric fundus first, and then spills into the gastric body like a waterfall

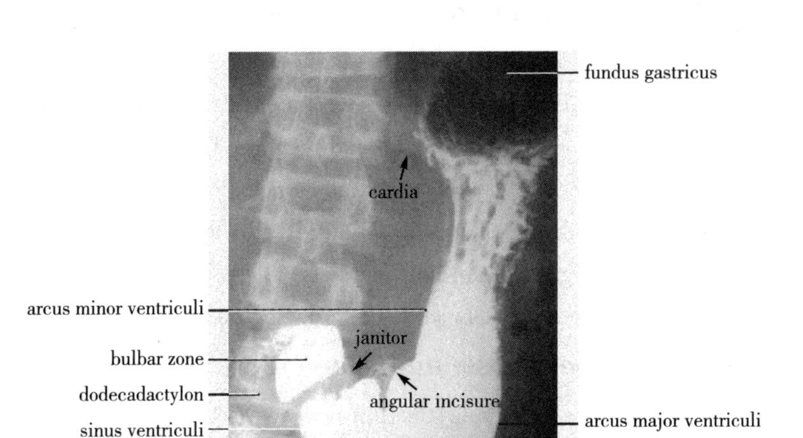

Fig 6-1-1 Gastric barium meal fluoroscopy

(Fig 6-1-2).

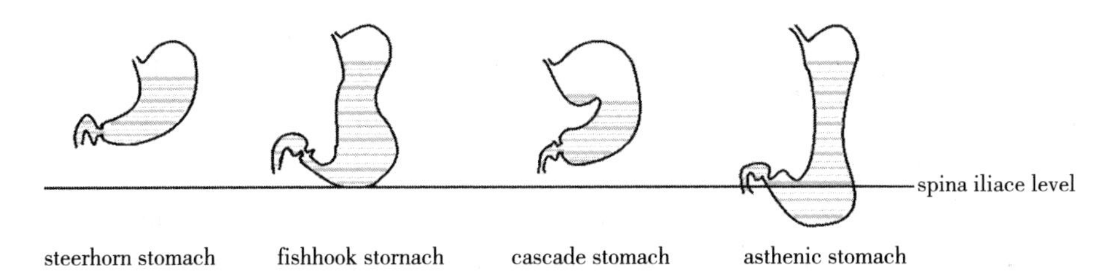

Fig 6-1-2 shapes of the stomach

(2) Contour of the stomach

On the lesser gastric curvature and gastric antrum greater curvature side, the contour of the stomach is smooth. The contour of gastric fundus and gastric body greater curvature always looks jagged because of the transversum and oblique mucosal folds.

(3) The mucous membrane of stomach

The mucous membrane image shows the strip transparent shadow and the linear high density of barium in the sulcus of mucous membrane. The mucous membrane of lesser gastric curvature is parallel and regular. The mucous membrane of greater gastric curvature is always irregular and thick due to prominent mucosal folds. The mucous membrane of gastric fundus is also thick and grid like. The mucous membrane of gastric antrum parallels to that of the lesser gastric curvature. Sometimes the mucous membrane of lesser gastric curvature is oblique.

(4) Gastric peristalsis and evacuation

Gastric peristalsis starts from the upper side of the stomach and moves forward to the pylorus regularly. Kinds of conditions can have an effect on gastric evacuation, such as the gastric tension, gastric peristalsis, function of pylorus, mental state and so on. The barium generally evacuates after 2~4 hours.

The entire duodenum appears as "C" shape and is divided into four parts including duodenal bulb, descendant duodenum, the ascending part and pars horizontalis duodeni. The duodenum wraps around the head of pancreas.

3 Small intestines

Oral barium small intestine radiography: the jejunum locates in the upper left abdomen. The circular mucosal folds appear as the feather. The boundary between jejunum and ileum is unclear. The ileum locates in the lower right abdomen and can be seen in the pelvis. The intestinal cavity of ileum is stenosis and the mucosal folds of ileum are small and shallow. The ileum contour is smooth. The terminal of ileum is upward to the right side and connected with the caecum. The oral barium takes 2~6 hours to reach the caecum. The small intestine can evacuate the barium after 7~9 hours.

4 Large intestines

In the colon gas barium double contrast radiography, the barium moves from the rectum and colon to the inner wall of the caecum. The main feature of the colon is the haustra coli, which is shown as several symmetrical bursiform humps

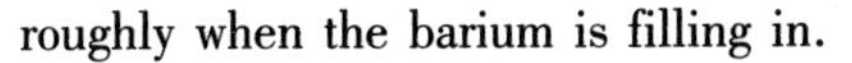

roughly when the barium is filling in.

The appendix can be seen in the barium meal and the colon gas barium double contrast radiography, which is located below the caecum as long strip shape. The caliber of appendix is homogeneous with neatly border and can be easily pushed. It does not mean pathological change when the appendix is not developed, is filled inhomogeneously or has defect due to the stercorolith.

Section 3 Basic imaging signs of esophagus and gastrointestinal tract diseases

1 Changes in cavity

(1) Lumen stenosis

The lumen narrows continuously to stenosis. The scope of lumen stenosis caused by inflammation is usually wide-raging and segmental; the scope of lumen stenosis caused by tumor is limited, the margin of which is irregular and the part parietal is stiff; the lumen stenosis caused by external pressure usually locates on one side, appears regular incisure or gression; the shape of stenosis caused by spasm can change. The shape will be recovered when spasm is relieved.

(2) Lumen dilation

The lumen can enlarge continuously to dilation. The common reason is the stenosis, obstruction or enteroplegia at the distal of the dilated lumen. The lumen dilation caused by intestinal obstruction usually appears as liquid and gas accumulation, which forms the ladder shape with air-fluid level, and is accompanied by hyperperistalsis. While the dilation caused by enteroplegia appears as the luminal dilation widely and is accompanied by bradydiastalsis.

2 Changes in contour

(1) Filling defect

It is caused by an occupying mass which can not be filled with barium; this may arise from the wall of the stomach or be due to mass which presses in from outside the stomach.

(2) Niche

The gastrointestinal outline coating with barium evaginates limitedly. It is the concave of parietal. The barium fills it and remains. It is caused by peptic ulcer or tumor necrotic ulceration. The ulcer appears as crater shape in axial view.

(3) Protrusion

Ulceration and diverticulum can usually result in a collection of barium outside the normal lumen.

3 Changes of mucosal rugae

The abnormity appearance of mucosal rugae is meaningful in detecting the early lesion and making the early diagnosis.

Destruction, interruption or disappearance of the mucosal rugae is usually caused by neoplasm.

Flat mucosal fold The stria between the mucosal rugae becomes unconspicuous. When the disease develops, the mucosal rugae can disappear. There are two common reasons leading to the result. The first one is malignant tumor, and the other is inflammation.

Convergence of the mucosal rugae is seen in healing ulcer, which is radial distribution.

Most of the widened and circuitous mucosal rugae are caused by inflammation. Varicosity is presented as widened and circuitous mucosal rugae too.

4 Functional changes

(1) Changes of tension

High tension always causes the lumen shrink, and low tension causes gastroptosis.

(2) Changes of peristalsis

Peristalsis may be strengthened or weakened. The hypoperistalsis is usually seen in obstructive atony or neoplastic infiltration of stomach. The hyperperistalsis is commonly due to ulcerative or inflammatory process.

(3) Changes of evacuation time

If the evacuation time is more than 4 hours, it will be seen as delayed. Two hours later after oral barium it will come to the cecum. It is slow when the time is more than six hours. It is seen as delayed discharge when the time is more than nine hours.

(4) Changes of secretion

Limosis results in hyper-secretion. With the increase of secretion, the barium disperses and the mucosal rugae can not be seen clearly.

Section 4 Common diseases of esophagus and gastrointestinal tract

1 Esophageal cancer

[**Pathology and clinical manifestations**]

The main symptoms of esophageal cancer include gradual disability of deglutition. Pathologically, squamous cell carcinoma is in the majority. Squamous Cell Carcinoma: Esophageal squamous cell carcinoma shows considerable regional variation in prevalence. Adenocarcinoma: Extensive associated dysplasia is commonly surrounding an esophageal adenocarcinoma. Many of these patients have a long history of gastroesophageal reflux, and gastric content has thus been implicated in carcinogenesis, but a specific carcinogen has not been identified.

[**Imaging appearances**]

(1) Radiography

Radiography features include: a) filling defect may be present in polypoid fungating form esophageal cancer; b) in ulcerating form, irregular niche in the inner contour of esophagus may be seen; c) in infiltrating form, limited abrupt narrowing of lumen may be seen; d) the mucosal rugae of esophageal carcinoma can be destroyed, interrupted or disappear; and e) The wall is rigid, and the peristalsis is weakened or disappears (Fig 6-1-3, Fig 6-1-4).

(2) CT

Irregular mass is present on CT, which can show the lymph node metastasis and metastasis to the lung.

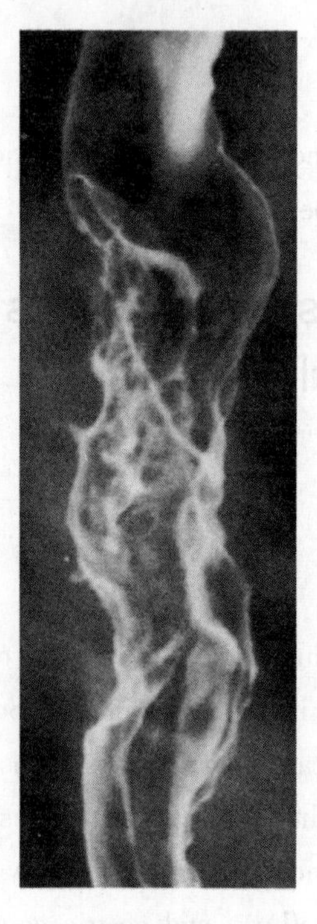

Fig 6-1-3

The radiography of the esophageal cancer

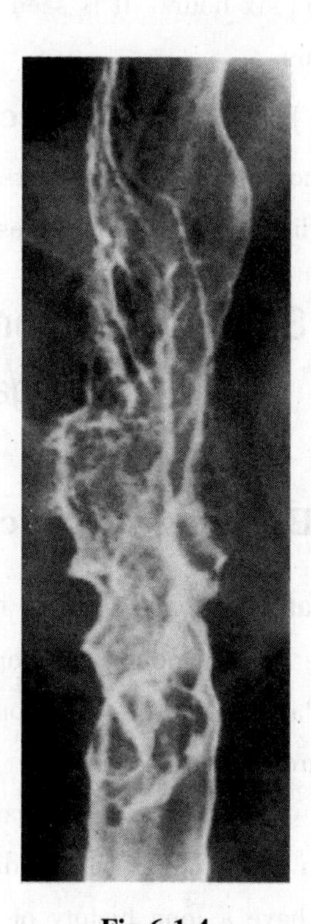

Fig 6-1-4

Irregular filling defect is seen in the middle portion of esophagus.

2 Esophageal varices

[Pathology and clinical manifestations]

In cirrhotic patients with portal hypertension, esophageal varices are the most common site for portosystemic shunting. Most varices eventually drain into

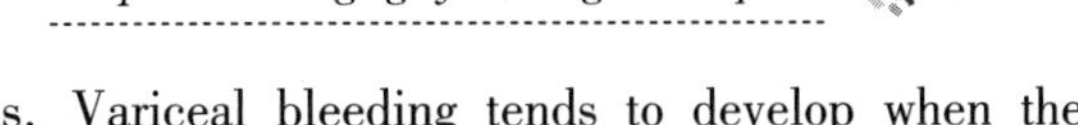

the azygos or hemiazygos veins. Variceal bleeding tends to develop when the portal pressure gradient is above 12mm Hg.

[**Imaging appearances**]

(1) Radiography

Radiography features include: a) early stage: The earliest changes maybe filling defects of a linear character a few centimeters long in the lower end of the esophagus. We can see the circular defects resembling bubbles of air sometimes. b) advancement stage: The lumen of esophagus becomes widened and slightly tortuous. The mucosa folds are possibly worm-like. It can present bead-like filling defects. Instead of smooth the profile of the esophagus becomes scalloped (Fig 6-1-5).

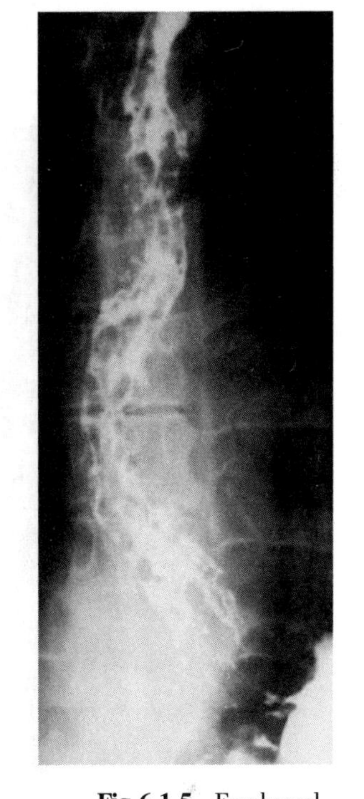

Fig 6-1-5 Esophageal varices

Bead-like filling defects are present.

(2) CT and MRI

The blood vessel around the lower part of esophagus is widened and proliferated, the veins of the portal vein are tortuously dilatated, and cirrhosis is present on both CT and MRI.

3 Gastric ulcer

[**Pathology and clinical manifestations**]

Ulcers typically present with intermittent epigastric pain, which occurs shortly after meals. Many patients have no gastric symptoms and present with gastrointestinal blood loss. Numerous medications induce gastric ulcers. Some nonsteroidal anti-inflammatory drugs are associated with giant gastric ulcers. Chemotherapeutic infusion into the hepatic artery for liver neoplasms is occasionally associated with gastric ulcerations. Some of these ulcers tend to be large.

[**Imaging appearances**]

The radiography of gastric ulcer are that: The niche or ulcer crater on the lesser curve which shows nipple or core shape is usually present. To the benign ulcer, it has the character of a surrounding halo zone which is due to edema. And it appears mucosal rugae line (1mm-2mm in width), necklace sign (0.5cm-1cm in width) and narrowing-neck sign (Fig 6-1-6). Because of scar formation the chronic ulcer may cause convergence of mucosal rugae.

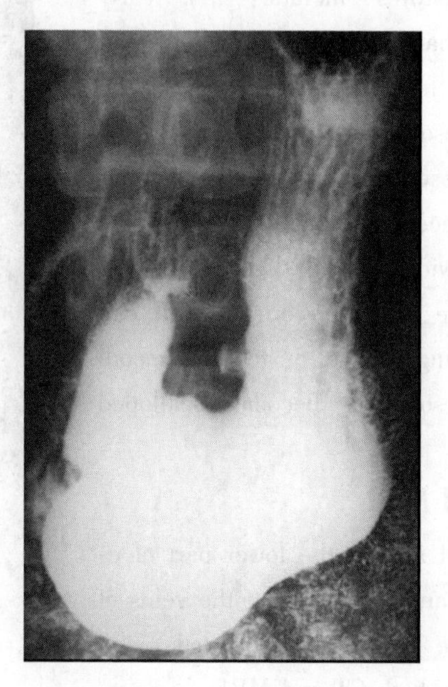

Fig 6-1-6 Gastric ulcer

Niche on the lesser curve which shows nipple shape is present.

3 Duodenal ulcer

[**Pathology and clinical manifestations**]

The discovery of Helicobacter pylori has modified our understanding of peptic ulcer disease pathogenesis. Duodenal bulb H. pylori colonization promotes bulbar gastric metaplasia, leading to further H. pylori infection, more inflammation, and further inability to neutralize gastric acid load. In some patients this cycle persists until an ulcer develops. Probably both bulbar gastric metaplasias and bulbar H. pylori colonization are necessary to develop a duodenal ulcer. Both the prevalence and the extent of gastric metaplasia and the amount of H. pylori in the duodenal bulb in patients with a duodenal ulcer are much higher than in those with a gastric ulcer or chronic gastritis. Eradication of H. pylori decreases the amount of acid entering the duodenum, and duodenal inflammation subsides.

[**Imaging appearances**]

Under radiography, Spasm and scarring may draw in the margins of the duodenal cap, distorting its shape and often producing a characteristic cloverleaf appearance. The ulcer niche may persist, reduce in size, become linear or a depression may persist at the site of ulceration. If the duodenum has become scarred it can be difficult to diagnose recurrent ulceration; thus, if there is a history of past duodenal ulceration, endoscopy is the preferred investigation. Occasionally, postbulbar ulcers develop, and are usually on the medial wall of the duodenal loop above the papilla. They are often associated with oedema and pronounced spasm which pulls in the opposing duodenal wall. Scarring from such ulceration may produce a permanent stricture of the postbulbar duodenum. A giant ulcer may replace the whole of the duodenal cap, and, when smooth margined, such ulcers may be mistaken for a normal cap. However, the giant ulcer will maintain its shape during a barium examination, whereas the normal cap can at times be seen to contract with peristalsis.

4 Gastric carcinoma

[**Pathology and clinical manifestations**]

Atrophic gastritis predisposes to the development of gastric carcinoma. A sequence of events may follow atrophic gastritis, with the development of intestinal metaplasia, then dysplasia and finally neoplasia. A past infection with H. pylori is an important initiator of this sequence of events. Adenomatous polyps also develop from mucosa affected by chronic atrophic gastritis and so many coexist with carcinomas, although in a minority of cases these polyps undergo malignant change themselves. Intake of nitrates may also be a risk factor as nitrates are converted to nitrosamines in the stomach; nitrosamines are known to be carcinogenic in animals. Conversely, diets rich in vitamin C prevent the formation of nitrosamines and are associated with a low risk of gastric carcinoma.

[Imaging appearances]

(1) Early gastric carcinoma

Radiography and CT: By definition these carcinomas are confined to the mucosa and submucosa, irrespective of whether or not regional lymph nodes are involved.

(2) Advanced gastric cancer

Radiographic findings: a) irregular filling defect, mostly seen in the fungating form gastric carcinoma; b) irregular niche: it can be primarily seen in ulcerating form. Niche is usually in the inner contour of stomach and looks like a half moon; c) in infiltrating form gastric carcinoma, the limited or intensive narrowing of lumen and rigidity of wall can be seen. When nearly the whole stomach is irregular and rigid, we call it leather stomach, which means it is in the advanced stage; d) mucosal rugae may be destroyed, interrupted or disappear; and e) peristalsis may be weakened or disappear (Fig 6-1-7).

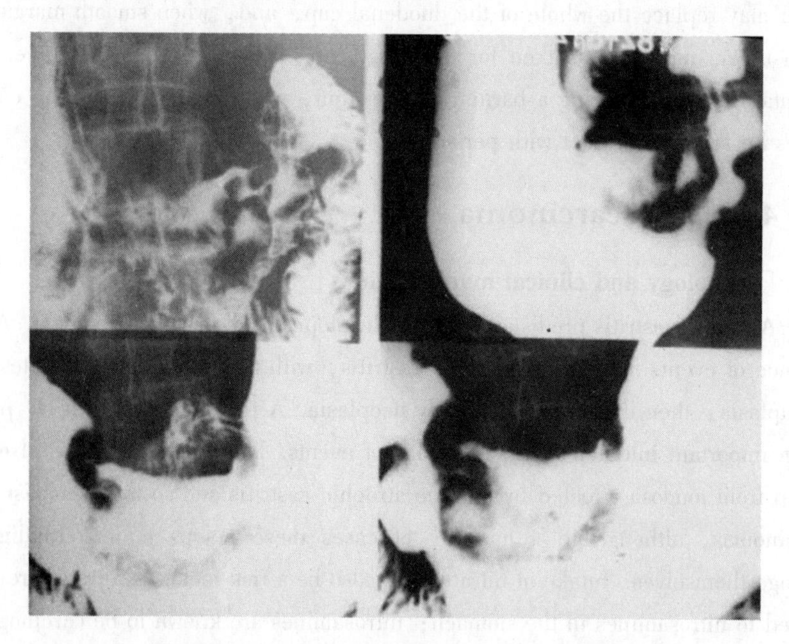

Fig 6-1-7 The radiography of the gastric carcinoma

Mucosal rugae are interrupted or disappear, and irregular niche is seen.

CT appearances: Polypoid mass, irregular ulceration and wall thickening may be present. CT plays an important role in observing gastric wall infiltrated, and far distance metastasis directly (Fig 6-1-8).

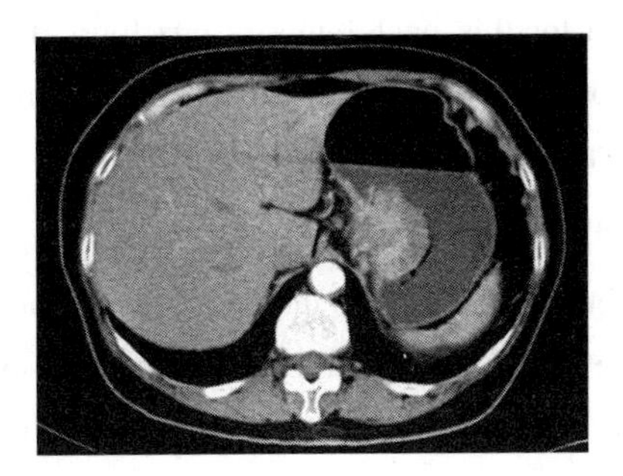

Fig 6-1-8 The CT imaging of the gastric carcinoma

Irregular mass is seen on this CT image.

Table 6-1-1 Differential diagnosis between benign and malignant ulcer of stomach

	Benign ulcer	Malignant ulcer
Contour of niche	Round or oval, smooth margin	Irregular, plat
Location	Exceed the contour of stomach	in the inner contour of stomach
Surrounding	mucosal rugae line, necklace sign and narrowing-neck sign; convergence of mucosal rugae	Irregular ulcer crater Destruction, interruption or disappearance of mucosal rugae
Wall of stomach	Soft and with peristalsis	Rigid and without peristalsis

5 Carcinoma of colon

[**Pathology and clinical manifestations**]

A number of studies show a correlation between meat consumption and colorectal cancer. Still, this topic remains controversial. Regular ingestion of aspirin or other nonsteroidal antiinflammatory drugs decreases the risk of colorectal cancer, although the length of time necessary before a reduction in risk occurs is debated.

Although not common, colorectal cancer does occur in young adults, with case reports describing even patients under 20 years of age. An association between Streptococcus bovis bacteremia and the presence of a colon carcinoma is well known. The reason for this bacteremia is puzzling, because bowel S. bovis colonization rates in those with colorectal cancer and controls appear similar.

[**Imaging appearances**]

(1) Radiography

Barium enemas detect most pedunculated, sessile and infiltrating colon and rectal carcinomas. The most important sign is the presence of filling defect. Other features include: colonic obstruction, fixation of the colon and change of the mucosa. When the carcinoma develops the annular scirrhous type and the lesion is limited to a very short part of the bowel, the filling defect may present the "napkin-ring" narrowing sign typically (Fig 6-1-9).

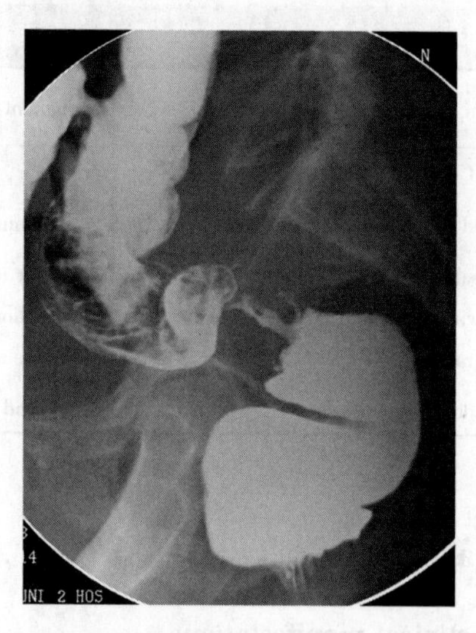

Fig 6-1-9 The radiography of the carcinoma of sigmoid

The filling defect is present

The relative roles of barium enema, flexible sigmoidoscopy, and colonoscopy are not established. Barium enema may miss a carcinoma in the rectum where the lesion is obscured in the dilated and filled cavity. A number of studies have shown a superiority of colonoscopy over barium enema.

(2) CT and MRI

CT and MRI can show the mass directly and show the enhancement of the mass; the expansion of the near-end lumen which is caused by the stenosis of the lumen is also present (Fig 6-1-10). Metastasis to lymph node and other organs can be demonstrated by CT and MRI. MRI can distinguish the fibrous tissue proliferation of rectum cancer post-operatively with the local recurrence of rectum cancer. Compared to the fibrous tissue proliferation, the local recurrence of rectum cancer shows hyper-intensity on T2WI and DWI.

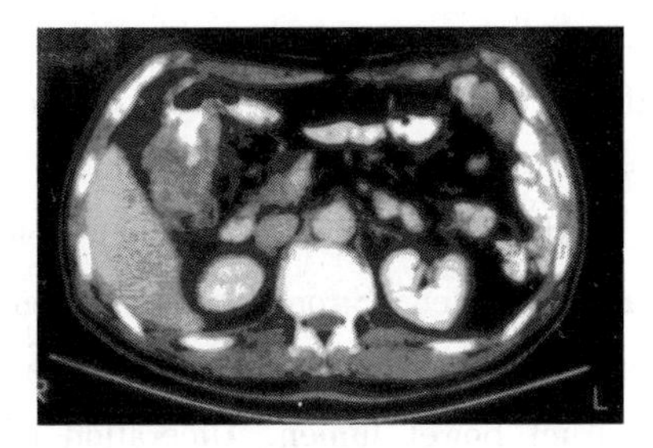

Fig 6-1-10 The CT imaging of the carcinoma of colon

Irregular mass is seen on this CT image.

6 Gastrointestinal stromal tumors

[**Pathology and clinical manifestations**]

Gastrointestinal stromal tumors occur most commonly in the stomach, followed by small bowel, then rectum, colon, and least often in the esophagus. The most common stromal tumor in the esophagus is a leiomyoma, and for clinical and prognostic purposes, whenever possible, it should be classified as such. Most stromal tumors originate from muscularis propria, with only a small minority from muscularis mucosa; most of the latter are in the colon and present as intraluminal polyps, although current evidence suggests that these colonic tumors are leiomyomas and not GISTs. Gastrointestinal stromal tumors' malignant potential is estimated based on their mitoses per high power field. Patient survival is significantly related to number of mitoses.

[**Imaging appearances**]

(1) Radiography

Filling defect can be demonstrated by barium meal, which has a sharp margin.

(2) CT and MRI

The imaging appearance of GISTs varies markedly. The tumors range from mostly exophytic, intramural, intraluminal to a dumbbell-shaped appearance. The tumors predominate in the gastric fundus and body. Small tumors have a sharp margin, tend to be mostly intraluminal and have a homogeneous density or intensity in unenhanced and contrast enhanced images; with growth, they become irregular in outline, have a larger extraluminal component and are more inhomogeneous in density or intensity. Large ones infiltrate adjacent organs. Presence of metastases establishes malignancy. When detected with CT, many appear large, bulky, and ulcerated. Stromal sarcomas tend to be solitary, multilobulated and mostly exophytic. Necrosis and hemorrhage are common. Interestingly, GISTs rarely obstruct bowel lumen. Ulceration of overlying mucosa is common with the larger ones, accounting for their propensity to bleed. Computed tomography and MRI readily outline the extraserosal extent of both benign and malignant varieties. Coronal and sagittal CT and MRI reconstructions are at times useful in establishing the organ of origin of large GISTs.

Postcontrast, these tumors have variable enhancement except in regions of necrosis.

Calcifications are rare. These stromal tumors rarely metastasize to lymph nodes, and the presence of enlarged adjacent nodes should suggest another diagnosis. Except when metastases are present, imaging cannot differentiate benign stromal tumors from malignant ones or other solid tumors such as neuroendocrine ones.

7 Crohn's disease

[**Pathology and clinical manifestations**]

Epidemiologic data for Crohn's disease patients suggest the presence of a recessive gene having high penetrance, in distinction to ulcerative colitis where a dominant or additive gene having low penetrance is more likely. Numerous investigators have searched for an infective etiology. Although a superimposed infection is not uncommon, identification of an infective etiology for Crohn's disease has not been fruitful and currently no convincing infective etiologic agent is established. Chronic abdominal pain is common, often being insidious in onset and progression. Some children present with growth retardation or simply delayed puberty. In a small minority of patients hepatobiliary or joint abnormalities manifest first. Especially in children, a blood count and erythrocyte sedimentation rate are almost always abnormal, and these tests appear reasonable with suspected Crohn's disease.

[**Imaging appearances**]

(1) Radiography

Crohn's disease and mild changes, including subtle aphthae and fistulas, are best seen with enteroclysis. It can detect cobblestone sign, strictures, obstruction, fistulas, and a phlegmon. We can not differentiate a phlegmon from an abscess. At times normal small bowel proximal to a diseased segment is somewhat dilated.

(2) CT and MRI

CT detects bowel wall thickening, increased enhancement of diseased bowel, mesenteric infiltration, fistulas, phlegmon, and abscesses in Crohn's patients. CT demonstrates submucosal and mesenteric fat deposition. A diffuse fibrofatty mesenteric infiltrate develops, with adjacent small bowel loops separated by this infiltrate. The normal sharp interface seen with CT between the bowel wall and its mesentery is lost, resulting in an irregular bowel contour. Enlarged mesenteric lymph nodes are common. In general, the involved lymph nodes are smaller than 10mm in diameter; larger ones should suggest a malignancy or other complication.

MRI: The use of oral and rectal contrasts and bowel distention aid in visualizing bowel wall thickening. One technique consists of oral contrast using 1000 mL of a 2.5% mannitol solution and imaging in axial and coronal planes using breath-hold T2-weighted half-Fourier acquisition single-shot turbo spin echo (HASTE) and contrastenhanced T1-weighted fast low-angle shot (FLASH) sequences; diseased bowel wall enhances considerably more than normal bowel. Inflammation, mesenteric involvement, sinus tracts, and abscesses are depicted by MR.

8 Intestinal obstructions

[**Pathology and clinical manifestations**]

Because of the high incidence of elective surgery the commonest cause of small-bowel obstruction in the developed world is adhesions due to previous surgery. Complete obstruction of the small bowel usually causes small-bowel dilatation with accumulation of both gas and fluid and a reduction in calibre of the large bowel. The amount of gas present in the large bowel depends on the duration and completeness or otherwise the small-bowel obstruction. It frequently takes several bowel movements to empty the large bowel entirely of gas and faeces. The commonest cause of large-bowel obstruction is carcinoma. Diverticular disease as a cause of obstruction has decreased in frequency since the introduction of high-fibre diets.

Mechanical obstruction of the small bowel may be caused by:

- Adhesions (75%) due to previous surgery
- Obstructed hernia—commonest cause in the absence of previous surgery
- Inflammation
- Small bowel volvulus
- Intussusception
- Malignancy
- Gallstone ileus—may be seen in elderly patients

Commonest causes of mechanical large bowel obstructioninclude:

- Malignancy
- Diverticular disease
- Volvulus
- Adhesions

[**Imaging appearances**]

The cardinal features of small bowel obstruction are dilated loops of small bowel (usually>3 cm in diameter) containing variable amounts of air and fluid with collapse of the large bowel. Small bowel obstruction can be difficult to differentiate from paralytic ileus. In the latter, the large bowel is also often dilated, and bowel sounds are absent. CT should be performed in all patients with suspected small bowel obstruction. A normal abdominal radiography does not exclude either diagnosis and CT is indicated if clinical concern persists. If the abdominal radiography is abnormal, then CT is indicated. In mechanical obstruction a transition zone from dilated proximal bowel to collapsed distal bowel should be sought (Fig 6-1-11).

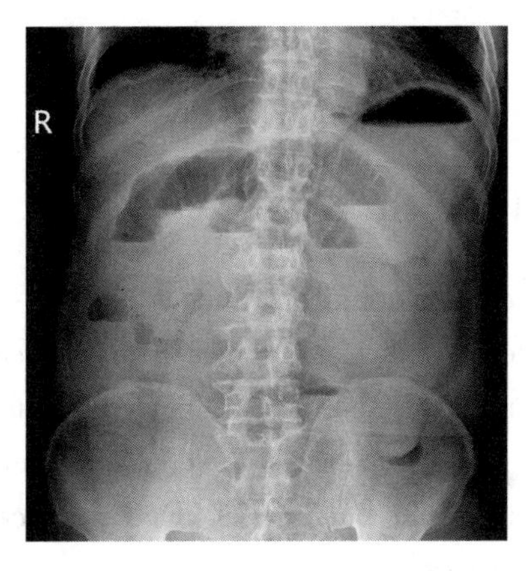

Fig 6-1-11 Radiography of the intestinal obstruction

Dilated loops of small bowel containing variable amounts of air and fluid plane with collapse of the large bowel are seen.

MDCT can often localize the level and cause of obstruction, differentiate between high and low grades of small bowel obstruction, and assess the presence of complications. In patients with paralytic ileus, pseudoobstruction can be seen (dilated large bowel with no obstructing cause).

A mechanical blockage of the bowel causes dilatation of proximal loops. The key to diagnosis is the identification of a transition point from dilated to collapsed bowel. This is often best visualized by starting at the rectum and working backwards (Fig 6-1-12).

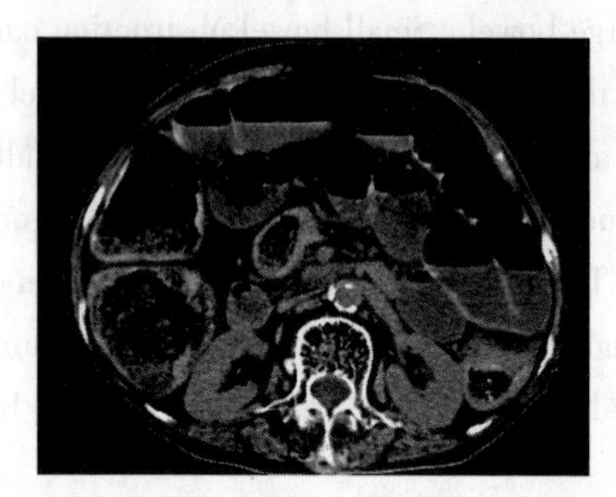

Fig 6-1-12 The CT imaging of the intestinal obstruction large amounts of air and fluid plane are seen.

9 Perforated peptic ulcers

[**Pathology and clinical manifestations**]

Ulcers on the anterior wall of the stomach or duodenum perforate into the peritoneal cavity, whereas those on the posterior wall perforate into the lesser sac or penetrate into the retroperitoneum and pancreas. The most frequent cause of a free peritoneal perforation is an anterior wall duodenal ulcer.

[**Imaging appearances**]

Free peritoneal air, although readily recognized below the diaphragm on an erect chest film, is only seen in 60% of perforated duodenal ulcers. Insufficient time may be allowed for the gas to collect under the diaphragm, pre-existing adhesions may prevent gas reaching the subphrenic space, or the perforation may seal before a significant amount of gas has entered the peritoneal cavity. Gastrografin can be used to study patients with a perforation, and the right lateral decubitus position best demonstrates leakage from duodenal and lesser curve gastric ulcers. Good mucosal detail is not obtained with gastrografin, so it may be difficult to recognize a perforated ulcer that has sealed. When the perforation is into the lesser sac a gas shadow or air-fluid level develops behind the stomach. Small volumes of free intraperitoneal gas from perforations can be demonstrated using

CT, which may be used in the context of diagnostic uncertainty in the acute abdomen. The site of the perforation itself is often not identified and has to be inferred. An antral ulcer may fistulate to the duodenal cap to give the appearance of a "double pyloric canal". Aspirin and non-steroidal anti-inflammatory drugs tend to produce ulcers on the greater curve, and these can fistulate to the colon or jejunum. Rarely, duodenal ulcers may fistulate into the common bile duct, causing cholangitis and air in the biliary tree.

Free intraperitoneal or retroperitoneal gas implies perforation (most commonly from a peptic ulcer). Pneumoperitoneum can also be caused by diverticulitis and can be present after a recent laparotomy. MDCT has a very high sensitivity and specificity for even small amounts (<2 ml) of free gas. Extraluminal gas may also form in a walled off collection anywhere in the abdominal cavity, forming a gas-fluid level (as in the diverticular abscess described later) or as small bubbles of gas trapped in solid material or sited in anti-dependent locations when the patient is supine for the CT examination (as in the example of necrotising pancreatitis seen later) (Fig 6-1-13).

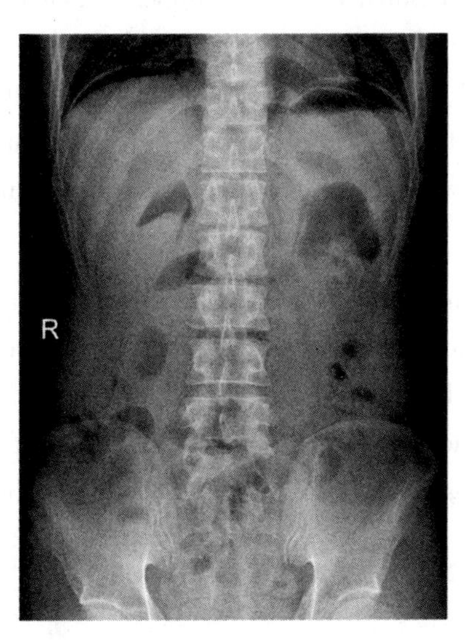

Fig 6-1-13 The radiography of the perforated peptic ulcers. Free peritoneal air is seen.

Lesson 2 Liver, biliary system, pancreas and spleen

Section 1 Liver

1 Imaging Methods

(1) Ultrasonography

Often ultrasound is the first line of investigation for suspected liver pathology and the decision to proceed to secondary investigative procedures is frequently determined by the findings of the initial ultrasound exam. Developing technology and techniques now result in improved diagnostic accuracy and are obviating the need for further radiology increasingly. Intraoperative and laparoscopic ultrasound, using high-frequency, direct-contact techniques, set the standard for liver imaging in many cases.

(2) CT

Plain CT provides a global view of the upper abdomen in axial sections enabling clear demonstration of the liver anatomy and adjacent structures. Enhanced CT scan is widely used for the detection of focal lesions and the delayed scan is widely used to observe the pattern of contrast enhancement in focal lesions. This technique is particularly helpful in the diagnosis of haemangiomas.

(3) MRI

MRI has the advantages of a range of contrast mechanisms and multiplanar imaging but continues to be less widely available and accessible than other liver imaging techniques. Although the major use of MRI in the liver is for targeted lesion detection and characterization, it may also be used effectively during the same examination for assessing the biliary duct system and hepatic vascular patency.

2 Normal imaging appearances

(1) Ultrasonography

On ultrasound the normal liver is a homogeneous, mid-gray organ. The echo of normal liver is the same as, or slightly higher compared to the cortex of the kidney. The smooth parenchyma of liver is interrupted by vessels and ligaments, which are hyperechoic, linear structures; the falciform ligament, which separates the anatomical left and right lobes. The ligamentum venosum separates the anatomical caudate lobe from the rest of the liver. Look at the inferior margin of the right lobe particularly, which should come to a point anterior to the lower pole of the right kidney.

(2) CT

Plain CT shows homogeneous density of liver, and veins are seen as tubes of lower density than the parenchyma. The three major hepatic veins are visible in the higher cuts as convergent on the intrahepatic vena cava, while the horizontally orientated main portal vein is seen in lower cuts. The porta hepatis is a cleft containing hepatic artery, portal vein and bile duct, and lies on the medial liver surface. Normal hepatic artery and biliary ducts are too small to be shown on conventional scanners. (Fig 6-2-1-A/B/C/D)

Plain CT (A) shows homogeneous density of liver, higher than that of

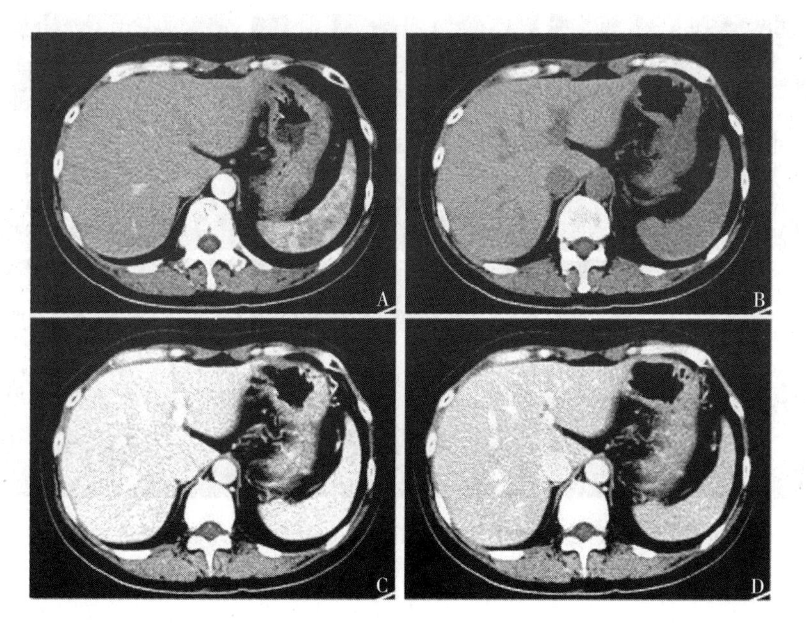

Fig 6-2-1-A/B/C/D Normal CT imaging appearances of liver and spleen

spleen. Enhanced CT (B, C) shows the enhancement intensity of liver increases gradually. Plain CT (A) shows homogeneous density of spleen, lower than that of liver. Enhanced CT shows the inhomogeneous significant enhancement on arterial phase images (B) and the density of spleen gradually reaches uniformity from venous phase images (C) to delayed phase images (D).

(3) MRI

The appearance of vessels varies widely on MRI depending on pulse sequence and on the use of artifact suppression techniques or contrast media. The bile ducts are best imaged using a dedicated MRI technique. In routine practice liver-spleen differences may be helpful as a simple guide to the efficacy of intrinsic T1 and T2 weighting. The liver has a T1-relaxation time shorter than that of other abdominal tissues except for fat and pancreas, while the T2-relaxation time of liver is shorter than most other abdominal tissues, including spleen. (Fig 6-2-2-A/B/C/D/E/F)

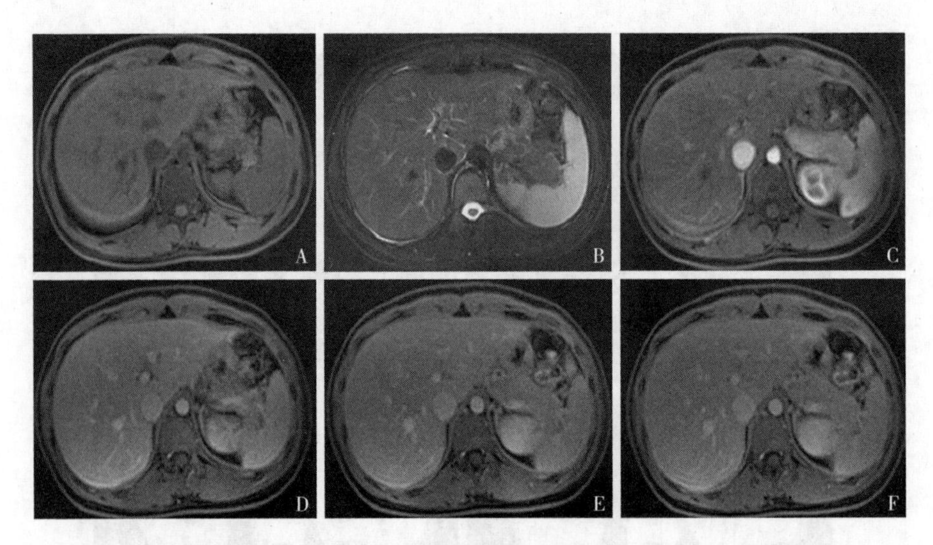

Fig 6-2-2-A/B/C/D/E/F Normal MRI appearances of liver and spleen

Plain MRI (A, B) shows moderate intensity signal in TIWI images,

higher than that of spleen and hypointensity in T2WI images, significantly lower than that of spleen. The appearances of enhanced MRI (C, D, E, and F) is similar with enhanced CT. Plain MRI shows the inhomogeneous signal of spleen, longer T1 signal in T1WI images and longer T2 signal than that of liver.

3 Imaging signs of liver

(1) Abnormality of hepatic size and shape

① ***Hypertrophy of liver***: It is common in diffuse hepatic disease and large hepatic mass. On US, CT and MRI, it shows the satiation of liver, and anteroposterior, transverse, and vertical diameters are beyond the normal range.

② ***Atrophy of liver***: It shows volume reduction of whole liver, often with deformation and wideness of hepatic hilum and fissure.

③ ***Change of hepatic shape***: It shows one lobe is hypertrophy and another lobe atrophy, causing disproportion of hepatic lobes.

(2) Abnormality of hepatic margin and outline

① ***Hepatic cirrhosis***: It can cause abnormality of hepatic margin and outline. US, CT and MRI all can show irregular hepatic margin and non-smooth surface.

② ***Hepatic mass***: It can highlight the liver surface, with the appearance of limited apophysis.

(3) Diffuse hepatic disease

The most common diseases are chronic hepatitis, hepatic cirrhosis, fatty liver, liver hemochromatosis etc.

1) CT

It shows the diffuse increase or decrease of density of whole liver, as well as mixed density with hyperdense and hypodense, and the edge may be well-defined or not.

2) MRI

Hepatic cirrhosis shows diffuse nodular seen as short T1 signal and long T2 signal; fatty infiltration can be seen as short T1 signal and long T2 signal; liver hemochromatosis can be seen as long T1 signal and short T2 signal.

(4) Focal hepatic lesion

Hepatic tumor, hepatic abscess and hepatic cyst show as focal hepatic lesion and they can oppress adjacent hepatic parenchyma, hepatic vessel and bile duct (the formation of so-called mass effect). US, CT and MRI can clearly show its size, number, shape and inner structure.

1) CT

On plain CT, focal hepatic lesion shows low density mass. On enhanced CT, cystic lesion shows no enhancement, or mere edge enhancement. Hypovascular hepatic mass lesion shows slight enhancement, and hypervascular hepatic mass lesion shows significant enhancement on arterial phase.

2) MRI

Its appearances is similar to CT appearances. Focal hepatic lesion can be seen as short or slightly short T1 signal, short T2 signal, and enhancement pattern is also similar to CT.

(5) Abnormality of hepatic vessels

US, CTA, MRA, and DSA all can clearly show abnormality of hepatic artery, hepatic vein and portal vein.

Abnormality of hepatic vessel position can be caused by oppression of large hepatic mass lesion to adjacent hepatic vessel, making it pulled straight and arc shift.

The enlargement and twist of hepatic vessel is most common in hepatic cirrhosis, causing dilation of portal vein trunk and the left and right main branches.

Hepatic vessel stenosis and obstruction or filling defection is caused by tumor thrombus of HCC.

The pathological blood vessel is common in malignant hepatic tumor, showing twisted and disordered neovascularization.

4 Diagnosis of diseases

(1) Hepatic Cysts

[**Pathology and clinical manifestations**]

Between 10% and 13% of the population have congenital hepatic cysts, either single or multiple. Clinical manifestation is related to the size, location, growth speed, combined with bleeding or infection, thus is often quite different. Small cysts are often asymptomatic; large cysts may be accompanied by the pain of right upper quadrant.

[**Imaging appearances**]

1) Ultrasonography

Although the appearances are often similar to those of a simple cyst, the diagnosis can be made by looking carefully at the wall and contents; the hydatid cyst has two layers to its capsule, which may appear thickened, separated or detached on ultrasound. Daughter cysts may arise from the inner capsule—the honeycomb or cartwheel appearance; thirdly, a calcified rind around a cyst is usually associated with an old, inactive hydatid lesion. The diagnosis of hydatid, as opposed to a simple cyst, is an important one as any attempted aspiration may spread the parasite further by seeding along the needle track if the operator is unaware of the diagnosis. (Fig 6-2-3)

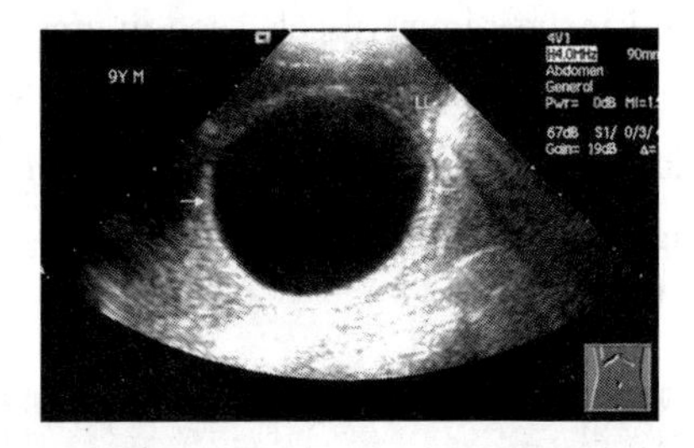

Fig 6-2-3 Hepatic cysts

Hydatid cyst demonstrates surrounding daughter cysts.

2) CT

The majority of hepatic cysts can be diagnosed by plain CT. Cysts less than 1 cm in diameter may be missed because of partial volume effects. The fluid of the minority cyst contains more protein components with high density or hemorrhage, which needs enhanced CT to differentiate it with liver lesions. (Fig 6-2-4-A/B/C)

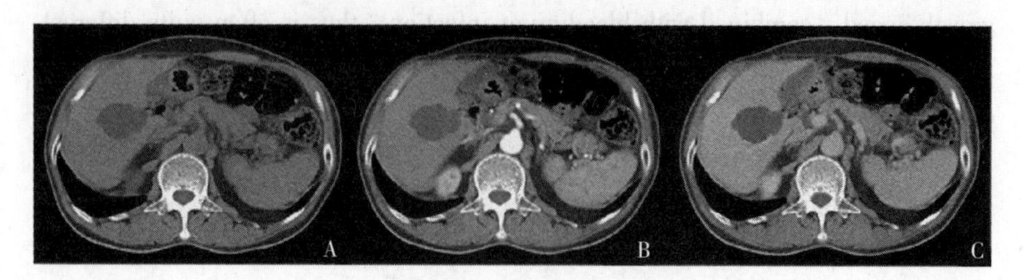

Fig 6-2-4-A/B/C Hepatic cysts

Plain CT (A) shows homogeneous low density, well-defined edge and enhanced CT shows no enhancement on arterial phase images (B) and venous phase images (C).

3) MRI

Hepatic cysts can be seen as long T1 signal and long T2 signal, and no enhancement with gadolinium. Small centrally placed cysts may be indistinguishable in T1WI images from vessels seen in cross-section, so their recognition always requires a contrast-enhanced acquisition. The presence of haemorrhage or infection within a cyst will alter its signal characteristics, typically producing shorter T1 signal and longer T2 signal. (Fig 6-2-5-A/B/C)

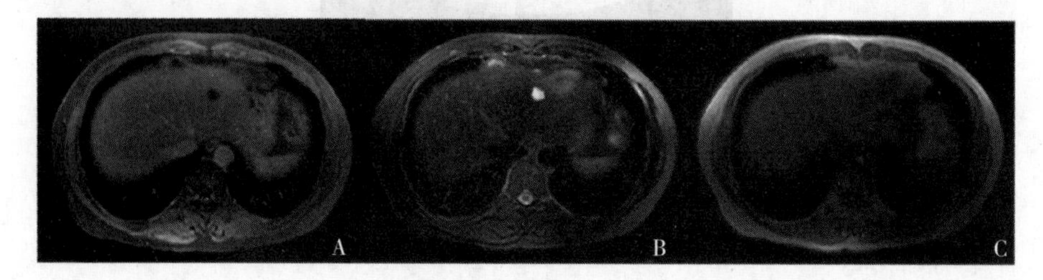

Fig 6-2-5 Hepatic cysts

Plain MRI (A, B) shows homogeneous long TI signal and long T2 signal, well-defined edge; Enhanced MRI shows no enhancement on arterial phase images (C).

(2) Hepatic abscess

[**Pathology and clinical manifestations**]

Hepatic abscesses can be divided into bacterial and amebic hepatic abscesses, and the former are more common. Typical clinical manifestations of pyogenic hepatic abscesses include liver pain and percussion pain, liver enlargement, body chills, fever (mostly remittent fever) and systemic failure, and anemia.

Hepatic pyogenic abscesses usually arise from portal pyaemia of whatever cause. The increasing number of chronically and transiently immunocompromised patients has led to a wider variety of underlying organisms with both fungal and mycobacterial abscesses. An initial local inflammatory reaction is followed by progressive central liquefaction with a surrounding inflammatory margin or "wall". The high right lobe is the commonest position. Gas may be present within them.

[**Imaging appearances**]

1) Ultrasonography

Usually, the pathological process of hepatic abscesses can be divided into three stages: early stage, abscess formation stage and abscess absorbed stage. It may display a variety of acoustic features.

In the early stage there is a zone of infected, oedematous liver tissue which appears on ultrasound as a hypoechoic, solid focal lesion. The border is indistinct. In the abscess formation stage, as the infection develops, the liver tissue becomes necrotic and liquefaction takes place. The abscess may still be full of homogeneous echoes from pus and can be mistaken for a solid lesion, but as it progresses, the fluid content may become apparent, usually with considerable debris within it. Abscess demonstrates posterior enhancement because they are fluid-filled. The boundary of an abscess is irregular and fuzzy. The abscess cavity disappears in the abscess absorbed stage. The local area changes into normal appearance. In some cases, it shows hyperechogenic change because of calcification. (Fig 6-2-6-A/B)

2) CT

Hepatic abscesses typically have ill-defined edge and are of low density.

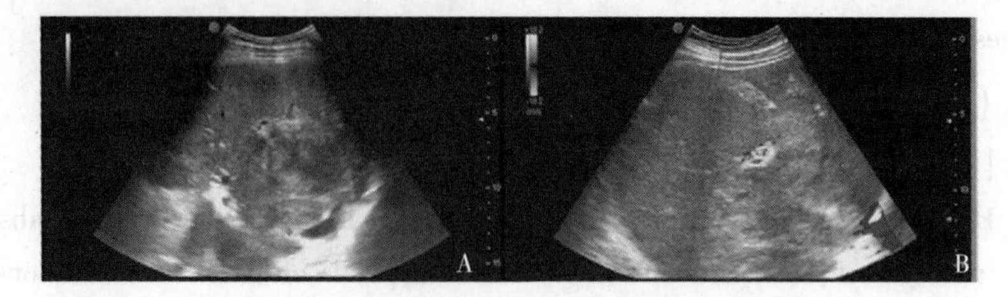

Fig 6-2-6-A/B Hepatic abscess

A: Hepatic abscess (abscess formation stage).

B: CDFI: there are some blood flow signals in the lesion.

Hepatic abscesses are usually low-density lesions with rim enhancement. When the centre of the abscess liquefies it may be of water attenuation and fails to enhance. (Fig 6-2-7-A/B/C/D)

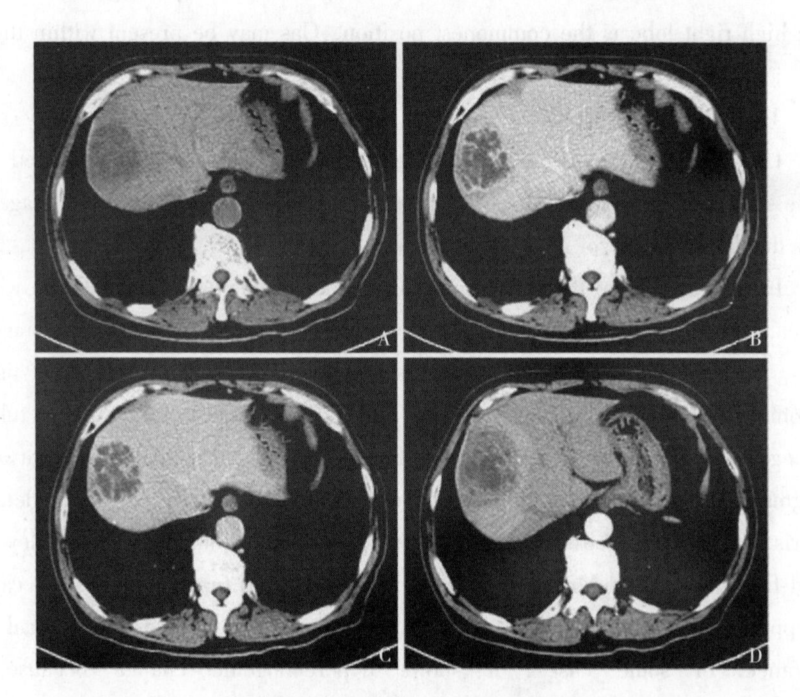

Fig 6-2-7-A/B/C/D Hepatic abscess

Plain CT (A) shows inhomogeneous low density with ill-defined edge. Enhanced CT (B, C, D) shows typical rim enhancement.

3) MRI

MRI findings overlap with necrotic metastases with an ill-defined lesion of long T1 signal, and long T2 signal, often with a higher signal outer edge. As the lesions liquefy the central signal decreases in T1WI images and increases in T2WI images. (Fig 6-2-8-A/B)

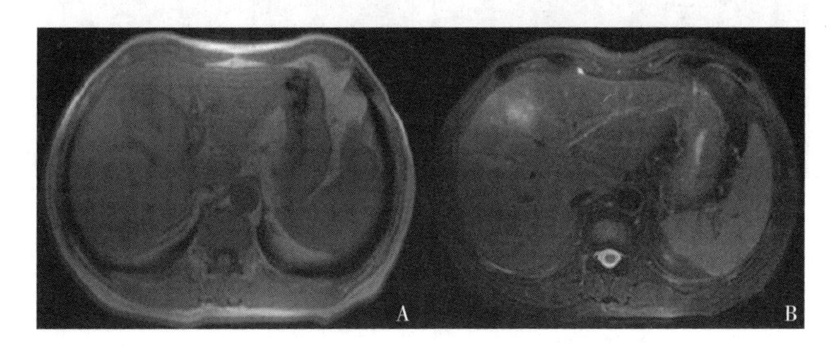

Fig 6-2-8-A/B Hepatic abscess

Plain MRI (A, B) shows an ill-defined lesion of long T1 signal, and long T2 signal.

(3) Hepatocellular carcinoma (HCC)

[**Pathology and clinical manifestations**]

HCC is the commonest primary malignant neoplasm of the liver. HCC is increasing in incidence worldwide, especially in those with hepatitis B, hepatitis C, cirrhosis and alcoholic liver disease. It may also complicate haemochromatosis and glycogen storage disease. Hepatic artery is the dominant blood supply. HCC appears as solitary or multiple masses, or as a diffusely infiltrating lesion of liver. Symptoms include right upper quadrant pain, weight loss, and fever. `

[**Imaging appearances**]

1) Ultrasonography

The ultrasound appearances of HCC vary from hypo-to hyperechogenic or mixed echogenicity lesion. Hypoechogenic and hyperechogenic types are usually seen clinically. The lesions may be solitary or multifocal. The solid masses show distinct border and the internal echoes are often heterogeneous. In large masses, the "Mosaic" pattern or "Nodule in Nodule" pattern are usually seen. The typical characteristic of HCC is periphery halo. It is thin hypoechogenic strip around the mass. (Fig 6-2-9-A/B)

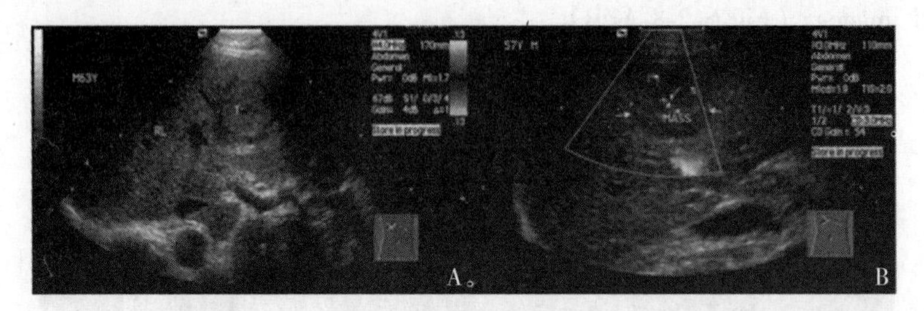

Fig 6-2-9-A/B HCC

A: Nodular type of HCC. B: CDFI: Blood flow signals are present in the lesion

2) CT

Plain CT may demonstrate focal or multi-focal HCC as ill-defined low-density lesions. The majority of HCC are hypervascular and enhance during the arterial phase with some lesions tending to merge with the background in the portal phase and others remaining of relatively low attenuation. Some lesions show a mosaic pattern of enhancement on enhanced CT with an enhancing grid-like pattern around central lower density areas. Arterial phase images may also allow the demonstration of arterial branches in tumor thrombus. The CT features of portal venous invasion by HCC include arterioportal fistulas, periportal streaks of high attenuation, and dilatation of the main portal vein or its major branches. Portal venous invasion is thought to be a specific feature of HCC. (Fig 6-2-10-A/B/C/D)

3) MRI

On plain MRI HCC is typically of long T1 signal, and inhomogeneous long signal in T2WI images, but not always with internal heterogeneity. Some lesions are of short signal in T1WI images, due probably to glycogen or fat accumulation. In enhanced T1WI images the enhancement patterns with gadolinium parallel with those for enhanced CT, with many lesions enhancing early in the arterial phase. The presence of a capsule of hypointensity in T1WI images

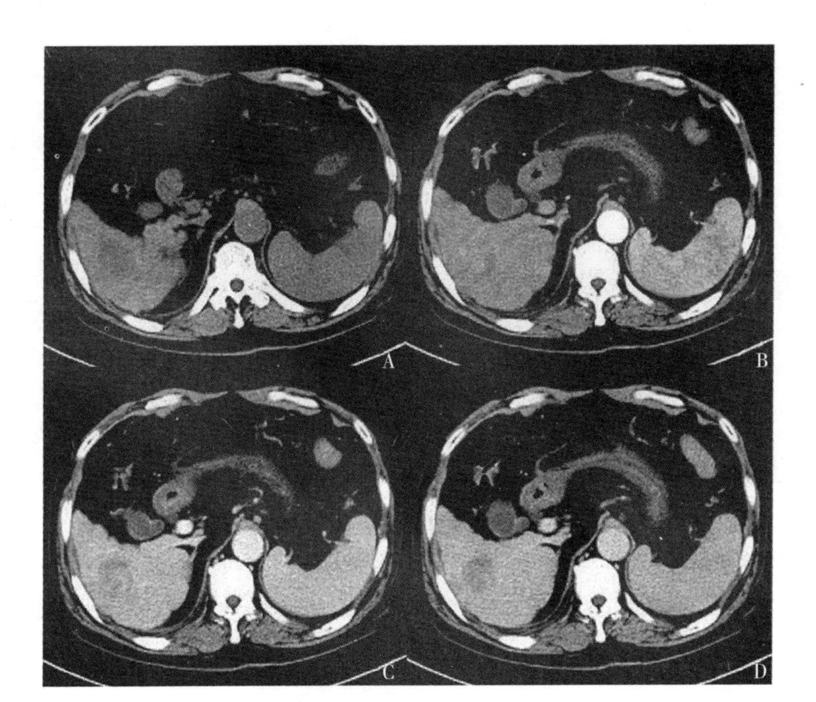

Fig 6-2-10-A/B/C/D HCC

Plain CT (A) shows HCC as low-density lesion, with ill-defined edge. Enhanced CT shows significant enhancement on arterial phase (B) and the enhancement intensity fast fades to that of hepatic parenchyma from venous phase images (C) to delayed phase images (D) (so-called sign of "fast in and out").

may be helpful. (Fig 6-2-11-A/B/C/D/E/F)

(4) Haemangioma

[Pathology and clinical manifestations]

Haemangioma is the commonest benign hepatic tumor. Females have 3.5~4 times higher rates of haemangioma than males. Multiple haemangiomas occur in up to 10% of cases. Most haemangiomas are asymptomatic, and they often show incidental findings on imaging. They are composed of vascular channels of varying sizes (cavernous to capillary), lined with endothelium, and often with

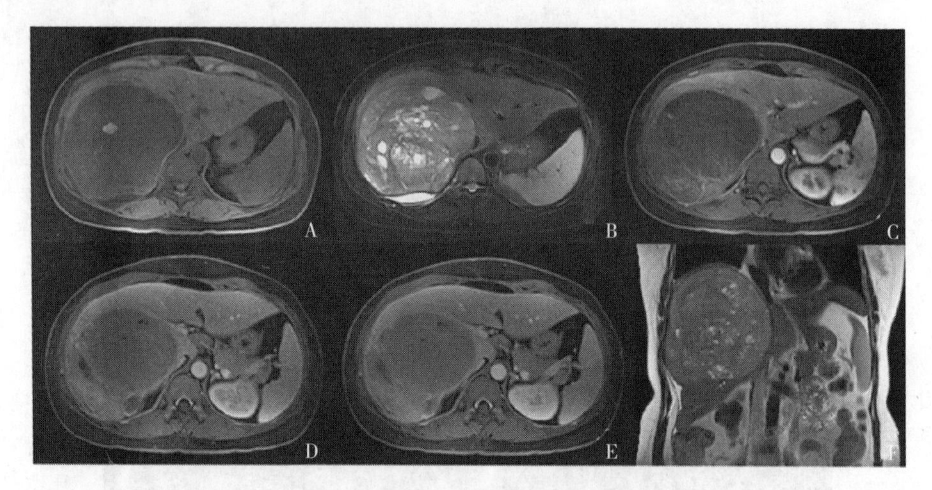

Fig 6-2-11-A/B/C/D/E/F HCC

Plain MRI shows long T1 signal in T1WI FS images (A) and inhomogeneous long signal in T2WI images FS (B). In enhanced T1WI images (C, D, E) the enhancement patterns with gadolinium parallel with those for enhanced CT. On coronal position, T2WI images show the lesion with low signal, well-defined edge.

intervening fibrous tissue of varying amounts.

[**Imaging appearances**]

1) Ultrasonography

The acoustic appearances of haemangiomas are various: hyperechogenic, hypoechogenic, mixed echoes and echo-free, and the majority is hyperechoic, rounded well-defined lesions. The internal echoes often present fine netlike or honeycomb appearance. Sometimes small vessels can see through the border. Because the blood within the haemangiomas is very slow-flowing, it is usually not possible to demonstrate flow with color or power Doppler and the lesions appear avascular on ultrasound.

Sometimes the hypoechogenic and mixed echo type of haemangiomas are difficult to be differentiated from hepatic carcinoma if the images are atypical. (Fig 6-2-12)

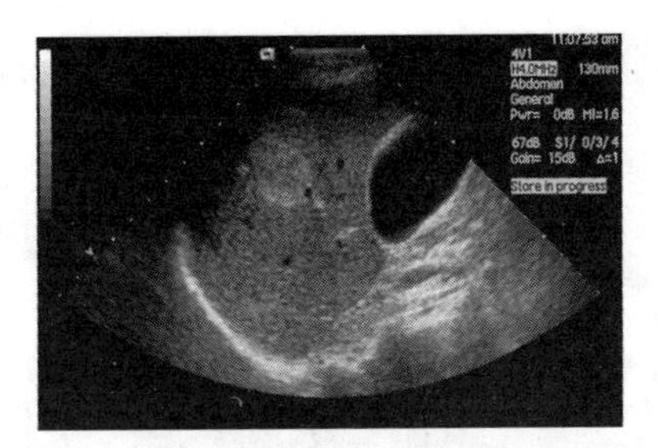

Fig 6-2-12 Haemangioma

A haemangioma is demonstrated in the anterior part of the right lobe of the liver.

2) CT

CT demonstrates a well-defined, lobular lesion with density similar to that of blood before enhancement. The pattern of enhancement is the lesion filling in centripetally and eventually merging with the background parenchyma. The time for complete in-filling has been applied as a diagnostic criterion, but the size of the lesion may influence this substantially, with larger lesions taking more than 10 minutes to opacify in some cases. (Fig 6-2-13-A/B/C/D)

Plain CT (A) shows homogeneous low density, with well-defined edge. Arterial phase images phase (A) shows peripheral nodular enhancement. The enhancement gradually fills in the lesion from the venous phase images to delayed phase images. Finally, the lesion has the same density with that of parenchyma of liver

3) MRI

MRI is now the most sensitive and specific imaging examination for the diagnosis of haemangioma. Haemangiomas are well-defined lesions with a lobular edge and homogeneous long T2 signal. On enhanced MRI typical haemangiomas have rapidly enhancing vessels at their periphery and those may be visible in arterial phase images. Over a period of several minutes the lesion will "fill in" centripetally to become isointensity with the adjacent parenchyma (Fig 6-2-14-A/B/C/D/E/F).

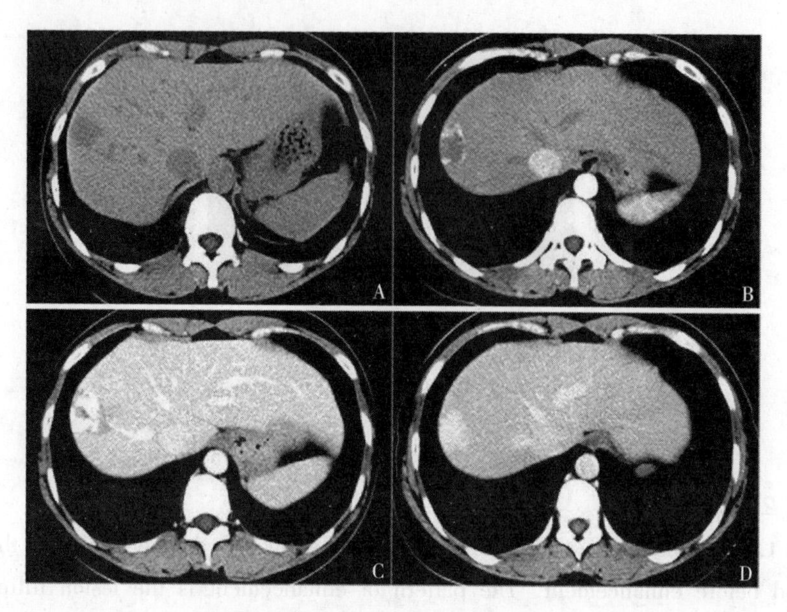

Fig 6-2-13-A/B/C/D Haemangioma

(5) Hepatic Metastases

[**Pathology and clinical manifestations**]

Metastatic involvement of the liver is a common event in the natural history of many primary malignancies involving many organ systems. Most secondary liver tumors are haematogenous in origin. Gastrointestinal tract tumors metastasize to the liver via the portal vein, and tumors elsewhere via the hepatic artery. There is evidence for blood flow separation in the portal vein as right colon primary tumors appear more likely to metastasize to the right lobe, whereas the lobar distribution appears equal for left colon tumors and for metastatic spread via the hepatic artery.

[**Imaging appearances**]

1) Ultrasonography

The acoustic appearances of liver secondaries are extremely variable. When compared with normal surrounding liver parenchyma, metastases may be hypere-

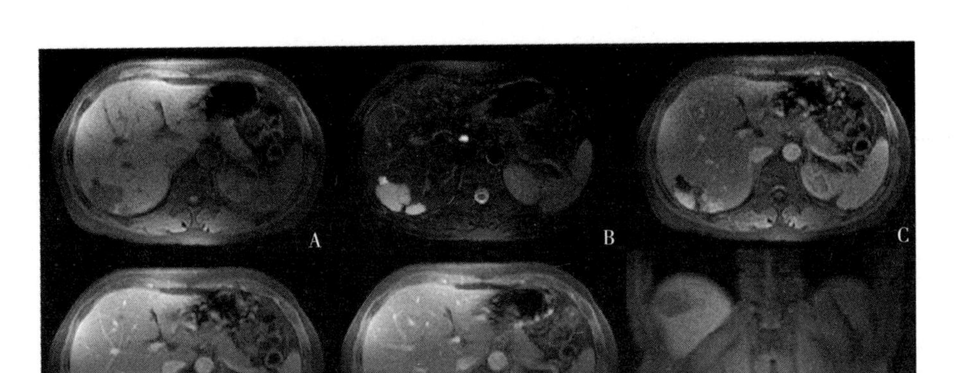

Fig 6-2-14-A/B/C/D/E/F Haemangioma

A well-defined lesion can be seen as long T1 signal in T1WI FS images, and long T2 signal in T2WI FS images (B) similar to that of fluid. A nodule-like enhancement at the periphery is visible in arterial phase image (C) and it enlarges with the time delay. Over a period of several minutes the lesion is "fill in" totally and becomes homogeneous high signal (E). On coronal position, T1WI FS images shows low signal, with well-defined edge.

choic, hypoechoic, isoechoic or of mixed pattern. In hyperechogenic type, the periphery halo is a little wider than that of HCC. It looks like the bull eyes or the ring of target, and therefore is called "Bull Eye Sign" or "Target Ring Sing". It is regarded as the typical sign of metastatic hepatic carcinoma. Sadly, it is not possible to characterize the primary source by the acoustic properties of the metastases. Metastases tend to be solid with ill-defined margins. Some metastases, particularly the larger ones, contain fluid as a result of central necrosis or because they contain mucin, for example from some ovarian primaries. Occasionally, calcification is seen within a deposit, causing distal acoustic shadowing, and this may also develop following treatment with chemotherapy. (Fig 6-2-15)

2) CT

Hepatic metastases are usually similar to, or slightly lower in density than that of adjacent liver on plain CT, but become of much lower density if they con-

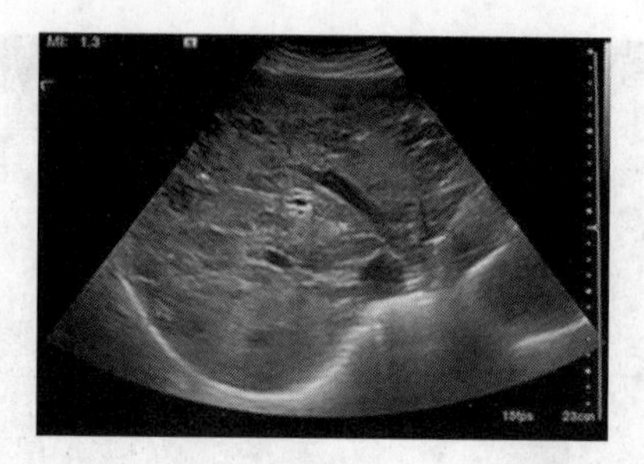

Fig 6-2-15 Metastatic hepatic carcinoma（"Bull Eye Sign"）

tain areas of necrosis or cyst formation. Even small lesions close to normal liver density should be made visible on good triple-phase CT. Hypervascular metastases such as those from endocrine or renal primary tumors are readily visible. The portal vein supplies 80% of liver blood input and on enhanced CT the contrast results in normal liver being enhanced by 150~190 HU. Hepatic metastases receive virtually all their blood supply from the hepatic artery and will thus show as negative defects.（Fig 6-2-16-A/B/C）

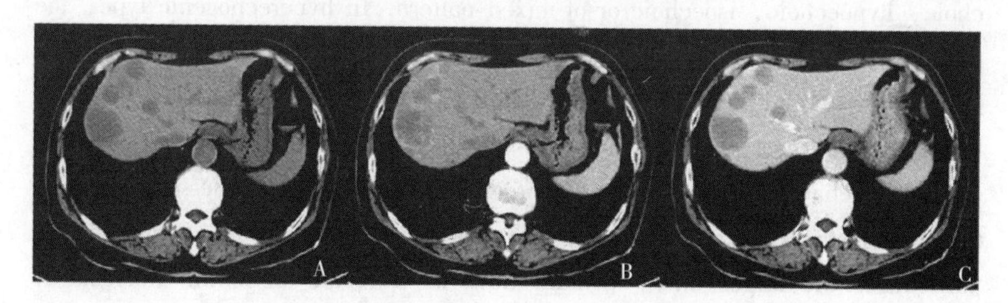

Fig 6-2-16-A/B/C Hepatic metastases

Plain CT（A）shows multiple lesions with slightly lower density than the adjacent liver. Enhanced CT（B, C）shows typical ring enhancement of lesions.

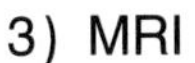

3) MRI

Most metastatic nodules can be shown as long T1 signal, and long T2 signal. Central necrosis occurs in a minority of metastatic lesions. Enhancement patterns of liver metastases are variable. Most lesions show fewer enhancements than the surrounding liver so they become more easily visible in T1WI images. About 10% of colorectal metastases show increased vascularity. The pattern of arterial phase enhancement with fairly rapid fading of the initial blush is typical of metastases from islet cell tumors and is seen in a substantial proportion of secondaries from phaeochromocytoma and carcinoid tumors.

(6) Hepatic Cirrhosis

[**Pathology and clinical manifestations**]

Cirrhosis is the endpoint of a wide variety of chronic disease processes, which cause hepatocellular necrosis leading to hepatic fibrosis and nodular regeneration. The most common finding in advanced cirrhosis is atrophy of the posterior segments (Ⅵ, Ⅶ) of the right lobe. Hypertrophy of the caudate (Ⅰ) lobe and of lateral segments of the left lobe (Ⅱ, Ⅲ) are frequently seen. Hepatic and portal system dynamics may alter radically in cirrhosis and in several different ways, with both increased overall hepatic blood flow (through intrahepatic arteriovenous shunts) and decreased hepatic blood flow (resulted from increased intrahepatic vascular resistance) recognized in advanced disease.

[**Imaging appearances**]

1) Ultrasonography

In cirrhosis bands of fibrous tissue are laid down in the liver parenchyma between the hepatic lobules. This distorts and destroys the normal architecture of the liver, separating it into nodules. The process may be micro nodular, which gives a generally coarse echo texture or macro nodular in which discrete nodules of 1 cm and above can be distinguished on ultrasound. The hepatocellular damage which causes cirrhosis gives rise to hepatic fibrosis, a precursor of cirrhosis. The fibrosis itself may have very little effect on the ultrasound appearances of the liver, but when advanced it is more highly reflective than normal liver tissue, giving the appearance of a "bright" liver often with a coarse texture. Unlike fatty change, which is potentially reversible, fibrosis is the result of irreversible damage to the liver cells. The picture is further complicated by the association of fibrosis with fatty change, which also increases the echogenicity. The acoustic attenuation properties of fibrosis, however, are similar to normal liver, so the ultrasound beam can penetrate to the posterior areas using normal TGC settings. The cirrhotic liver tends to shrink as the disease progresses. However, it may be normal in size, or may undergo disproportionate changes within different lobes. In some patients the right lobe shrinks, giving rise to relative hypertrophy of the caudate and/or left lobes. This is likely to be due to the venous drainage of the different areas of the liver. (Fig 6-2-17)

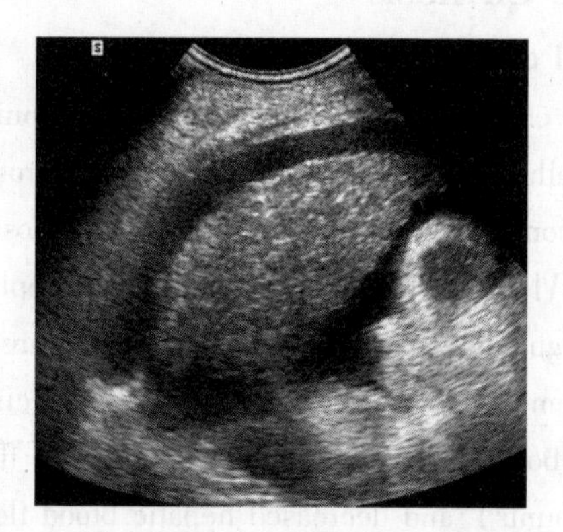

Fig 6-2-17 Hepatic cirrhosis

Macronodular cirrhosis in a patient with primary biliary cirrhosis. Cirrhotic nodules are demonstrated throughout the peripheral hepatic substance with a lobulated liver outline. Ascites is also present.

2) CT

The early stage of cirrhosis is not detectable on plain CT. Hepatic parenchyma enhances irregularly. Splenic enlargement and widening of splenic and portal veins with attendant varices and collaterals secondary to portal hypertension are common. Underlying fat in the liver may confuse the enhancement pattern and small hepatomas can be missed. Note that a "normal" parenchymal appearance on CT may sometimes be seen in the presence of a widespread infiltrate. Hepatic parenchymal density may also increase with iodine deposition in patients treated with amiodarone and by increased glycogen content in those with glycogen storage disease. Reduced liver density occurs in fatty infiltration, which may be diffuse or regional circular areas of parenchyma spared by fat. It may be reversible. Infiltration by sarcoid or amyloid does not affect the parenchymal CT value. With hepatic venous thrombosis (Budd-Chiari syndrome), enhanced CT shows typical hypertrophy and bright enhancement of the caudate lobe, the remainder of the liver being of low density due to congestive edema, and the hepatic veins failing to obtain contrast media. (Fig 6-2-18-A/B/C/D).

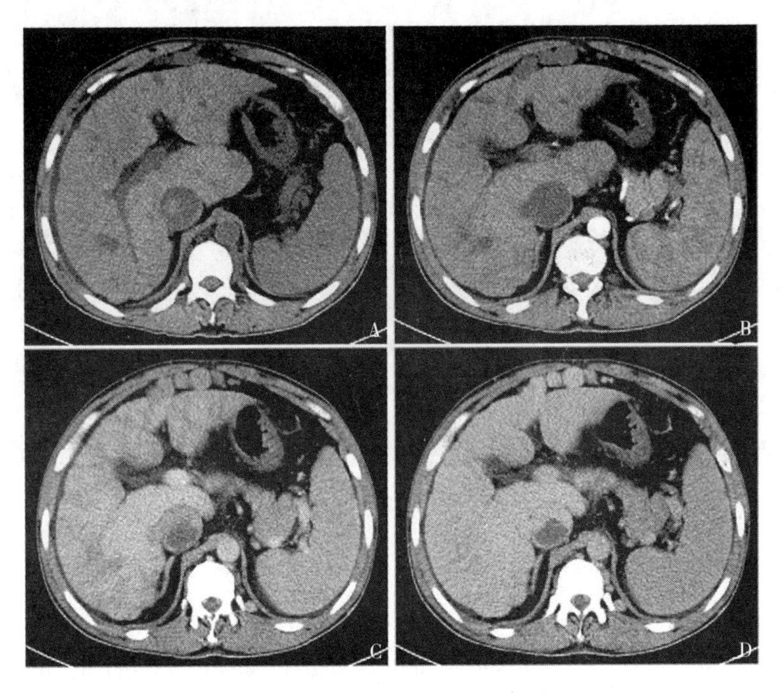

Fig 6-2-18-A/B/C/D Hepatic cirrhosis

Plain CT shows the inhomogeneous density of hepatic. Enhanced CT (B, C, D) shows typical hypertrophy and bright enhancement of the caudate lobe, the remainder of the liver being of low density.

3) MRI

MRI is also relatively insensitive to the changes of early cirrhosis and there are no specific changes of parenchymal signal in T1WI or T2WI images. MRI delineates the morphological changes of advanced cirrhosis but can also provide noninvasive assessment of portal vein patency along with flow direction and bulk flow volume estimation. The liver architecture in macronodular cirrhosis is well shown on MRI. Bands of fibrosis produce slightly shorter T1 signal, and heterogeneous early enhancement on enhanced MRI. (Fig 6-2-19-A/B/C/D/E/F)

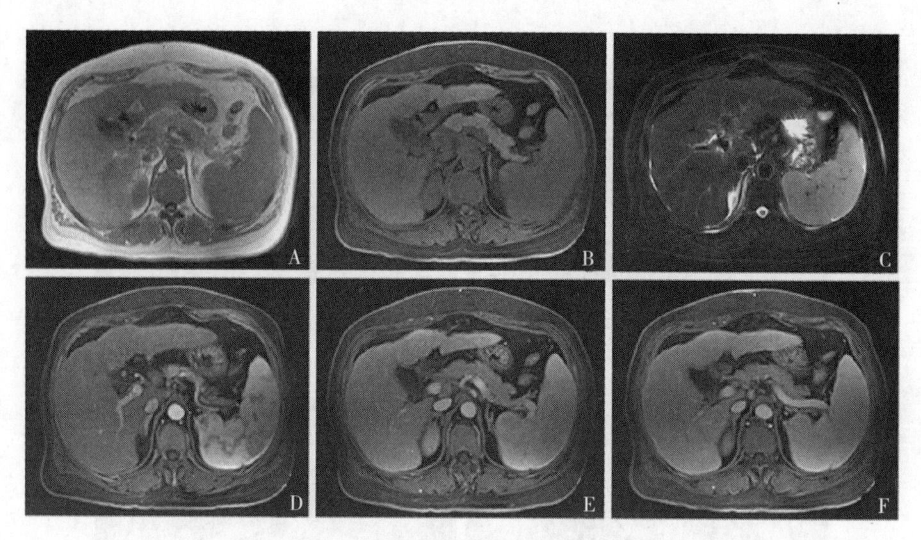

Fig 6-2-19-A/B/C/D/E/F Hepatic Cirrhosis

Plain MRI (A, B, C) shows no specific changes of parenchymal signal. Enhanced MRI (D, E, F) shows fibrosis slightly shorter T1 signal, heterogeneous early enhancement in arterial phase images and continuing enhancement in delayed images.

Section 2 Biliary system

1 Imaging Methods

(1) Radiography

①Plain film is of limited value for assessing biliary diseases, but may demonstrate gallstones.

②PTC and ERCP (Endoscopic Retrograde Cholangiopancreatography) ERCP and PTC have become the primary methods of direct cholangiography and have developed considerable therapeutic potential. ERCP offers the ability to examine the upper gastrointestinal tract, the papilla of Vater and the pancreatic duct.

(2) Ultrasonography

Ultrasonography is an essential first-line investigation in suspected gallbladder and biliary duct disease. It is highly sensitive, accurate and comparatively cheap and is the imaging modality of choice.

(3) CT

Plain CT assumes a secondary role in the assessment of the biliary tree. CT can demonstrate gallstones and stage malignant biliary obstruction in potentially operable patients. In cholangiocarcinoma, CT is useful in evaluating the extent of sectoral or segmental duct involvement and in detecting lobar atrophy.

(4) MRI

MRCP (Magnetic resonance cholangiopancreatography) is becoming established as a non-invasive alternative for evaluating the biliary tree. There is evidence that MRC may be diagnostic in non-dilating biliary disorders. The combination of conventional MRI with MRCP has the potential to produce a complete morphological view of the liver and biliary tract system by a single non-invasive means.

2 Normal imaging appearances

(1) Ultrasonography

The gallbladder is divided into the neck, the body and the fundus. The gallbladder appears as an echo-free, pear-shaped structure. The wall of gallbladder is thin and smooth. In a fasting patient, the thickness is normally 3 mm or less. The length is less than 8.0 cm and the width is less than 3.5 cm.

(2) CT

The cholecyst is located inside the left segment of the hepatic lobe, below the lumen of the watery density within the cholecyst fossa. The capsule wall is smooth, with a clear edge between the surrounding structures. (Fig 6-2-20-A/B/C/D)

Plain CT (A) shows homogeneous watery density of cholecyst and

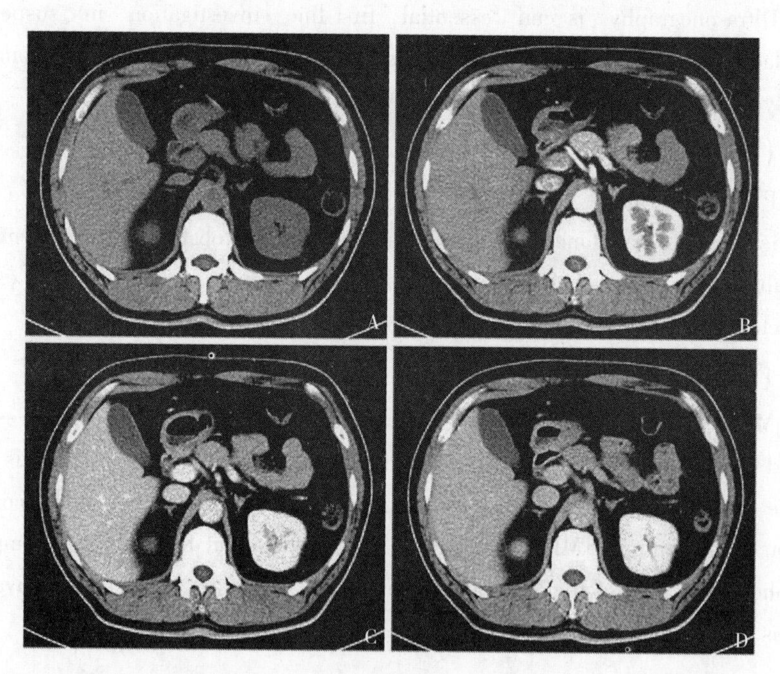

Fig 6-2-20-A/B/C/D Normal imaging appearances of cholecyst

enhanced CT (B, C, D) shows no enhancement of cavity of cholecyst and liner enhancement of cholecyst wall.

(3) MRI and MRCP

Bile can be generally shown as homogeneous long T1 signal in T1WI images and long T2 signal in T2WI images. MRI is helpful in judging the thickness of cholecyst wall.

The entire bile duct system appears as a branch, so it can also be called the biliary tree. MRI can only show the common hepatic duct, the left and right hepatic ducts and it is difficult to show normal branch of intrahepatic bile ducts. Bilious intrahepatic bile ducts sometimes can be characterized by round dot on the thin layer of MRI or low long T1 signal and long T2 signal. MRCP can display normal intrahepatic bile ducts and 3~4 branches. The hepatic duct is 0.4~0.6 cm in diameter, and forms the common bile duct after merging with cystic duct. The common bile duct is 0.5 to 0.8 cm, usually no more than 1 cm, in diameter. (Fig 6-2-21-A/B/C)

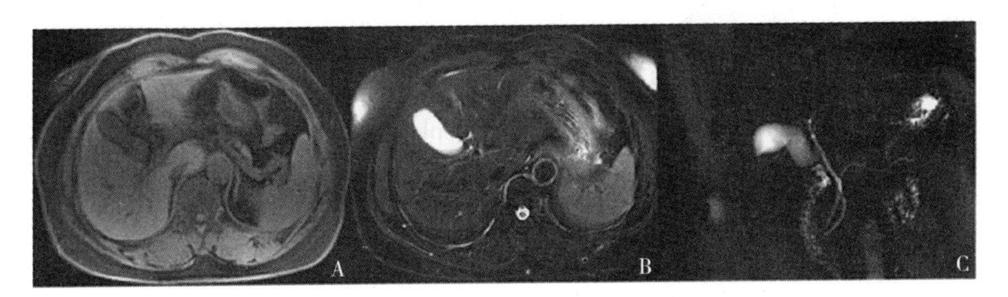

Fig 6-2-21-A/B/C Normal imaging appearances of cholecyst

Plain MRI (A, B) shows inhomogeneous signal in cholecyst with low signal in T1WI images, and high signal in T2WI images. MRCP shows inhomogeneous high signal with well-defined edge of cholecyst.

3 Imaging signs of biliary system

(1) Abnormality of cholecyst location, size and number

① ***Enlargement of cholecyst***: Common in cholecystitis and obstruction of biliary system, US, CT and MRI show that the diameter of axial imaging of cholecyst is larger than 5cm.

② ***Cholecyst shrinking***: With thickening of the cholecyst, it can be seen in chronic cholecystitis. If cholecyst wall is thicker than 3mm, it can be called thickening of the cholecyst. Annular thickening is common in cholecystitis. On enhanced CT thickening of cystic wall shows hierarchical shape or homogeneous enhancement. Focal thickening of cystic wall is common in cholecyst tumor or tumor-like lesions.

③ ***Abnormality of cholecyst location, and number***: Ectopic cholecyst means cholecyst is not in the fossa for cholecyst. Besides, double cholecysts and absence of cholecyst can be found. All above are congenital anomalies.

(2) Calcification of biliary system

It is usually associated with calculi. On plain radiography cholecystolithiasis always shows the low density of center and the high density of margin. On CT calculi of cholecyst and bile duct always show single or multiple high density shadow in cholecyst or dilatated bile duct. In MRI images the majority of calculi of cholecyst and bile duct are hypointensity signal in T1WI images and T2WI images, but some calculi of cholecyst and bile duct show high signal in T1WI images. In T2WI and MRCP images these calculi show round or polygonal hypointensity filling defection in the high signal bile.

(3) Dilatation of biliary tract

(4) Obstruction and narrowness of biliary tract

It can be congenital and posteriority dilatation of biliary tract. Congenital one shows focal spindle and cystic dilatation of intrahepatic bile duct and extrahepatic bile duct, which connect with normal bile duct.

(5) Filling defection

Cholecystolithiasis, calculus of bile duct and tumor of cholecyst and bile duct can cause filling defect.

4 Diagnosis of diseases

(1) Congenital dilatation of the bile duct

[**Pathology and clinical manifestations**]

Ⅰ type: It is a rare or simple type, not companied with congenital cirrhosis of the liver but often accompanied by cholelith, cholangitis and liver abscess. Patients are often with symptoms of fever or abdominal pain. Sepsis and liver abscess often lead to death. A few cases can result in bile duct carcinoma.

Ⅱ type: It is a common type, often with the combination of congenital hepatic fibrosis, fewer cholangitis and bile duct stones. In childhood, the symptoms often appear, such as the enlargement of the liver and the spleen, and gastrointestinal bleeding and esophageal varices. Liver failure and portal hypertension often leads to death.

Ⅲ type: It shows the dilation of the common bile duct, which protrudes to the end of the duodenum cavity.

Pathology appearance: The expansion of intrahepatic bile duct links intrahepatic bile ducts, forming traffic bile duct cyst. Some people think that Caroli's disease and renal cystic disease belong to a class of diseases of bile duct and kidney collecting tubule, characterized by different degrees of expansion.

[**Imaging appearances**]

1) ERCP and PTC

Intrahepatic bile duct cystic expansion and left and right lobes are often affected. Common bile duct often expands but with no obvious obstruction.

2) Ultrasonography

The common bile duct is dilatation, which appears anechoic, and connecting with the hilar bile duct. (Fig 6-2-22)

3) CT

On plain CT, a clear demarcation between the intrahepatic cystic dilatation

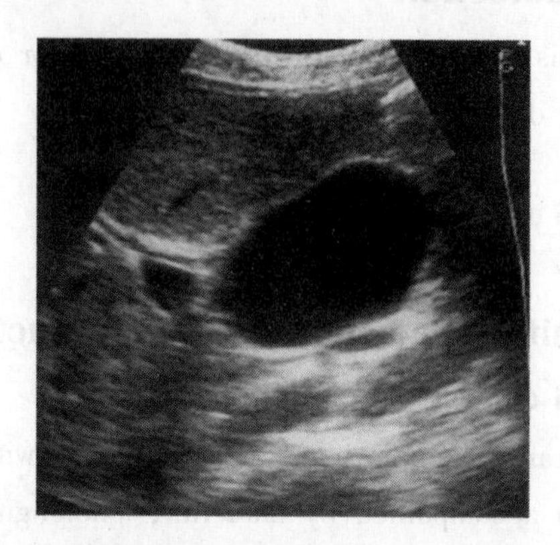

Fig 6-2-22 The common bile duct is dilatation

of bile duct is striped, branching and spindle low density with diffuse involvement of the liver or a segmental distribution. Cystic structure can link with mildly expanded bile duct. Low density in high density shadow is bile duct stone. Ⅱ type also shows liver cirrhosis and portal hypertension.

On enhanced CT, striped low density lesion is with no reinforcement, but after the injection of biligrafin, enhancement and the low density area is a spindle, branching high-density shadow, which can explain the relationship between it and biliary system.

4) MRI

The morphological characteristics of MRI and CT are similar, showing the circular or elliptic long T1 and long T2 signal with different sizes and sharp edge and no enhancement performance.

Intrahepatic bile duct dilation is multiple, arranging as a string of beads in MRCP images or high signal of lotus root shape with visible normal bile duct connected with each other.

(2) Cholecystitis

[**Pathology and clinical manifestations**]

This is inflammation of the cholecyst and may be acute or chronic. It is usually associated with stones. Clinical symptoms are often atypical, including abdominal distension discomfort, abdominal ache, indigestion and so on. Physical signs include the limited tenderness of right epigastrium and positive Murphy sign.

[**Imaging appearances**]

1) Ultrasonography

The gallbladder of the simple cholecystitis may be a little enlarged and the gallbladder wall is thickened greater than 3 mm. This is not in itself a specific sign, but characteristically the thickening in acute cholecystitis is symmetrical, affecting the entire wall. There is an echo-poor "halo" around the gallbladder as a result of oedematous changes in purulent and gangrenous cholecystitis. And the gallbladder is enlarged. There are some debris-like echoes in gallbladder, which indicates the accumulation of purulence. In the above two types, the images of gallbladder wall often show "Double Layer" signs, which are caused by edema of gallbladder wall. (Fig 6-2-23)

2) CT

CT is not a routine examination method of acute cholecystitis. As is caused by cholecyst contraction, Plain CT often shows narrowness of cholecyst, as well as thickening by cholecyst seeper. The cholecyst wall thickens homogeneously or not, with calcification sometimes. Enhanced CT shows thickening of cholecyst wall of homogeneous enhancement. (Fig 6-2-24)

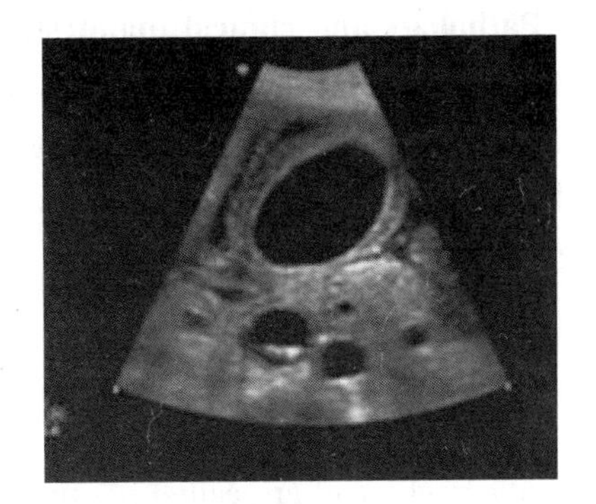

Fig 6-2-23 Cholecystitis

oedematous, thickened gallbladder wall

3) MRI

MRI is relatively easy to show enlarged cholecyst, and the thickening of cholecyst wall. Thickening of the cholecyst wall by edema can be seen as long T1 signal and long T2 signal. Within the cholecyst, bile moisture increases, seen as long T1 signal and long T2 signal.

The cavity of gall bladder narrows, and cholecyst wall thickens homogeneously, but the thickness is rarely more than 5 mm. Enhanced MRI shows moderate enhancement of cholecyst wall.

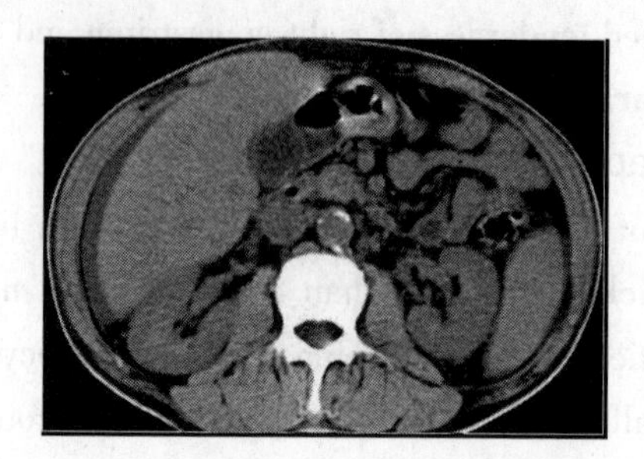

Fig 6-2-24 Cholecystitis

Plain CT shows narrowness of cholecyst and homogeneous thickening of cholecyst wall.

(3) Cholelithiasis

[**Pathology and clinical manifestations**]

Cholelithiasis is a common disease, including cholecystolithiasis and calculus of bile duct. The densest stones are almost pure calcium carbonate and are often described as mulberry stones. However, the majority of stones have mixed constituents.

[**Imaging appearances**]

1) Radiography

Small high density nodules on the right upper abdomen may be seen in the plain radiography and are called positive stones. Negative stones are invisible on the plain radiography. Sole or multiple filling defects, which are round or in other shapes in the cholecyst or biliary tract, may be present in the PTC or ERCP.

2) Ultrasonography

There are three classic acoustic properties associated with stones in the gallbladder: they are highly reflective within the cavity, mobile with changing of body position and cast a posterior acoustic shadow. There are also four types of atypical gallstones: a) Gallbladder full of stones: the typical sign is "WES", which means the wall, echo and shadow. The gallbladder cavity is full of strong echo masses; b) Stone located in neck of gallbladder; c) Sand-like stone, which are often accumulated on the posterior wall in a strip shape; and d) Stone within the wall. (Fig 6-2-25)

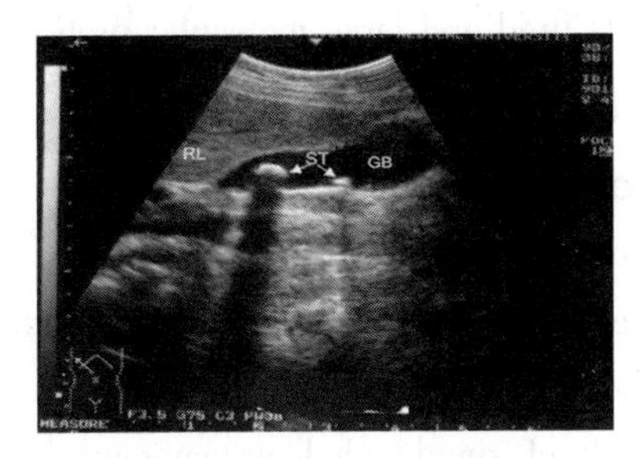

Fig 6-2-25 Cholelithiasis

Longitudinal section images of the gallbladder containing stones with strong distal acoustic shadowing.

3) CT

Gallstones may be shown as high intensity, isointensity or low density in the cholecyst with different levels of calcium on plain CT and annular or multiplayer stones can appear. (Fig 6-2-26-A)

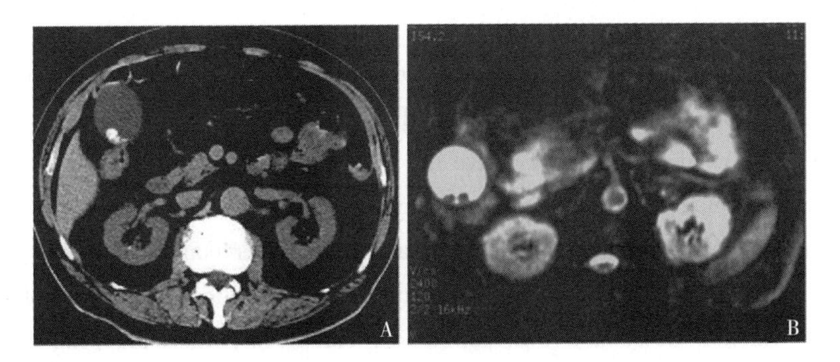

Fig 6-2-26-A/B Gallstone

Plain CT (A) shows high intensity in the cholecyst with slight enlargement of cholecyst. Plain MRI shows low signal on T2WI (B).

4) MRI

Gallstones mostly show obliteration of the signal or short T1 signal, long T2 signal. Many investigations have shown that the signal of gallstones is highly related to the content of its lipid and large molecular protein. (Fig 6-2-26-B)

(4) Tumor of biliary system

1) Carcinomas of the cholecyst

[**Pathology and clinical manifestations**]

Most carcinomas of the cholecyst are discovered after cholecystectomy for symptoms relating to cholecyst disease. When the excision of the tumor appears to be complete, as a result of simple cholecystectomy, further investigation and surgery are usually not necessary. However, patients in whom the tumor has spread outside the cholecyst should be managed as described below for cholangiocarcinoma. When carcinoma of the cholecyst presents clinically, it is usually diagnosed at a late stage. When it has either metastasized to the liver or spread to the porta hepatis, it causes obstructive jaundice. The radiological assessment for such a tumor is similar to that used for cholangiocarcinoma of the bile duct; 90% of cases have gallstones and concomitant chronic cholecystitis is common. The porcelain (calcified) cholecyst is especially prone to malignant transformation and prophylactic cholecystectomy is warranted in this condition even when the patient is asymptomatic.

[**Imaging appearances**]

①***Ultrasonography***: Cancer of the gallbladder is usually associated with gallstones and a history of cholecystitis. Most often the gallbladder lumen is occupied by a solid mass which may have the appearance of a large polyp. The wall appears thickened and irregular and shadowing from the stones may obscure it posteriorly. A bile-filled lumen may be absent, further complicating the ultrasound diagnosis. In a porcelain gallbladder (calcification of the gallbladder wall), which is associated with gallbladder carcinoma, the shadowing usually obscures any lesion in the lumen, making the detection of any lesion present almost impossible. Doppler may assist in differentiating carcinoma from other causes of gallbladder wall thickening, but further staging with CT is usually necessary. Ultrasound may also demonstrate local spread into the adjacent liver.

(Fig 6-2-27)

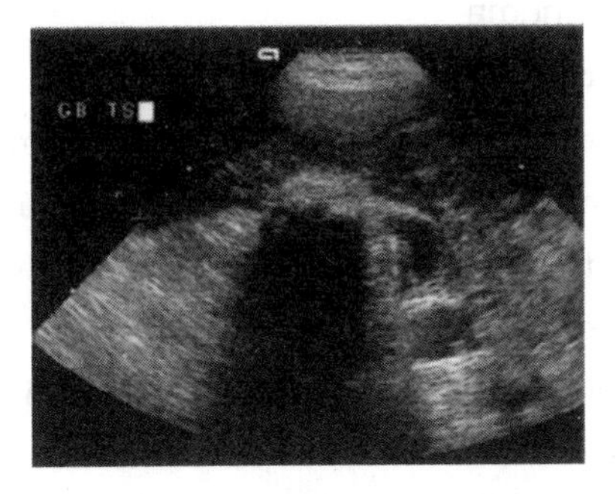

Fig 6-2-27 Carcinomas of the cholecyst

Gallbladder carcinoma, containing stones, debris and irregular wall thickening.

②***CT***: The cholecystic carcinoma is mostly shown soft tissue density, and high reinforcement with long duration. We can observe manifestations of dilatation of choleccyst or bile duct, direct invasion of the liver, metastasis of the liver or lymph nodes (Fig 6-2-28).

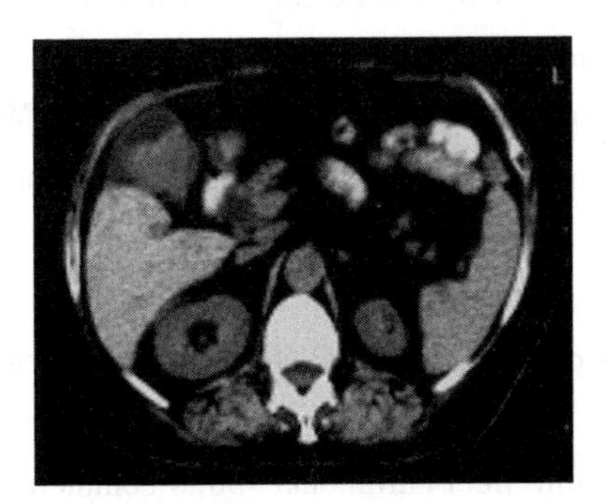

Fig 6-2-28 Common bile duct carcinoma

Plain CT shows soft tissue mass in the gallbladder.

③***MRI***: Cholecystic carcinama can be seen as hypointensity or isointensity on T1WI and high signal on T2WI. On enhanced MRI, enhancement is clear with long duration.

2) Cholangiocarcinoma

[**Pathology and clinical manifestations**]

Histologically, the tumors are characterized by a marked scirrhous reaction, with clumps of carcinoma cells surrounded by fibrous tissues resulting in a malignant stricture. The tumors are slow growing but are locally invasive with involvement of the hepatic artery and portal venous system. The tumor has to be distinguished from peripheral cholangiocarcinoma arising from peripheral bile ducts. These tumors are distinct in their clinical presentation and course, with the peripheral type only complicated by jaundice at a later stage, whereas, in hilar or extrahepatic tumors, biliary obstruction is an early appearance. Distant metastatic spread is not a major feature.

[**Imaging appearances**]

①***Ultrasonography***: It is obviously easier to recognize from an ultrasound point of view when it occurs in and obstructs the common duct, as the subsequent dilatation outlines the proximal part of the tumor with bile. Cholangiocarcinoma may occur at any level along the biliary tree and is frequently multifocal. A cholangiocarcinoma is referred to as a Klatskin tumor when it involves the confluence of the right and left hepatic ducts. These lesions are often difficult to detect on both ultrasound and CT. They are frequently isoechoic, and the only clue may be the proximal dilatation of the biliary ducts. Multifocal cholangiocarcinoma may spread to the surrounding liver tissue and carries a very poor prognosis for long-term survival. In a liver whose texture is already altered by diffuse disease it may be almost impossible to identify these lesions before they become large. A pattern of dilated ducts distal to the lesion is a good clue. (Fig 6-2-29)

②***CT***: Common bile duct carcinoma shows common bile duct at the bottom of the lesion and intrahepatic bile ducts show dilation, the sudden obstruction in the dilation site. Some cases in the intermitting position have visible lumen soft tissue mass. On enhanced CT mass shows slight to moderate enhancement.

Intrahepatic cholangiocarcinoma shows low density lesion inside liver, intra-

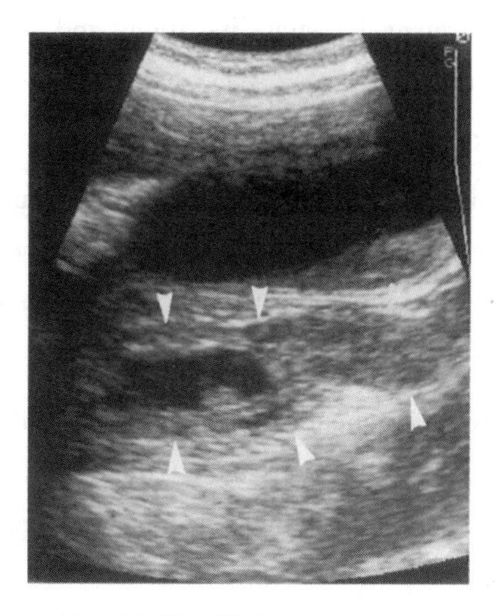

Fig 6-2-29 Cholangiocarcinoma

The distal CBD has a thickened wall (arrowheads),

and the lumen is filled with tumor at the lower end.

hepatic bile ducts dilation in corresponding area. The density of lesion is still lower than that of normal liver on enhanced CT.

③***MRI***: Bile duct contorts area lump. On TIWI, signal is lower than the liver parenchyma, a slightly high signal on T2WI. On enhanced MRI, lump shows moderate arterial enhancement with a longer duration. MRCP shows not only dilatation of bile duct but also the end of the visible dilatation of bile duct tumors with long T1 signal and inhomogeneous long T2 signal.

Section 3 Pancreas

1 Imaging Methods

(1) ERCP

It allows assessment of the biliary tree, upper gastrointestinal tract and pancreatic ducts, as well as certain therapeutic procedures, such as sphincterotomy, stone removal, stmt insertion and cyst drainage, to be performed when appropriate.

(2) Ultrasonography

US as the first choice in the pancreatic imaging is valued in diagnosis of pancreatic diseases. Before taking the US exam, patients should empty their stomach, and drink lots of water throw the window of the stomach or the left kidney.

(3) CT

CT is the mainstay of pancreatic imaging, being able to demonstrate focal masses within the gland, calcifications, duct dilatation, cysts, abscesses and associated abnormalities in upper abdominal organs, lymph nodes and peripancreatic vascular structures. CT is a useful tool for guiding percutaneous pancreatic biopsy and cyst aspiration or drainage.

(4) MRI

MRI can now be considered to be of major value in pancreatic diseases, particularly in the detection and staging of tumors, and in the prospective demonstration of surgical anatomy.

MRCP is very accurate in the diagnosis of choledocholithiasis, pancreatic duct abnormalities and pancreatic tumors and has the advantage of being non-invasive to patients.

2 Normal imaging appearances

(1) ERCP

ERCP can show the picture, such as shape, branch, diameter, intraluminal abnormalities of pancreas.

(2) Ultrasonography

The echogenicity of the normal pancreas alters according to age. In a child or young person it may be quite bulky and relatively hypoechoic when compared to the liver. In adulthood, the pancreas is hyperechoic compared to normal liver, and becomes increasingly so in the elderly, and tends to atrophy.

(3) CT

On plain CT pancreas is shown as the density of the uniform soft tissue. On enhanced arterial phase imaging pancreas is shown as homogeneous significant enhancement because of the abundant blood supply. On portal venous phase imaging degree of enhancement of pancreas gradually decreases. CTA can clearly show anatomy picture of peripancreatic arteries, veins. Normal pancreatic duct is not easy to show and with the use of 1 ~ 2mm thickness scanning technology, appearance rate of pancreatic duct on CT will greatly increase. (Fig 6-2-30-A/B/C/D)

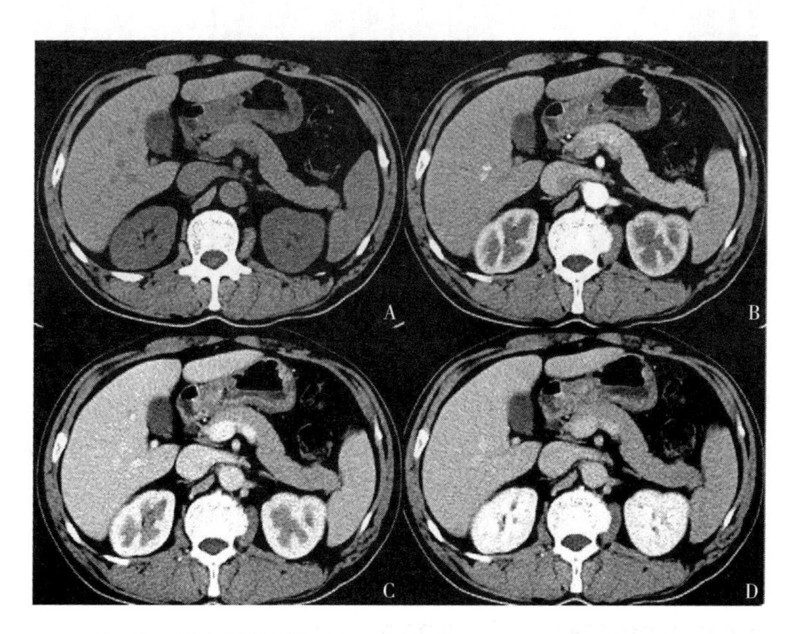

Fig 6-2-30-A/B/C/D Normal imaging appearances of pancreas
Plain CT (A) shows homogeneous density lower than that of liver, and enhanced CT (B, C, D) shows homogeneous enhancement.

(4) MRI

Plain MRI shows gray-white dilatation on T1WI and gray-black signal on T2WI. Duct is shown as elongated strip shadow and on thin T2WI the duct is easier to be shown.

MRCP can show the picture, such as shape, branch, diameter, intraluminal abnormalities of pancreas. (Fig 6-2-31-A/B/C/D)

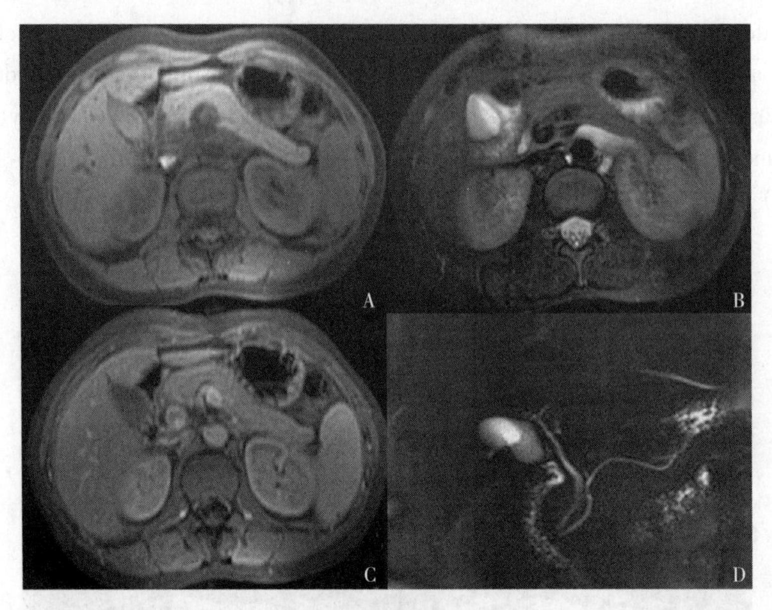

Fig 6-2-31-A/B/C/D Normal imaging appearances of pancreas

Plain MRI (A, B) shows homogeneous intensity on T1WI and on T2WI similar to that of liver. Enhanced MRI (C) shows slightly enhancement similar to that of liver. MRCP (D) shows the outline and pipe diameter of the pancreatic duct.

3 Imaging signs of pancreas

(1) Abnormalities of pancreatic size and shape

Diffuse enlargement of pancreatic parenchyma showing enlargement of whole gland, including pancreatic head, pancreatic neck and pancreatic body, is always common in acute pancreatitis. Diffuse atrophy of pancreatic parenchyma is always common in chronic pancreatitis and atrophy of pancreatic parenchyma of old people. Focal enlargement of pancreatic head is always common in pancreatic tumor.

(2) Abnormalities of pancreatic parenchyma

All pancreatic diseases can cause abnormality of pancreatic parenchyma. A-cute haemorrhage and necrotic pancreatitis on plain CT are shown as parenchyma of low density and high density of acute haemorrhage. MRI shows inhomogeneous signal. On enhanced CT and on enhanced MRI necrotic area is shown as no enhancement. Pancreatic cyst is shown as low density on plain CT, long T1 signal and long T2 signal on plain MRI. Pancreatic tumor is shown as lower density of mass than adjacent pancreatic tissues on plain CT, and long T1 signal and longT2 signal on plain MRI. Enhanced scan shows that enhancement is not significant, but adjacent pancreatic tissue is enhanced significantly.

(3) Abnormalities of pancreatic duct

These include dilatation of pancreatic duct, narrowing of pancreatic duct, and calcification of pancreatic duct. Dilatation of pancreatic duct means obstruction of pancreatic or chronic pancreatitis. On CT and MRI, it is shown as inhomogeneous thickness, tubular or beaded low density and long T1 signal, long T2 signal. MRCP can clearly show the shape of pancreatic duct dilatation. Calcification of pancreatic duct is common in chronic pancreatitis, shown as high density on CT.

(4) Abnormalities of peripancreatic space and vessels

They are mainly in pancreatitis and pancreatic carcinoma. On US, plain CT and plain MRI acute pancreatitis is shown that pancreatic edge is rough or obscure because of edema of surrounding tissue, exudation and ethmyphitis. Pancreatic carcinoma can invade adjacent tissues and main vessel and can also cause diminishment of surrounding fat and dislocation, embedding, irregular stenosis and occlusion of adjacent vessels.

4 Diagnosis of diseases

(1) Pancreatitis

1) Acute pancreatitis

[**Pathology and clinical manifestations**]

The majority of cases of acute pancreatitis can be attributed to an excessive alcohol intake or to gallstones. Serum markers have been identified for the diagnosis of pancreatic necrosis and these include α1-protease inhibitor, α2-macroglobulin, complement factors C3 and C4, and C-reactive proteins.

[**Imaging appearances**]

①***Ultrasonography***: Mild acute pancreatitis may have no demonstrable features on ultrasound, especially if the scan is performed after the acute episode has settled. In more severe cases the pancreas is enlarged and hypoechoic due to oedema. In acute hemorrhagic pancreatitis, the internal echoes are hyperechogenic and heterogeneous. The main duct may be dilated or prominent. As the condition progresses, digestive enzymes leak out, forming collections or pseudocysts. These are most frequently found in the lesser sac, near the tail of the pancreas, but can occur anywhere in the abdomen—within the pancreatic tissue itself, anywhere in the peritoneal or retroperitoneal space or even tracking up the fissures into the liver—so a full abdominal ultrasound survey is essential on each attendance. Usually ascites and pleural effusion can be shown in acute hemorrhagic pancreatitis. (Fig 6-2-32)

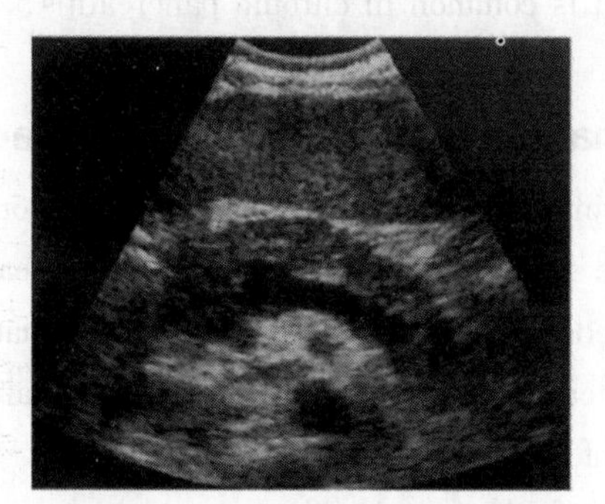

Fig 6-2-32 Acute pancreatitis

The pancreas is hypoechoic and bulky with a lobulated outline.

②***CT***: Diffuse or focal glandular enlargement and focal areas of reduced density within the gland may be shown. Inflammation of the peripancreatic fat will produce ill-defined strands of soft-tissue density within the fat although preservation of the fat around the superior mesenteric artery is usual. Enhanced CT is useful for showing the degree of pancreatic necrosis, which is a predictor of mortality and morbidity. Complications of acute pancreatitis are also demonstrated—fluid collections of water density and they tend to occur in the anterior pararenal spaces or lesser sac but less commonly in the peritoneum. Heterogeneously increased density collections may be due to haemorrhage, necrotic tissue or secondary infection. Secondary infection to form abscesses significantly increases the mortality of acute pancreatitis. Pseudoaneurysms of the duodenum, spleen or other arteries may occur and can be demonstrated on enhanced CT. Fibrous encapsulation of pancreatic or penpancreatic fluid collections results in persistence of the collection as a pseudocysts. (Fig 6-2-33-A)

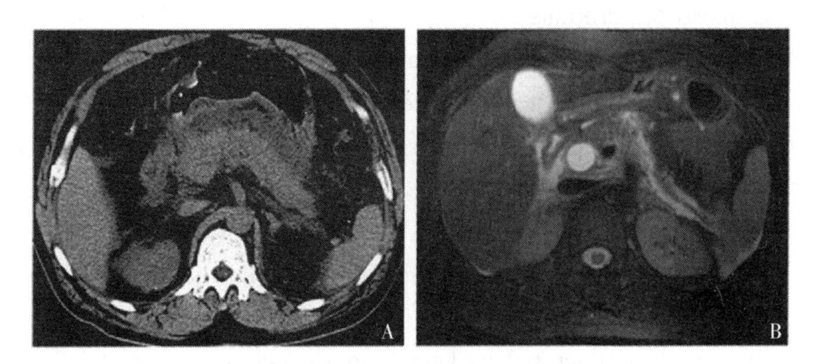

Fig 6-2-33 Acute pancreatitis

Plain CT (A) shows enlargement of pancreas, ill-defined strands of soft-tissue density in peripancreatic fat. A T2WI FS image (B) shows exudates and fluid collections within and around the pancreas with high signal intensity and the edge of pancreas is ill-defined.

③***MRI***: Edema of the pancreas causes diffuse signal reduction on T1WI and reduced enhancement on enhanced MRI. In more severe cases T1WI may show peripancreatic edema as areas of hypointensity extending into the fat surrounding the gland, best shown on T1WI without fat suppression. Dynamic scan showing a mass within the pancreatic acquisition is a sensitive method for demonstrating the presence and extent of pancreatic necrosis, shown as areas of diminished or absent parenchyma enhancement. Exudates and fluid collections within or around the pancreas can be shown in T1WI images, but are also well shown on T2WI, where they appear as areas of high signal intensity. T1WI also give a clear distinction between the fluid and solid components of localised exudates and pseudocysts. This may be useful in patients who are candidates for percutaneous drainage of pancreatic collections, which often appear as areas of homogeneous low density on CT even when the collection is mostly solid. Gas within the pancreas produces areas of signal void, and oral gadolinium contrast may be helpful when searching for fistulous connections with the upper gastrointestinal tract. (Fig 6-2-33-B).

2) Chronic pancreatitis

[**Pathology and clinical manifestations**]

It develops mostly from acute pancreatitis with chronic persistence or recurrent attack. Clinical manifestations are characterized by the recurrent abdominal pain with varying degrees of pancreatic exocrine and endocrine disorders.

[**Imaging appearances**]

①***ERCP***: ERCP has the advantage of providing detailed images of the duct system. Findings in chronic pancreatitis include dilatation or multifocal narrowing of the main pancreatic duct and its lateral side-branches, intraductal filling defects representing protein plugs, areas of calcification, and narrowing of the intrapancreatic segment of the common bile duct.

② ***Ultrasonography***: The pancreas becomes abnormally hyperechoic. This should not be confused with the normal increase in echogenicity with age. The gland may be atrophied and lobulated and the main pancreatic duct is frequently dilated and ectatic, with a beaded appearance. Calcification may be identified in the pancreatic tissue, both on ultrasound and on a plain radiography, and there may be stones in the duct. Obstruction of the duct can cause pseudocyst formation. (Fig 6-2-34-A/B)

③***CT***: Glandular enlargement or atrophy, irregular dilatation of the pan-

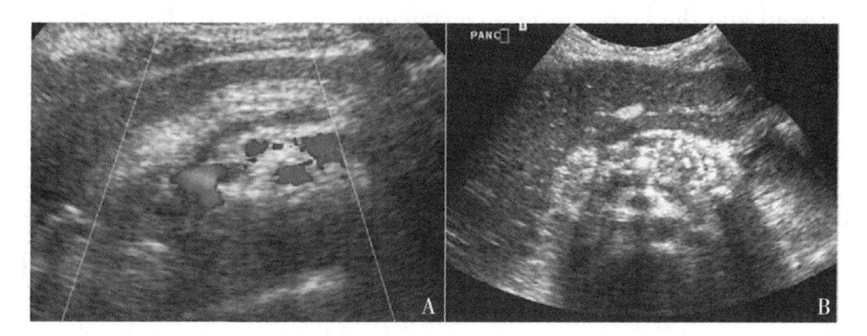

Fig 6-2-34-A/B Chronic pancreatitis

A: the pancreas is hyperechoic compared with the liver and has a heterogeneous texture with a lobulated outline. B: Calcification of the pancreas.

creatic duct ("chain of lakes" appearance), dilatation of the common bile duct, and calcifications in the pancreatic duct and tissue may all occur. Chronic pancreatitis may involve the entire gland or be focal; the latter can be difficult to be distinguished from pancreatic carcinoma. (Fig 6-2-35)

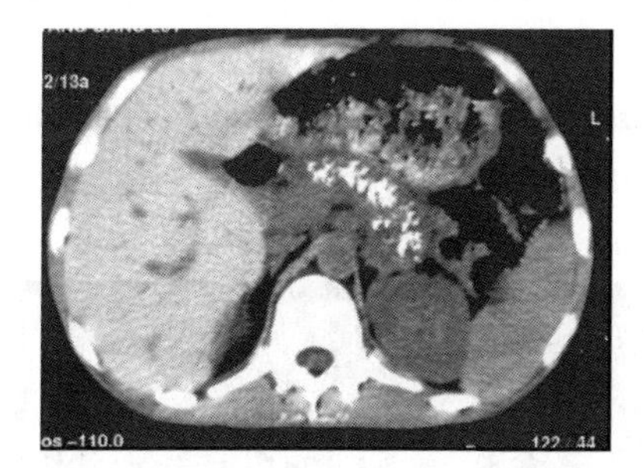

Fig 6-2-35 Chronic pancreatitis

Plain CT shows dilatation of the pancreatic duct and irregular calcifications in the pancreatic duct and tissue occur.

④ ***MRI***: Generalized or localized dilatation of the pancreatic duct and pseudocysts either within or adjacent to the gland can be seen as a areas of long

T1 signal and long T2 signal. Calcifications within the pancreas appear as areas of signal void and therefore are less conspicuous than on CT. The development of MRCP may obviate the need for ERCP in many patients in the future.

(2) Pancreatic carcinoma

[**Pathology and clinical manifestations**]

Most tumors arise in the head of the pancreas, usually presenting with jaundice, anorexia and weight loss, with upper abdominal pain penetrating through to the back.

[**Imaging appearances**]

1) Ultrasonography

Direct signs: a) The pancreas is enlarged locally. In diffusely infiltrative type, the pancreas is enlarged diffusely with irregular margin. b) Localized solid mass can be imaged in pancreas. The internal echoes are usually hypoechogenic. c) The mass is shown with indistinct border and irregular margin. d) Posterior acoustic attenuation can be seen. And e) CDFI shows blood flow in the mass.

Indirect signs: a) The most obvious secondary feature of carcinoma of the head of pancreas is the dilated biliary system. b) The dilation of pancreatic duct can be seen sometimes. c) The mass can oppress the vessels or organs around the pancreas. And d) A thorough search for lymphadenopathy and liver metastases should always be made. (Fig 6-2-36)

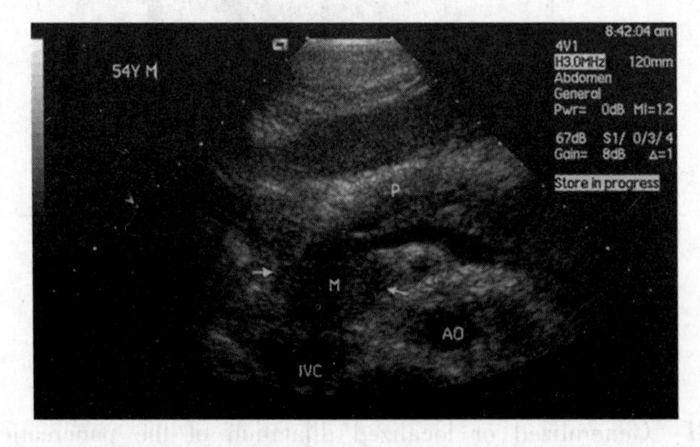

Fig 6-2-36 Tumor in the head of the pancreas (arrows), confirmed by CT

2) CT

The tumors are usually less vascular than normal pancreas, thus they produce a focal mass of lower density than the surroundings, and thick septa and irregular calcification are frequently seen in gland on enhanced CT. Obstruction occurring in the pancreatic head and dilatation of the common bile duct may be seen. Obstruction with inhomogeneous dilatation of the distal pancreatic duct in the absence of duct calculi and atrophy of the distal gland are also characteristic CT findings. Extension beyond the gland to produce vascular obstruction can be identified on enhanced CT and is present in the majority of patients at diagnosis. (Fig 6-2-37-A/B/C/D)

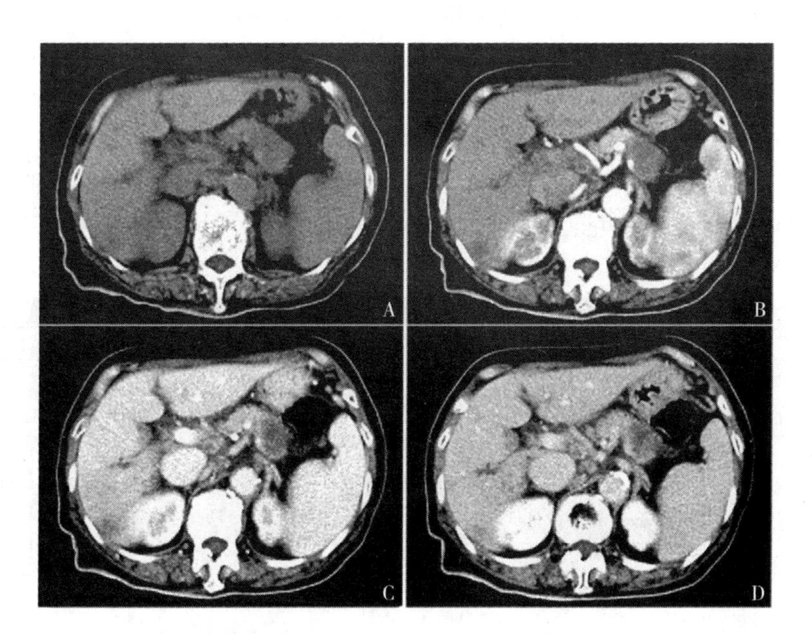

Fig 6-2-37-A/B/C/D Pancreatic carcinoma

Plain CT (A) shows slightly low density than the surroundings. Enhanced CT (B, C, D) shows inhomogeneous lower density than the adjacent with thick septa.

3) MRI and MRCP

Adenocarcinoma can be seen as an area of hypointensity in fat-suppression T1WI images. The signal intensity in the tumor is typically less than that shown in chronic pancreatitis, which is also high signal in T1WI images. Carcinoma usually has more well-defined edge and fewer enhancements with gadolinium than an inflammatory mass in chronic pancreatitis. If the remainder of the gland is normal, then the diagnosis is clear-cut, but in cases where the tumor has obstructed the main duct, causing distal pancreatitis, the distinction may be more difficult. Local staging requires visualisation of the edge of the tumor in relation to the duodenum, the posterior wall of the stomach, the main veins of the portal system, and the origin of the superior mesenteric artery. This can usually be achieved in axial images but for optimum demonstration of the relation of the pancreas to the superior mesenteric vein and the lower end of the portal vein, direct corona or oblique corona images are helpful. In T1WI images, carcinoma may be isointense or show signal which is slightly higher or slightly lower than that of normal pancreas.

In MRCP images the pancreatic and bile ducts can be clearly shown. The pancreatic duct anatomy can be shown in patients with tight strictures or total obstruction of the main duct where ERCP is unsuccessful or shows only the distal part of the duct system. MRCP is also suitable for patients in whom gastric or previous pancreatic surgery renders the endoscopic approach impractical. (Fig 6-2-38-A/B/C/D/E/F)

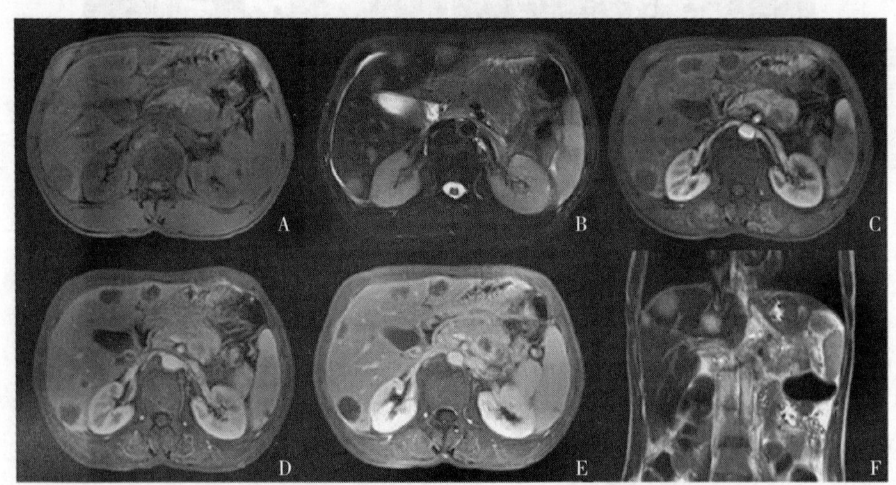

Fig 6-2-38-A/B/C/D/E/F Pancreatic carcinoma

T1WI FS images (A) and T2WI FS images (B) show the lesion as lower signal than that of normal pancreas with ill-defined edge. Arterial phase images (C) show multiple metastasis of liver and spleen. Enhanced MRI (C, D, and E) usually shows arcinoma with more well-defined edge and fewer enhancements and the enhancement is similar to that of enhanced CT. On coronal position (F), T2WI FS images show the lesion of tail of pancreas with low signal and ill-defined edge.

Section 4 Spleen

1 Imaging Methods

(1) Ultrasonography

US usually is the first choice in diagnosing the splenic diseases. The two-dimensional ultrasound can measure the size of spleen accurately. Abscess, infarction, tumor can be found by US.

(2) CT

Thin-layer and multi-phase scan is conducive to show all small lesions. CT examination can determine the presence and extent of disease, and by other ancillary clinical examination, the nature of lesions may be inferred.

(3) MRI

It is a supplement of US and CT. MRI is better than CT in showing diffuse splenic diseases (such as lymphoma and splenic hemangioma).

2 Normal imaging appearances

(1) Ultrasonography

The normal spleen has a fine, homogeneous texture, with smooth margins and a pointed inferior edge. It has similar echogenicity to the liver but may be slightly hypo-or hyperechoic in some subjects.

(2) CT

On CT the long axis of the spleen should not exceed 11 cm. Splenic parenchyma is homogeneous density on plain CT with a similar density to blood in nearby aorta. On enhanced CT the spleen may show homogeneous swirls of contrast. Enhanced CT can demonstrate the configuration and patency of the splenic and portal veins. The relatively greater perfusion of the spleen is illustrated by intense early enhancement after gadolinium, with capillary phase images producing the serpiginous pattern also seen on spiral CT, which coalesces to form a more inhomogeneously diffuse enhancement in equilibrium phase images.

(3) MRI

MRI may provide a useful additional date in a minority of cases. Compared with the normal liver, the spleen is shown as a longer T1 signal and a shorter T2 signal probably because of its greater blood volume. The spleen is also shown moderate uptake of SPIO particles with resulting loss of signal from the normal parenchyma in T2WI images.

3 Imaging signs of spleen

(1) Abnormality of splenic number, size, and shape

Number of spleen increases, including accessory spleen and polysplenia, and number of spleen decreases, including absence of spleen. Density, signal and enhancement pattern of varied spleen are the same as normal spleen.

Enlargement of spleen is shown with the values of respective diameters exceeding the normal. US, CT, and MRI all can find abnormality of splenic shape. For example, splenic mass lesions can cause change of splenic margin, and the splenic rupture can cause abnormality of splenic shape and the irregular outline.

(2) Abnormality of splenic parenchyma

Calcification of spleen is shown as high density on CT and hypointensity on MRI. Acute haematoma of splenic trauma is shown as high intensity on CT and heterogeneous signal on MRI. CT and MRI appearances of splenic cysts are the same as cysts of other positions. Primary and metastatic tumors are shown as low density on CT, and hypointensity in T1WI images, high signal in T2WI images. Enhanced CT and enhance MRI can improve detection of splenic tumor, but it is difficult to have an accurate diagnosis.

4 Diagnosis of diseases

(1) Splenic trauma

[**Pathology and clinical manifestations**]

Splenic trauma may follow blunt or penetrating injuries and may be spontaneous or iatrogenic. Injury to the spleen can take the form of laceration, intrasplenic haematoma, subcapsular haematoma or infarction.

[**Imaging appearances**]

① ***Ultrasonography***: The laceration may appear as a subtle, hyperechoic line within the spleen immediately after the injury. A frank area of haemorrhage, easily identifiable on ultrasound, may not develop until later.

② ***CT***: Splenic haematoma and laceration may be isodense to splenic parenchyma on plain CT. Splenic laceration is shown as an irregular linear area of hypodensity on enhanced CT. An intrasplenic haematoma is shown as a hypodense area of nonperfused spleen on enhanced CT. A subcapsular haematoma is shown as a crescentic collection of fluid that distorts the underlying spleen. Perisplenic haematoma may have a multilayered or onion skin appearance if there are repeated episodes of bleeding. Pseudoaneuyrsm formation can occur after trauma and appears as a focal, well-circumscribed area of vascular enhancement within the splenic parenchyma. (Fig 6-2-39)

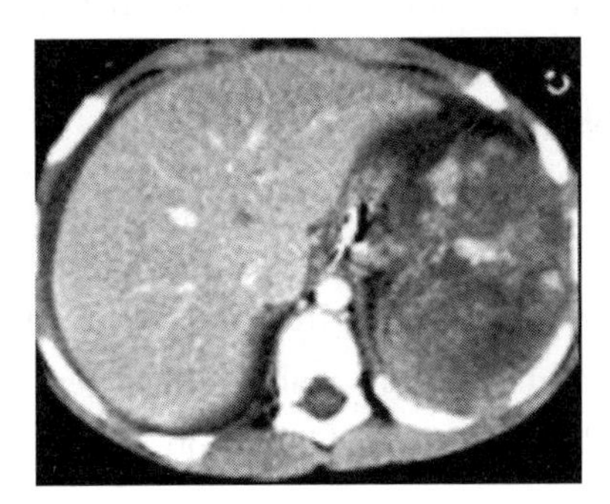

Fig 6-2-39 Splenic trauma

Splenic laceration appears as an irregular linear area of hypodensity and intrasplenic

haematoma appears as a hypodense area of nonperfused spleen on enhanced CT.

3) MRI

The performances of MRI and CT are the same, just like the hematoma of MRI signal intensity with varying hematoma duration.

(2) Splenic tumor

1) Splenic hemangioma

[**Pathology and clinical manifestations**]

Haemangioma is the most common primary benign neoplasm of the spleen. Most lesions are detected incidentally.

[**Imaging appearances**]

①***CT***: On plain CT splenic hemangioma is shown as homogeneous low density or isodensity mass with a well-defined edge; some masses are shown as cystic low density in the area, with a few calcium rings. On enhanced CT the solid part begins to emerge from the edges of the nodular reinforcement. As time elapses, the enhanced scope expands to the center and finally into isointensity with clear border. The CT manifestations are of specificity.

②***MRI***: On plain MRI the lesion is shown as hypointensity or isointensity on T1WI and high signal on T2WI. On enhanced MRI appearances are similar to enhanced CT.

2) Splenic lymphoma

[**Pathology and clinical manifestations**]

It is a common malignant splenic tumor. It can be systemic lymphoma involving the spleen and can also originate from the spleen; Generally in pathology, diffuse lesions can be small nodules, multiple lumps or single mass model. Oppressing gastrointestinal and other neighboring organs can have symptoms such as abdominal distension, nausea, vomiting etc.

[**Imaging appearances**]

①***CT***: On plain CT it is shown as single or multiple low density lesions, with ill-defined edge. On enhanced CT lesion is shown as slightly irregular enhancement, but the density is still lower than normal splenic tissue and the display of the edge is more well-defined.

②***MRI***: It is shown as round single or multiple sizes, oval-shaped mass of unclear border with the same or lower heterogeneous signal on T1WI and slightly higher heterogeneous signal in T2WI images. On enhanced MRI lesions are slightly enhanced, and are shown as the well-defined edge and map-like hypointensity area compared with significantly enhanced splenic parenchyma.

3) Spleen metastases

[**Pathology and clinical manifestations**]

Metastases in the spleen are unusual. The most common primary sites for splenic metastases are the breast, lung and melanoma.

[**Imaging appearances**]

①***CT***: CT performance can be single, multiple or confluent lesions. The appearances on plain CT and enhanced CT are lower density lesions than the surrounding splenic parenchyma with edge well-defined or not, or they can be thick-walled cystic lesions. Partial lesions can not be detected on plain CT but can be shown as low density lesions on enhanced CT.

②***MRI***: It is not easy to find lesions in TI-weighted images, and the signal of lesions is slightly higher in T2-weighted images. Slight and moderate enhancement appears in lesion on enhanced MRI, compared with obvious enhancement of spleen parenchyma. Cystic lesions can be shown as long T1-and long T2-relaxation time.

Chapter 7

Imaging of the urogenital system

The urogenital system can be detected with different imaging methods, including plain films, intravenous urography, ultrasound, CT, MRI, and nuclear imaging. They have different diagnosis values and limitations. Thus, in different clinical situation, reasonable methods should be used.

Lesson 1 Imaging of the Urogenital System

Section 1 Kidney and ureter

1 Imaging Methods

(1) Radiography

1) X-film

The standard plain radiographic imaging of the urinary tract is the KUB (kidney-ureter-bladder), which consists of a full length abdominal film and an upper abdominal film. The KUB is most usefully employed as part of an intravenous urogram (ⅣU) or to follow up a previously proven calculus.

2) Intravenous urography

Intravenous urography, including excretory urography and retrograde urography, is mainly used to detect the inner wall and cavity of kidney pelvis, calices, ureter and bladder.

①***Excretory urography***: It is also named as intravenous pyelography. After intravenous injection of iodine-containing contrast agent, almost all of glomerular filtration is discharged by the calices, pelvis and ureter, bladder, urinary tract and therefore ⅣP can show not only the form, but also a general understanding of renal excretory function. Generally, iodine-containing contrast agent has renal toxicity, thus this method is not appropriate for patients with kidney insufficiency.

② ***Retrograde urography***: Put the catheter into the ureter with cystoscopes and inject the iodine-containing contrast agent through the catheter, the kidney pelvis, calices and ureter will develop. But it is an invasive method and is appropriate for the patients with contraindication of intravenous pyelography and those who fail to achieve ideal imaging results with other methods.

(2) Ultrasonography

US is the most commonly used method in the urinary system. Most diseases in the urinary system can be found and given an exact diagnosis. Sometimes the gas in the colon may influence the result.

(3) CT

CT of the urinary system is the most important and also the most commonly used method.

①***Plain CT***: It is the routine method and can diagnose certain diseases definitely, such as calculus, simple cyst and polycystic kidney, etc.

②***Enhanced CT***: The majority of the urinary system diseases, including congenital lesions, inflammation, tumors, trauma and even renal artery diseases, need enhanced scan to further define the extent and characteristics of lesion. After bolus injection of contrast agent and scan at different delay time, three phases of enhanced imaging can be obtained, namely cortical phase, nephrographic phase and excretory phase.

(4) MRI

MRI is an important complementary approach for the urinary system besides the CT and ultrasound examination; it contributes to the diagnosis and differential diagnosis of diseases.

①***Plain MRI***: It a routine method, including axial T1WI and T2WI, and coronal and/or sagittal sequences if necessary. Fat-suppression sequence is in favor of the diagnosis of the lipidic lesions.

②***Enhanced MRI***: After injection of the contrast agent Gd-DTPA, the different phase enhanced images of kidney and ureter can be obtained with the application of fast sequence. This method is not appropriate for patients with kidney insufficiency.

③***MRU***: MRU utilizes the water imaging method: the pelvis, calices, ureter and bladder filled with urine are high signal, while the surrounding construction is extremely low signal, which is similar to the ⅣP imaging. It is always used for detecting the urinary obstruction.

2 Normal imaging of urinary system

(1) Radiography

1) KUB film

On anteroposterior films, kidneys are bean-shaped with sharp edge. Adult kidney is about 12～13cm in diameter, and about 5～6cm in width.

2) Intravenous urography

In excretory urography, the imaging appearances of the kidney, ureter, bladder vary over time. 1～2 min after the injection of contrast agent, the contrast agent concentrates in glomerular and tubular renal parenchyma. This period is called renal parenchymal phase. 15～30 minutes after injection, calyces and pelvis will develop.

Calyces are divided into renal minor calycles and renal major calycles. There is a great difference in the number and form between minor and major calycles. Each side insists of 2～4 major and 6～14 minor calycles.

Renal minor calycles are in an "egg cup" shape, and the infundibulum is connected to the major calycles. There is a cup-like depression at the top of the fornices, from where the papilla of pyramid breaks into. Renal major calycles have tubular edges, and they are connected to one or several renal minor calycles at the apex. They have a long tubular neck and the basilar is connected to the pelvis.

(2) Ultrasonography

Normal ultrasound appearances of the kidney: the cortex of the normal kidney is slightly hypoechoic when compared to the adjacent liver parenchyma, although this is age-dependent. In young people it may be of similar echogenicity

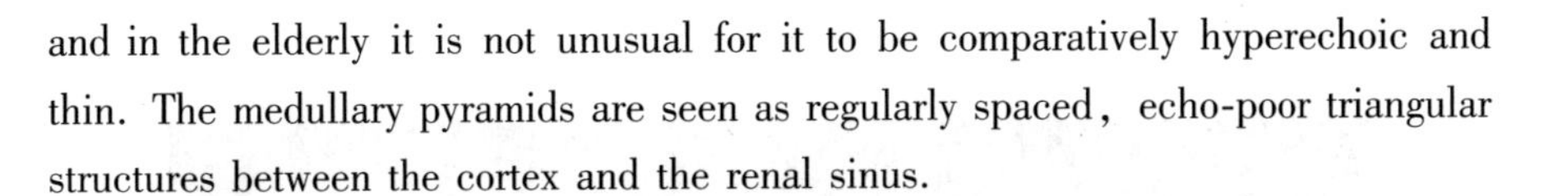

and in the elderly it is not unusual for it to be comparatively hyperechoic and thin. The medullary pyramids are seen as regularly spaced, echo-poor triangular structures between the cortex and the renal sinus.

(3) CT

In axial images, the kidney is circular or oval soft tissue density shadow with a well-defined edge; the fat in renal sinus is extremely low density; and the renal pelvis is watery density.

In multi-phase enhanced scanning images, the enhanced performance of cortex varies from the scan time. Cortical period (1 min after injection): renal vascular and renal cortex are significantly enhanced, while medulla is not strengthened obviously. The significantly enhanced part of renal cortex between the medullary pyramids is called "Bertin columns." Parenchymal phase (2~3 min after injection): the cortex is of the similar degree enhancement with the medulla. Excretory phase (5~10 min after injection): the degree of renal parenchyma is reducing, while the calycles and pelvis are significantly enhanced. (Fig 7-1-1-A/B/C/D)

On plain CT imaging, the kidney is tissue density shadow with a well-defined edge; the fat in renal sinus is extremely low density (A). The signal of the cortex is slightly higher than the medulla on T1WI (B) and the signal of medulla is equal to or slightly higher than the cortex on T2WI (C-D).

(4) MRI

The signal of the cortex is slightly higher than the medulla on T1WI. It can be more obvious on fat-suppressed image, and the signal of medulla is equal to or slightly higher than the cortex on T2WI (Fig 7-1-1). The enhanced performance of kidney cortex is similar to the CT enhanced scan.

3 Imaging signs of kidney and ureter diseases

(1) The abnormality of kidney number, size, shape and location

The changes of kidney number, size, shape commonly occur in congenital dysplasia. The change of shape is most common; the minority is congenital variation, and the majority is pathological change, always combined with the change

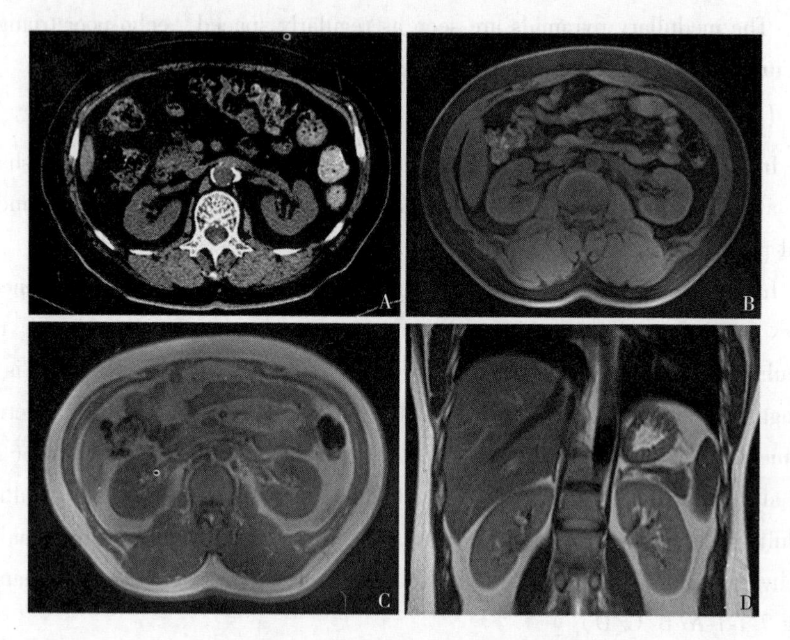

Fig 7-1-1-A/B/C/D Normal kidney

of kidney size.

(2) The abnormality of kidney echo, density, signal and enhancement

CT or MRI can show the lesion with abnormal echo, density, or signal which commonly can be found in a variety of kidney tumors, cysts, infection and hematoma. The performances of different lesions are varied with different pathological characteristics, which are used as diagnosis evidences.

(3) The abnormal calcification

The abdominal plain films, especially CT, can detect the abnormal calcification in kidney and ureter easily, while MRI is insensitive of calcific lesions. The abnormal calcification in kidney can be found in renal tuberculosis or renal tumors; the calcification in pelvis, calices and ureter is the common performance of urinary calculi, and also the primary diagnosis evidence.

(4) The abnormality of pelvis, calices and ureter

The commonest performance is the pelvis, calices and ureter dropsy and extension mainly caused by obstruction.

4 Diagnosis of diseases

(1) Congenital lesions and variants of kidney and ureters

[**Pathology and clinical manifestations**]

Congenital lesions and variants of kidney and ureters are common, which is related to the complex procedure of the embryo development.

[**Imaging appearances**]

1) Duplication of renal pelvis and ureter

The unilateral kidney is divided into two sections, which are connected to the independent kidney pelvis and ureter. The ⅣU imagings can show the independent pelvis and ureters. The duplicated ureter can be mutually fused.

2) Renal agensis

It is also known as solitary kidney, and the solitary kidney frequently shows compensatory hypertrophy.

3) Horse-shoe kidney

The kidneys are low lying, with their upper poles pointing superlaterally, and lower poles pointing inferomedially. The upper poles are usually at the same height. The pelvicalyceal systems point anteriorly and show fullness or some degree of stasis.

[**Diagnosis**]

The ⅣU can detect and diagnose the congenital lesions and variants of kidney and ureters, while US, CT, MRI can not only further diagnosis definitely, but also aid in studying the shape and relationship between the abnormal kidney and ureters.

(2) Calculus of kidney and ureters

Urinary calculus occurs in everywhere of the urinary tract, mostly in kidney pelvis, calices and bladder. The ureter calculi are caused by the upper urinary tract descending.

[**Pathology and clinical manifestations**]

Renal calculus is the commonest urinary calculi, and always occurs in unilateral kidney. The clinical performance is hematuria and radiating pain of hypogastric region and perineal region. The calculi consists of some kinds of chemical composition, mainly calcium oxalate, calcium phosphate, and lithate, etc.

[**Imaging appearances**]

90% of the calculi, named radiopaque calculus, can be shown on radiography, while 10% of the calculi, called radioparent calculus, are invisible on plain imagings. The difference lies in the different components of the calculi.

1) Kidney calculus

Over 90% of calculi are radiopaque on KUB imagings. They are highly radiopaque and round, ovalis or staghorn shaped shadow, particularly calcium phosphate calculus. They always demonstrate filling defects in kidney pelvis. The calculus is punctiform or massive high-level echo in renal sinus on US imagings.

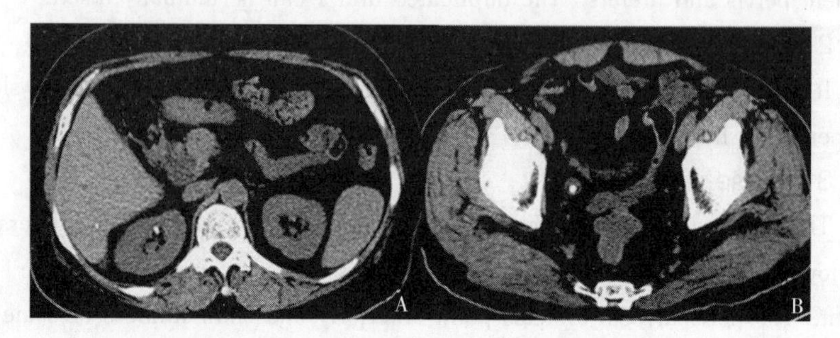

Fig 7-1-2 A/B The calculus of the renal system

The calculus of kidney and ureter are highly radiopaque and round shaped shadow on CT imagings.

2) Ureteral calculus

Ureteral calculus is several millimeters long, and in long-round shape. The long axis is parallel with the longitudinal axis of the ureter, and is always located at the 3 physiological narrow zones. It can cause ureter wall swelling, abrased wounds, and proximate hydroureterosis and hydronephrosis (Fig 7-1-2-A/B).

[**Diagnosis**]

KUB scan is the first screening method of choice. CT is the most accurate method. When it is difficult to diagnosis, CT scan is the best choice.

(3) Tuberculosis

[**Pathology and clinical manifestations**]

Urinary tuberculosis can involve kidney, ureter and bladder, and are always secondary to tuberculosis in other regions. 7% ~ 8% of the pulmonary tuberculosis are accompanied by renal tuberculosis. Ureter and bladder tuberculosis always develops from kidney tuberculosis. When the kidney is calcified totally, we name it autonephrectomy.

[**Imaging appearances**]

1) Radiography

The classical features can be shown on IVU. In early stage, the kidney pelvis has eroded edge. The kidney pelvis and calices are destructed and deformed, combined with empyema and dilation in pelvis and calices, thus it is poor visualization on excretory urography films. The ureter tuberculosis is looks like irregular beads or stiffness.

2) Ultrasonography

US can demonstrate the hydronephrosis and the calcification, but there are many kinds of kidney tuberculosis, and the US imaging is not atypical.

3) CT

CT will demonstrate hydrocalycles and/or hydronephrosis, which may contain a considerable amount of debris, areas of calcification and parenchymal loss. Bacilli pass into the bladder, which also becomes inflamed and subsequently contracted.

4) MRI

The signal of the tuberculosis is poorly distinctive, and MRU can show the morphologic change of urinary system.

[**Diagnosis**]

The clinic performance of kidney tuberculosis is uncharacteristic. The primary evidence is from serological testing, bacteriological analysis and radiological study. KUB and CT are the general methods.

(4) Renal Cysts

[**Pathology and clinical manifestations**]

Renal cysts are one of the cystic lesions of the kidney, and are always divided into simple cysts and adult polycystic cysts. Simple renal cysts are extremely common. They emerge in adulthood, increase in frequency with age, and are present in 25%~50% of subjects over the age of 50. The vast majority of simple renal cysts are asymptomatic. They have a thin fibrous wall lined with cuboidal epithelium and contain clear serous fluid. Adult polycystic cysts are an autosomal dominant inherited disease, and are always combined with polycystic liver and spleen.

[**Imaging appearances**]

Simple renal cysts On CT and MRI scan, the lesion is watery density and signal, and it is not enhanced on enhanced scan.

Adult polycystic cysts The two kidney are enlarged and lobulated with multiple cysts of unequal sizes, and the density and signal characteristics are similar to simple cysts (Fig 7-1-3-A/B/C/D).

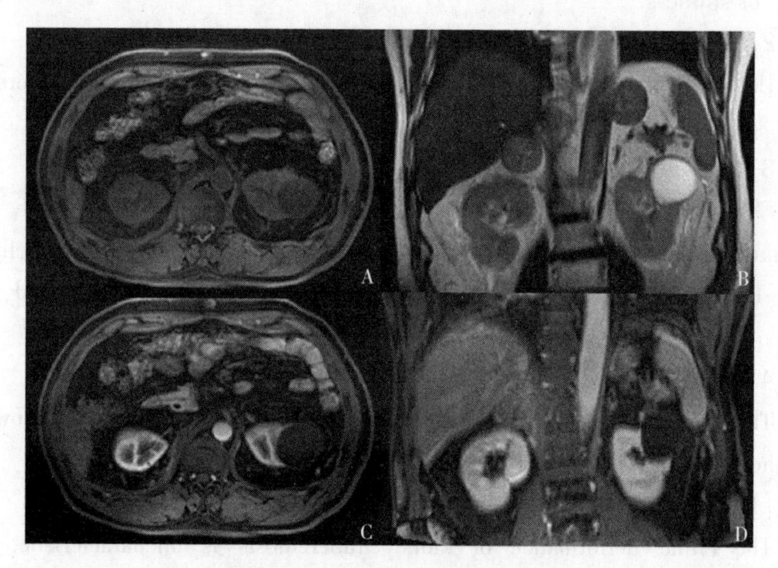

Fig 7-1-3-A/B/C/D Renal cysts

The signal of renal cysts is similar to water: long T1 signal (A) and long T2 signal (B), and it is not enhanced on enhanced MRI (C-D).

[**Diagnosis**]

The US is the first choice of radiological methods. It is easy to distinct simple renal cysts and adult polycystic cysts with characteristic performances.

(5) Angiomyolipoma

[**Pathology and clinical manifestations**]

These are benign hamartomas consisting of varying proportions of angioid, myoid and lipoid tissues. They may be extremely vascular and contain small aneurysms with a predilection to bleed as the mass enlarges. Classically they have been described as large at presentation but increasingly small angiomyolipomas are being identified incidentally on ultrasound or CT.

[**Imaging appearances**]

1) Radiography

ⅣU generally is normal when the lesions are small, and shows one or more non-specific masses when larger.

2) Ultrasonography

Because the contrast between the hypoechoic renal parenchyma and the hyperechoic angiomyolipoma is so great, very small lesions a few millimetres in diameter can be easily recognized.

3) CT and MRI

They will demonstrate some fat in over 90% of cases. CT shows areas of low density, and MRI shows high signal on T1WI and T2WI. The amount of fat, however, is extremely variable. The non-fatty areas of the lesions are intensely vascular and show marked enhancement with intravenous contrast. Acute haemorrhage may be seen on CT as areas of high density within the lesion and in the perinephric space. Blood and blood breakdown products may be seen on MRI, with complex signal appearances. In the subacute phase there is usually high signal on T1 and T2-weighted sequences (Fig 7-1-4-A/B/C/D).

Plain MRI shows multiple purely fat-density angiomyolipoma of the left kidney (A-B). Enhanced MRI shows complex signal of the lesions (C-D).

[**Diagnosis**]

It mainly relies on imaging studies to determine adipose tissue, which is the

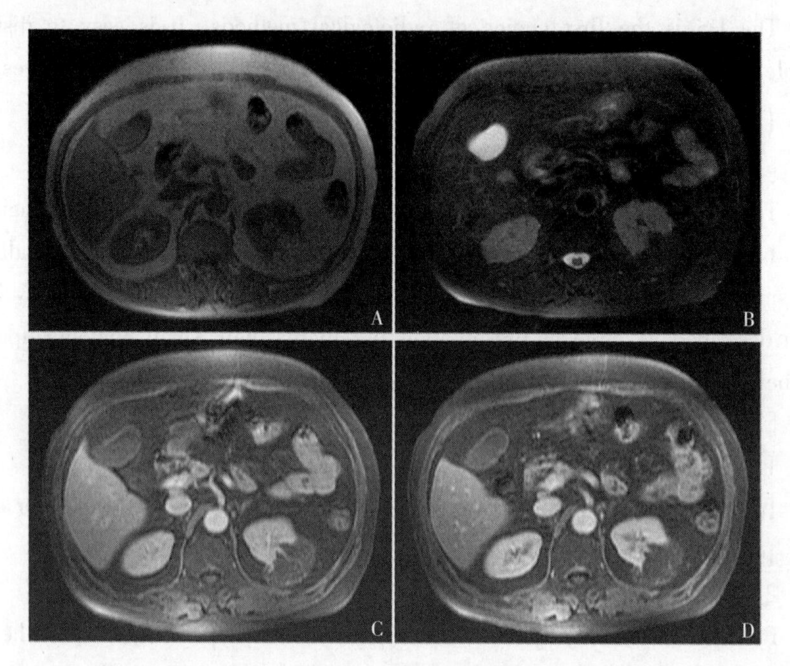

Fig 7-1-4-A/B/C/D Angiomyolipoma

only reliable basis.

(6) Renal cell carcinoma

[Pathology and clinical manifestations]

Renal cell carcinoma accounts for approximately 85% of adult renal malignancies. Advanced renal cell carcinoma has a wide variety of symptoms, usually related to metastases and/or tumor bulk. More commonly they present as haematuria or as an incidental mass on CT or ultrasound of the abdomen for some other conditions. Renal cell carcinoma may metastasize to bone, brain, lung, liver and soft tissues. Sometimes the metastatic disease is the presenting symptom.

[Imaging appearances]

1) Radiography

The ⅣU is the traditional modality used to investigate haematuria. Large tumors may be visible as soft-tissue masses on the preliminary plain films. Up to

10% of renal cell carcinomas show some calcification on plain films.

2) Ultrasonography

The kidney is normal or enlarged locally according to the different sizes of tumors. The solid mass can be seen in renal parenchyma. Its border is usually well-defined. The renal sinus can be oppressed by the mass. The internal echoes differ from different sizes as listed below. Mass in small size: hyperechogenic. Mass in mid size: hypoechogenic. Mass in large size: mixed echogenic. CDFI can show blood flow in it (Fig 7-1-5-A/B). Metastasis signs: Carcinoma embolus can be seen in renal vein and inferior vena cava.

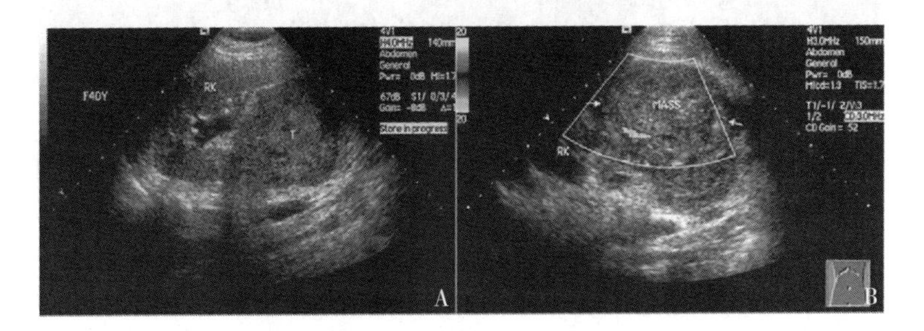

Fig 7-1-5-A/B The renal carcinoma

A. The RK is almost completely replaced by a large renal carcinoma.

B. CDFI: multidirectional blood flow within it

3) CT

Generally, smaller tumors appear more homogeneous and well defined. They are becoming more heterogeneous, containing more substantial areas of necrosis and becoming less well defined as they enlarge. On CT they are usually isodensity or hypodensity compared to normal renal tissues, occasionally hyperdensity. They enhance variably with intravenous contrast but almost always less than normal renal tissue. Cystic degeneration, hemorrhage, necrosis, calcification and other structures within the kidney can be seen. Especially necrosis is most common, even if the tumor is small (Fig 7-1-6-A/B/C/D).

4) MRI

On MRI, they appear as intermediate signal on the T1WI, high signal on

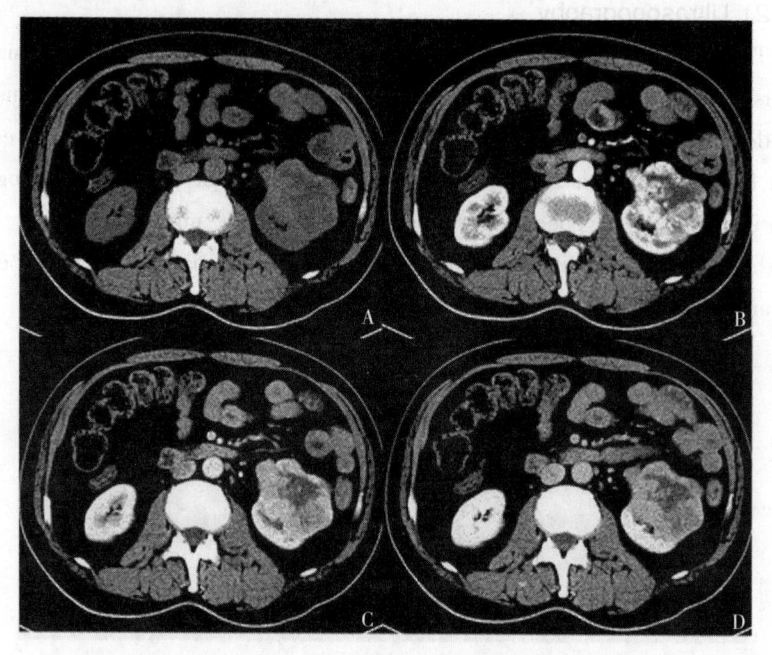

Fig 7-1-6-A/B/C/D Renal cell carcinoma of the right kidney

On plain CT they are usually isodensity or hypodensity compared to normal renal tissues（A）. On enhanced CT，the tumor is enhanced unevenly in cortical phase（B-D）.

STIR and variable but often intermediate to high signal on T2WI. In 10%～15% of cases the tumor is predominantly cystic but evidence of malignant tissue is still commonly apparent in the form of enhanced soft-tissue areas within the walls. Occasionally renal cell carcinoma is predominantly infiltrating，showing obliteration of normal renal architecture on ultrasound，MRI and CT with little mass effect（Fig 7-1-7-A/B/C/D/E/F）.

(7) Renal pelvic carcinoma

[**Pathology and clinical manifestations**]

Renal pelvic carcinoma is transitional cell carcinoma occurring in kidney pelvis and calices. It is a rare malignancy originating from the medulla at its interface with the renal pelvis. The mean age of occurrence is 20 and it is virtually

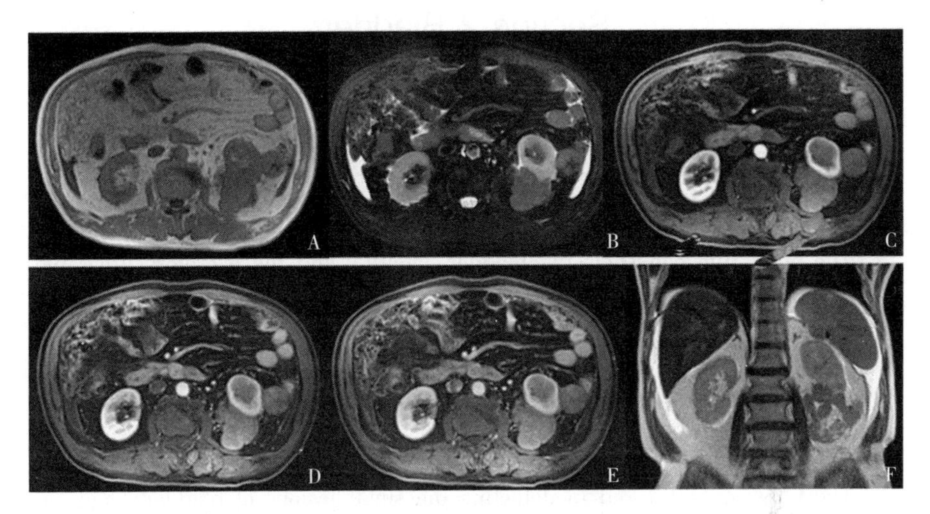

Fig 7-1-7-A/B/C/D/E/F Renal cell carcinoma

The carcinoma is intermediate signal on T1WI (A) and T2WI (B. F). The tumor is significantly enhanced in cortical period and the intensity is similar to the cortex (C). It will become clear quickly (D-E). There are nonenhanced regions within the tumor on enhanced MRI, which are the zones of necrosis.

confined to patients with sickle-cell trait or haemoglobin SC disease. It is extremely aggressive with a poor prognosis, invading into the renal pelvis and showing early involvement of the lymphatic and vascular structures.

[**Imaging appearances**]

Radiologically it behaves as an invasive transitional cell carcinoma, showing an ill-defined heterogeneous central mass, which involves the renal sinus and is associated with dilated calyces. There may be satellite nodules within renal parenchyma and early distant metastases.

Section 2 Bladder

1 Imaging Methods

(1) Radiography

The plain film can show the bladder calculi, and the excretory urography can diagnosis the bladder lesions.

(2) Ultrasonography

The US can show the calculi, tumor and most of the bladder lesions.

(3) CT

The CT scan is favored in detecting the small lesions of bladder, and can clearly show the range and adjacent structures of the lesions. On multiple-phase enhanced scanning imagings, it can evaluate the enhanced performance of lesions and can further show the shape of lesions on delay-phase.

(4) MRI

MRI is the complementary method of US and CT scan. MRU also can be used to detect the bladder lesions.

2 Normal imaging of urinary system

(1) Radiography

The cystography can show the size and shape of bladder. The filling bladder is round and well-defined over the symphysis, with iso-density.

(2) Ultrasonography

When the bladder is distended with urine, the walls are thin, regular and hyperechoic. The walls may appear thickened or trabeculated if the bladder is insufficiently distended, making it impossible to exclude a bladder lesion. The ureteric orifices can be demonstrated in a transverse section at the bladder base.

(3) CT

The bladder is elliptical when it is engorged, and is square or round in watery density. The bladder wall is uniformly thin in soft tissue density, and the exterior and interior edges are sharp. In the early period, the wall of bladder is strengthened, while in the delay period, the bladder is filled with high-density contrast agent, and the interior wall is sharp-edged.

(4) MRI

Intravesical urine is rich in free water, shown as a uniform low signal on T1WI and high signal on T2WI. Bladder wall signal is similar to the muscle, above and below the cavity of the urine signal on T1WI and T2WI respectively. On T2WI, since the artifacts from chemical shift, there are a high signal line and a low signal line on both sides of the bladder wall. Due to the contrast agent concentrating in the bladder, the strength of the urine signal will increase, but it will turn to low signal when it reaches a certain concentration of the contrast agent.

3 Imaging signs of kidney and ureters diseases

(1) The abnormality of bladder size and shape

The big bladder is always caused by the urethral obstruction, while the little bladder is caused by bladder inflammation and tuberculosis.

(2) Vesical thickening

The diffuse thickening is always caused by varied inflammation and chronic obstruction. The localized thickening is commonly caused by tumors and certain kind inflammations.

(3) The masses in bladder

The free masses or the masses connected with bladder wall are the common performance, which can be calculi, cruor or tumors.

4 Diagnosis of diseases

(1) Malignant bladder tumors

[Pathology and clinical manifestations]

There are rare and usually mesenchymal in origin. Bladder cancer is the commonest malignancy of the urinary tract and represents roughly 4% of all malignancies; 95% originate from the urothelium and 4% are of non-epithelial origin. Chronic irritation of any sort is associated with an increased risk of urothelial metaplasia and malignancy, particularly squamous cell carcinoma. This is seen on schissomiasis, recurrent cystitis, especially with calculi, neurogenie bladder and long-term catheterisation. Adenocarcinoma is related particularly to urachal remnants and bladder exstrophy.

[**Imaging appearance**]

1) Radiography

The vast majority of bladder carcinoma present with haematuria. ⅣU is used in initial investigation of the urinary tract. It may be focal, linear, punctate or coarse. On contrast films bladder cancer may be seen as irregular filling defects, which may be associated with focal or asymmetrical wall thickening.

2) Ultrasonography

Irregular solid mass in cauliflower-like or papillary shapes can be seen projecting into the lumen from the inner wall. They may appear as single or multiple. The surface of mass is usually not smooth and the internal echo is heterogeneous. It does not move with changing of body position. The degree of infiltration may be determined. CDFI shows blood flow in the mass (Fig 7-1-8).

Cystoscopy is regarded as the most exact diagnosing method for bladder tumors; however, it is an invasive examination. So ultrasonography is still re-

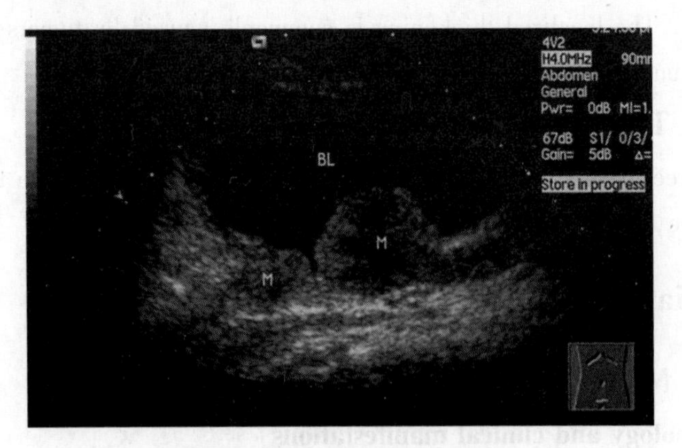

Fig 7-1-8 Tumors of urinary bladder

garded as the first choice for diagnosis of urinary bladder tumors.

3) CT and MRI

As the density and signal of the bladder tumor are neither similar to the urine in the bladder nor to the fatty tissue surrounding the bladder, it is easy to find the mass developed in the cavity and the localized thickening caused by the tumor (Fig 7-1-9-A/B/C).

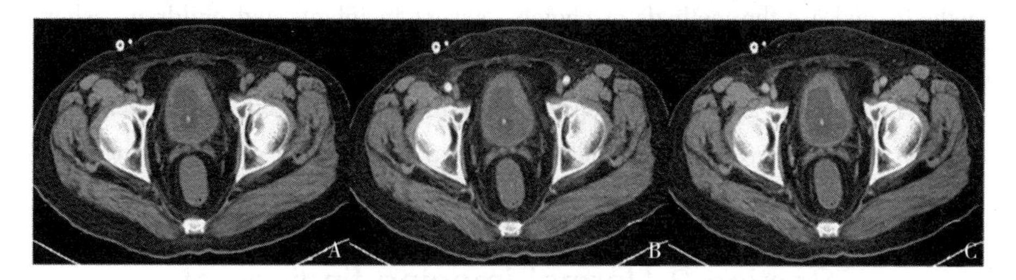

Fig 7-1-9-A/B/C The bladder tumor

On plain CT, the bladder wall is localized thickening and the density is different to the urine in the bladder and the fatty tissue around the bladder (A). On enhanced CT, the tumor is enhanced obviously (B-C).

[**Diagnosis**]

Most bladder tumors are intra-cavity polypoidal or papillary masses. They can be diagnosed with the clinical performances. The CT and MRI scan can show the tumor range and detect the metastatic lesions, and they are used in tumor staging and the clinical treatment protocols.

Lesson 2 Imaging of the Adrenal Glands

The adrenal glands are, despite their small size, among the most important and vital organs in the body. The adrenal glands lie just above the kidneys and are composed of a cortex and arise with the sympathetic nervous system. Both cortex and medulla secrete hormones. Three main groups of hormones are secreted by the adrenal cortex.

Primary adrenal lesions are divided into functional and non-functional. Primary adrenal masses into are divided benign and malignant to benign adenomas, which are the most common non-functional adenomas.

Section 1 Imaging methods

MRI and spiral CT are now the most widely used and important imaging method, and are the methods of choice, except in infants and children, where ultrasound may be preferred as a simpler primary investigation. Isotope scanning, simple radiography and needle biopsy are used less widely, but can be helpful in selected cases. Many other methods have been used in the past, but these are now obsolete or used only in special circumstances.

Section 2 Normal imaging findings of the adrenal glands

1 Ultrasonography

US as an inspection method for the adrenal glands isn't sensitive to little lesions.

2 CT

The normal adrenal glands are isodensity similar to the tissue. The right lobe of the liver lies on its right lateral aspect, and the right crus of the diaphragm on its medial aspect. The left adrenal gland is a little lower in position, its lower pole lying anteromedial to the upper pole of the left kidney. The left crus of the diaphragm is medial to it and the spleen lateral to its upper pole. The right gland appears as an elongated, slightly curved structure pointing backward and laterally. The left gland is more easily identified, resembling an arrowhead pointing anteromedially. It should be noted that, unlike the conventional anatomical descriptions, both glands are not in direct apposition to the kidneys, but may be separated by a centimeter or more of fatty or areolar tissue.

3 MRI

The intensity of normal adrenal glands is the same as or slightly higher than that of liver parenchyma and obviously lower than the fatty tissues around the adrenal glands (Fig 7-2-1-A/B/C/D/E/F).

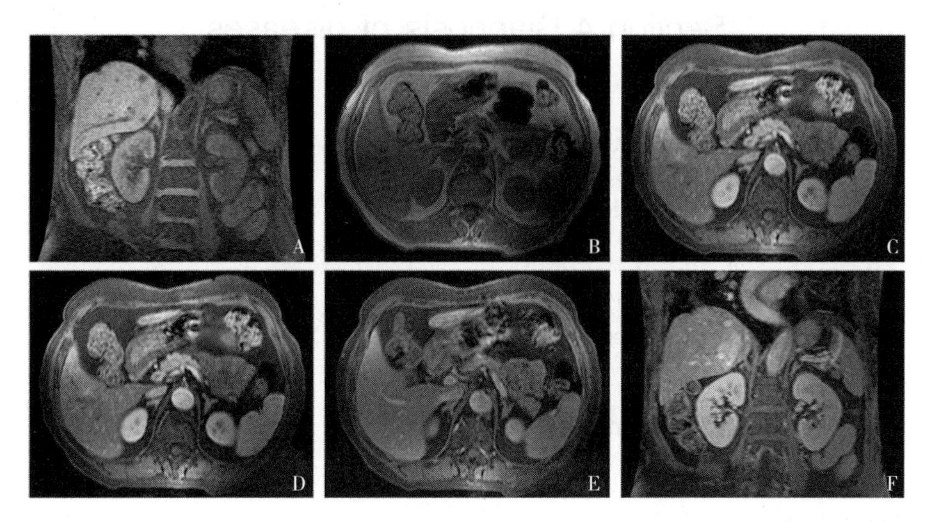

Fig 7-2-1-A/B/C/D/E/F Normal adrenal glands

The intensity of normal adrenal glands is the same as or slightly higher than that of liver parenchyma and obviously lower than the fatty tissues around the adrenal glands. Plain MRI (A-B), Enhanced MRI (C-F).

Section 3 Imaging signs of kidney and ureters diseases

1 The change of adrenal glands' size

The adrenal glands are always bilaterally and diffusely enlarged while the echo, density and signal are similar to the normal adrenal glands. When the adrenal glands atrophy, the size will decrease.

2 The masses of adrenal glands

The majority of the masses are tumors, and there are multiple nodules in adrenal glands when the adrenal glands are hyperplasia.

Section 4 Diagnosis of diseases

1 Adrenal cortical hyperplasia

[**Pathology and clinical manifestations**]

Adrenal hyperplasia can occur at any age, more common in young adults and significantly more in women than men.

[**Imaging appearance**]

(1) Ultrasonography

The both sides of the adrenal glands are enlarged. The internal echoes are homogeneous.

(2) CT and MRI

CT is the first choice of imaging method for the diagnosis of adrenal hyperplasia. MRI is better than CT in determining tissue components within the adrenal lesions, thus it is a necessary complement to CT examination.

Adrenal hyperplasia symmetry diffusely and uniformly increases, with smooth edges, normal shape, and uniform density.

[**Diagnosis**]

Adrenal hyperplasia may not cause significant changes in shape, and only microscopic tissues can be seen. There are corresponding endocrine clinical manifestations of hyperthyroidism. Therefore, the sensitivity of the adrenal hyperplasia imaging is not high.

2 Adrenal adenoma

[**Pathology and clinical manifestations**]

According to whether they cause clinical endocrine disorders, adrenal cortical adenomas (adrenocortical adenomas) are divided into nonfunctioning adrenocortical adenomas and functional adrenal cortical adenomas.

[**Imaging appearance**]

(1) Ultrasonography

Homogeneous hypoecho round-like mass is present, with well-defined border.

(2) CT

Clear boundary, uniform density of round or oval soft tissue mass; the mass shows equal density or density close to water. Enhanced scan shows homogeneous or heterogeneous enhancement (Fig 7-2-2-A/B/C/D).

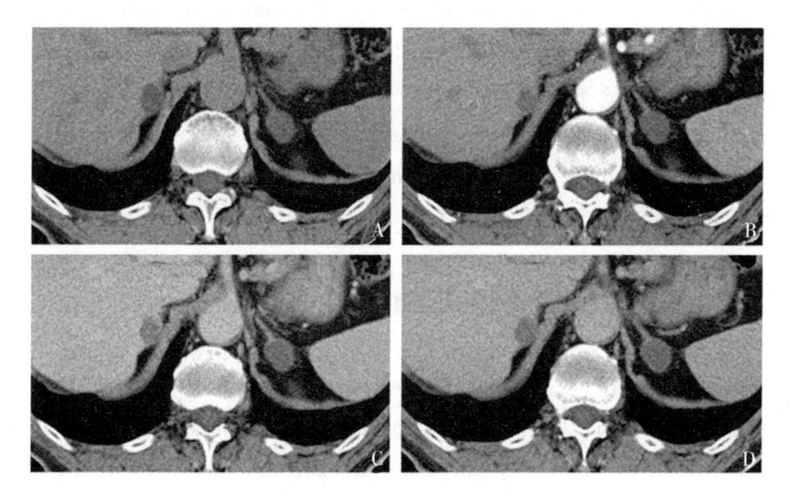

Fig 7-2-2-A/B/C/D The adrenal adenoma

There are two adenomas within the bilateral adrenal glands. On plain CT imagings, the adenoma is round soft tissue mass within the adrenal gland and the density is similar to water (A), On enhanced CT imagings, the adenoma is enhanced and becomes clear quickly (B-D).

(3) MRI

On T1WI and T2WI, the signal of adenoma is similar with or slightly higher than that of the liver. As the tumor has some lipid, the signal will attenuate in fat suppression sequence.

3 Adrenal metastases

[**Pathology and clinical manifestations**]

The adrenal gland is one of the incidental metastasis regions, and metastases always come from the lung carcinoma, breast cancer, gastric cancer and renal cell carcinoma. The adrenal metastases are bilateral.

[**Imaging appearance**]

Ultrasonic examination, CT and MRI The adrenal metastases are shown as masses in the bilateral adrenal glands. They are round or segmented, and the echo, density and signal are even or uneven. The masses are even or uneven enhanced on CT and MRI scanning.

[**Diagnosis**]

For the patients with definite diagnosis of tumors, adrenal metastases should be considered when there are masses founded in the adrenal glands. Convertional chest CT scans should be taken.

Lesson 3 Female Genital System

The genital system is mainly composed of the uterus, adnexal structures, vagina and pudendum. The uterus is located in pelvic cavity, posterior to the bladder and in front of the rectum. The adnexal structures, including ovaries, fallopian tubes, and ovarian vessels, are connected to the uterus by the broad ligament. Imaging examination has important value in discovering the genital system diseases and in determining the lesion's position, size, scope, etc.

Section 1 Imaging methods

1 Radiography

(1) Hysterosalpingography

It is used to display the uterus and fallopian tube cavity by injecting iodine contrast medium through the cervix. It can also evaluate the patency of fallopian tube.

(2) Pelvic arteriography

The uterine artery and ovarian artery angiography is rarely used in disease diagnosis, but in the interventional therapy of diseases.

2 Ultrasonography

Ultrasonography is a preferred and most commonly used method in the female genital system.

3 CT

The radiation dose of CT examination is high, so it is not suitable for preliminary investigation and conventional imaging for most women of childbearing age. However, postmenopausal women or women with pelvis larger mass may use CT examination.

(1) Plain CT

Plain CT is conventionally used when the bladder is filled with urine.

(2) Enhanced CT

Enhanced CT is often performed after finding lesion by plain CT, followed with the contract medium intravenous injection. It can be usually used to determine the origin of masses, differentiate diagnosis of benign or malignant masses, and show the lesion's character, position and the relationship with adjacent tissues.

Patients who are allergic with iodine agent can not do this detection.

4 MRI

Plain MRI is a conventional method to get T1-and T2-weighted images of axial, coronal and sagittal sections. T2-weighted examination is very important, which can help to determine the location and the origin of the masses.

Multiple phase enhanced MRI examination is often performed after finding lesions by plain scan, and the contract medium injected to intravenous is Gd-DTPA.

Section 2 Normal imaging findings of the female genital system

1 Ultrasonography

The internal echo of cervix is a little higher than that of the body. The uterine cavity is a thin line of strong echo and is surrounded by endometrium.

2 CT

(1) Plain CT

Uterine body is transversely oval or circular with clear border, and its density is similar to that of soft tissues before enhancement. The center area of the body is uterine cavity with lower density.

Cervix is well-defined, transversely spindle, below the uterine body, and its density is similar to that of soft tissues and the transverse diameter is usually less than 3cm. The bilateral ovaria of women of childbearing age are low density structures that are located at both sides of the uterus.

(2) Enhanced CT

After intravenous enhancement with the iodine contract medium, the myometrium becomes obviously homogeneously enhanced. (Fig 7-3-1-A/B/C/D)

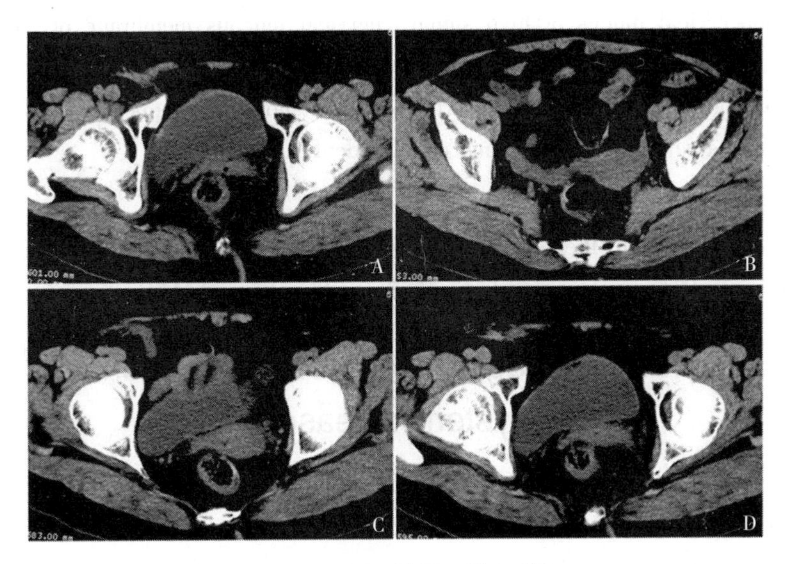

Fig 7-3-1-A/B/C/D Plain CT

Normal uterus of a young woman is transversely oval with clear border and its density is similar to that of soft tissues.

3 MRI

(1) Plain MRI

1) T1WI

The uterine body, cervix and vagina are clearly displayed on T1WI, charactered by homogeneous low signal.

2) T2WI

T2WI, especially sagittal scan can clearly display the anatomy of the cervix, vagina and the uterine body. From inside to outside, there are three layers of signals of the uterine body: the endometrial and uterine secretions lie at innermost, showing T2WI high signal; the inner layer of the myometrium, also called combined zone, is located in the middle, showing thinner low signal; the outside layer of the myometrium is located at the external side, showing intermediate signal. Cervical from inside to outside is divided into four layers, which are the endocervical mucus of high signal, cervical mucous membrane of medium signal, cervical fiber matrix of low signal, and tunica muscular cervical uteri of medium signal. Pre-menopausal normal ovarium shows low signal on TIWI, and follicles charactered by high signal can be identified on T2WI.

(2) Enhanced MRI

Combined with the low degree of enhancement, the endometrium and uterine muscle become obviously homogeneously enhanced.

Section 3 Imaging signs of female genital system diseases

1 Abnormal uterine

(1) Uterine size and shape abnormalities

It is easy for US and MRI to find uterine size, shape changes. Simple uterine size or shape abnormality is rare, mainly for various types of congenital anomalies, such as infantile uterus, bicornuate uterus, double uterus, and may be associated with cervical change. Uterine size and shape abnormalities are often associated with abnormal uterine masses.

(2) Uterine masses

Uterine masses show intrauterine focal abnormal echo, density or signal intensity lesions, and are often associated with uterine size, shape changes. Uterine masses are found in various benign and malignant tumors, among which the ones with clear boundary and containing calcium, or showing low signal on T2WI tend to be benign uterine leiomyomas, and the ones with unclear boundary or moderate signal on T2WI may indicate malignant uterine tumors.

2 Pelvic masses

Female pelvic masses often come from the ovary. Ultrasonic examination, CT or MRI examination of ovarian masses often has some characteristics, which not only can further confirm the masses from the ovary, and can infer its properties. For example, round or oval masses with thin and uniform wall, as well as watery density or signal are often ovarian cysts of various types. Mixed mass density or signal with fat low density or high signal is the performance feature of ovarian cystic teratoma.

Section 4 Diagnosis of diseases

1 Uterine leiomyoma

Uterine leiomyoma is composed of smooth muscles and fibrous stromas. It is the most common benign tumor of female genital system.

[**Pathology and clinical manifestations**]

Uterine leiomyomas are mainly formed by the proliferation of uterine smooth muscle cells, and often occur in 30 ~ 50 year-old women of childbearing age, with the incidence rate of 20% ~ 30%. Fibroids are often multiple and of unequal sizes. Uterine leiomyomas occur mainly in the uterine body, and can be divided into submucous leiomyomas, myometrial leiomyomas and subserous leiomyomas. Common symptoms include menorrhagia, long and short intervals of menstruation. Malignancy is rare, with the incidence below 1%.

[**Imaging appearances**]

(1) Ultrasonic examination

The uterus is normal or enlarged according to different sizes of uterine leiomyoma. Most uterine leiomyomas appear as hypoechogenic masses and are well defined. Cystic degeneration, hemorrhage, necrosis and calcification can be present in the lesion. Blood flow is present in CDFI.

(2) CT

① Uterine volume increases, and the performance may be lobulated;

② Un-enhanced fibroids' density is equal to or slightly lower than normal uterus;

③ On enhanced imaging, fibroids may have varying degrees of enhancement, and the intensity is lower than normal uterus;

④ About 10% of uterine leiomyomas' calcification mainly occur in the degenerated fibroids of postmenopausal women.

(3) MRI

① T1WI signal is similar to the signal of normal uterine muscle;

② On T2WI, uterine leiomyomas show a typical low signal with clear boundary, which apparently contrasts with the uterine muscle;

③ If the fibroid degenerates, there will be uneven signal within the tumor: cystic changes make T2WI show high signal; myxoid change by T1WI signal slightly increases.

④ On T2WI, fibroids can be sometimes surrounded by annular high signal, which represents the expansion of the lymphatic vessels, veins, or edema.

[**Diagnosis**]

As a conventional screening method, US can find most uterine tumors, but it can not accurately locate the position of the tumors. CT examination, in addition to detecting calcification, lacks representative characteristics to diagnose uterine leiomyoma.

MRI is now the most sensitive and specific imaging examination for the diagnosis of uterine leiomyoma, and it can detect tumors less than 3mm in diameter.

2 Endometrial carcinoma

[**Pathology and clinical manifestations**]

Endometrial carcinoma is a common gynecologic malignancy, and its incidence rate is only second to cervical carcinoma in China. Women in their fifties and sixties are most commonly affected. The vast majority are adenocarcinoma in pathology. Risk factors are related to increased estrogen states and include early menarche, late menopause, estrogen replacement therapy, obesity, ovulation failure, and nulliparity. Postmenopausal bleeding is the most common presenting symptom. Other symptoms include vague pelvic pain caused by increasing uterine size.

Clinically, according to the aggressive scope it is divided into four phases:

Phase Ⅰ: tumor confined to the uterus body

Phase Ⅱ: tumor invading to the cervix

Phase Ⅲ: tumor invading outside the uterus, but limited to the true pelvis tissues

Phase Ⅳ: tumor invading to the bladder, bowel or occurrent distant metastases

(1) Ultrasonography

In the early stage, the thickening endometrium has no typical signs; in the advanced stage, the endometrium is thickened obviously. The hyperechogenic area in irregular shape in muscular layer or the focal hyperechogenic mass can be seen. Blood flow is present in CDFI in most cases.

(2) CT

CT imaging of endometrial cancer often shows a mass with endometrial enhancement, and fluid within the endometrial canal. But small lesions can not be found by CT.

(3) MRI

① Lesions are confined to the uterine body. T1WI shows equal signal, and most lesions on T2WI show high signal. Combined belt with integrity is the most important sign for evaluating the degree of myometrial invasion.

② IA tumors are confined to the endometrium, and the endometrial will appear normal or widened.

③ For IB tumors, the combined belt will be interrupted or discontinuous; abnormal signals may invade abnormal muscle, but only 50% of the depth of the muscle.

④ As to phase Ⅱ tumors, the depth of myometrial invasion can be more than 50%, but the outer portion of normal myometrium remains complete. For phase Ⅲ or Ⅳ endometrial uterine cancer, in addition to displaying the surrounding organs such as the rectum, bladder involvement, the most important part is the evaluation of pelvic or para-aortic lymph node involvement.

⑤ For enhanced MR, the strengthening of endometrium is uneven and is obviously below the marked enhancement of the muscle.

[**Diagnosis**]:

Diagnosis of endometrial cancer mainly relies on curettage and cytology. The purpose of imaging is to determine the scope of the tumor, to observe the treatment effect and to determine whether the tumor recurs.

3 Cervical carcinoma

Cervical cancer is the most common cancer in female genital system in China. Human papilloma virus (HPV) is considered closely related to the occurrence of cervical cancer.

[**Pathology and clinical manifestations**]

Cervical cancers belong to malicious tumors which usually occur in the squamous epithelium and columnar epithelial cells at the junction of the cervix and vagina or cervix endometrial transitional zone. Women aged forty-five to fifty-five are often affected. And contacted vaginal bleeding is the main symptom of cervical cancer. Lymphatic metastasis is the conventional way of transference.

Cervical cancer stage:

Phase Ⅰ tumor is entirely confined to the cervix tumors.

Phase Ⅱ tumor extends beyond the cervix, but does not infiltrate to the pelvic wall and 1/3 of the vagina.

Phase Ⅲ tumor infiltrates to the pelvic wall and over 1/3 of the vagina.

Phase Ⅳ tumor extends beyond the true pelvis or infiltrates bladder and rectum.

(1) Ultrasonography

The cervix is thick and irregular. If liquid or purulence is present in the lesion it will show echo-free. Blood flow is present in CDFI in most cases.

(2) CT

①***Phase*** Ⅰ: When the tumor is small, CT can not detect it. Larger tumors may manifest as increased cervix, with its diameter often over 3.5cm.

②***Phase*** Ⅱ: The cervix is enlarged and its periphery is irregular or unclear, the density of parametral adipose tissue is increased, or even a mass can be observed.

③***Phase*** Ⅲ: Tumor infiltrates the pelvic wall, and enlarged lymph nodes can be found in the pelvis.

④***Phase*** Ⅳ: When the tumor infiltrates the bladder or rectum, the wall of the bladder or rectum is thickened, their surrounding fat spaces are disappeared, and even mass can be found. The retroperitoneal lymph node may be enlarged or other organ metastasis may happen.

(3) MRI

① ***Tumors show high signal on T2WI.***

② ***Phase I_A*:** there may be no signal or abnormal signal in cervix, and the low signal ring is complete.

③ ***Phase I_B*:** the cervix may be enlarged associated with abnormal signal, and the low signal ring is complete.

④ ***Phase* Ⅱ$_A$:** the lesions extend beyond the cervix and infiltrates to the upper 1/3 of the vagina, and vaginal fornix disappears.

⑤ ***Phase* Ⅱ$_B$:** the abnormal signal appears at tissues surrounding cervix, and normal cervical stroma disappears completely.

⑥ ***Phase* Ⅲ$_A$:** the performance of Ⅱ A tumor extends to the lower 1/3 of the vagina.

⑦ ***Phase* Ⅲ$_B$:** the performance of Ⅱ B tumor extends to the pelvic wall or leads to ureter obstruction.

⑧ ***Phase* Ⅳ$_A$:** the normal low signal of bladder or rectum wall disappears, especially in the sagittal T2WI.

⑨ ***When pelvic lymph node's diameter is more than1cm, it is considered abnormal.***

⑩ ***In dynamic enhanced MRI*,** tumors show obvious enhancement early and the signal is higher than that of the normal cervical tissue; then the signal decreases gradually, and later enhanced signal is lower than that of normal cervix. (Fig 7-3-2-A/B/C/D)

[**Diagnosis**]

Early diagnosis relies on clinical examination and cervical liquid-based cytology. Imaging is mainly used for staging of the cervical cancer, determining the infiltrated range, and deciding whether there is a clear parametrial invasion, pelvic wall or surrounding organ invasion and lymph node metastasis.

MRI is the preferred imaging in determining cervical cancer periodization.

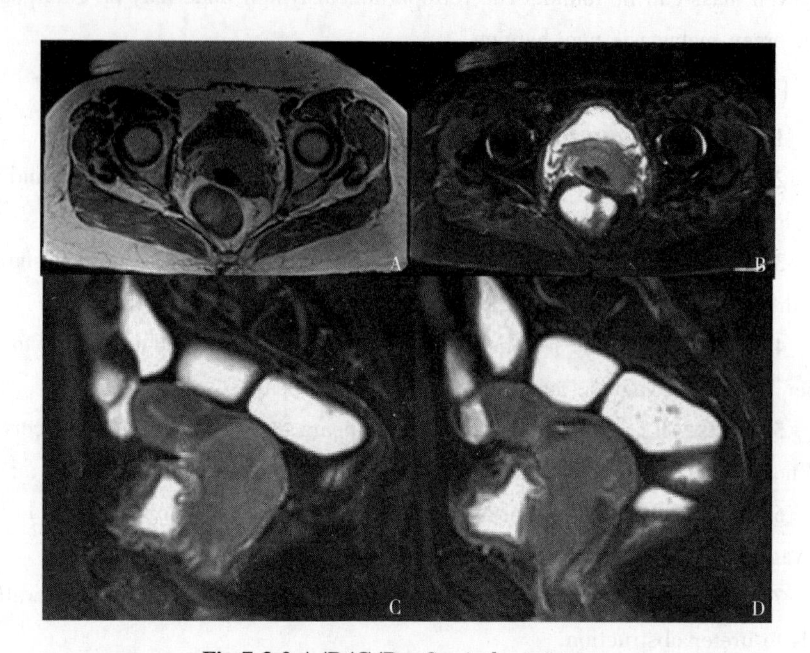

Fig 7-3-2-A/B/C/D Cervical carcinoma：

The cervix is enlarged; the signal of the lesion is lower on T1WI and higher on T2WI than normal cervical tissue. The lesion extends to lower 1/3 of the vagina.

4 Ovarian cysts

[Pathology and clinical manifestations]

Ovarian cysts include simple cysts and functional cysts; most cysts are unilateral, only few of them are bilateral.

The size of cysts is varying. The wall of unilocular cyst is thin and without separation. However, the polycystic ovaries are bilateral-polycystic. Clinically, ovarian cyst is often asymptomatic; functional cysts may lead to abnormal menstruation. The clinical performance of polycystic ovaries is hairiness and infertility.

(1) Ultrasonography

Well-defined border, thin and smooth wall, and echo-free are present in

US. It is usually unilateral in follicular cyst, corpus luteum cyst, and bilateral in flavin cyst. The internal echoes may not be pure because of the hemorrhage.

(2) CT

① The typical manifestations of ovarian cyst are the homogeneous water density mass in uterine adnexa or uterine rectum lacunae, round or oval, which has a thin wall, smooth and clear with even density.

② Polycystic ovary shows bilateral ovarian enlargement with multiple cystic low density lesions in it.

(3) MRI

① Lesions show homogeneous long T1 and long T2 signals, with clear boundary and thin wal; meanwhile,, the diameters of most lesions are less than 5cm.

② When cyst is accompanied by hemorrhage, T1WI shows high central signal and low edge signal, while T2WI shows high signal.

③ Polycystic ovary shows obvious increase of bilateral ovarium. Within the ovary there are many circular long T1 and long T2 signals follicular with thick wall; on T2WI, fibrous tissue has low signal.

[**Diagnosis**]

Using CT and MR, it is easy to find ovarian cyst based on the features mentioned above. However, it is difficult to determine the type of the cyst.

5 Ovarian carcinoma

[**Clinical and pathological**]

Ovarian carcinoma is the most common malignant tumor of ovary, and is mainly divided into serous cyst adenocarcinoma and mucinous cyst adenocarcinoma, with the former being the most common type. Clinically, ovarian cancer often has no symptoms at the early stage, and it is already at advanced stage when found. The clinical manifestations are rapid growth abdominal mass, bloody ascites, emaciation, anemia, and fatigue performance, etc.

(1) Ultrasonic examination

Irregular mass is present, and blood flow is present in CDFI in most cases.

(2) CT

The direct signs:

① Large pelvic mass, lobulated, and unequal size.

② Lesions are composed of cystic and solid components; the cystic part has intervals and the cystic wall is uneven; the solid component shows soft tissue density.

③ Enhanced examination reveals that the tumor has intervals; the cystic wall and solid part are significantly enhanced.

Tumor spreads in the pelvis:

① Uterus, bladder and bowel are violated; their boundary is not clear; the fat gap around them disappears or becomes vague.

② The wall of bladder or bowel thickens;

③ Ureteral involvement causes upper ureter and renal pelvis dilatate.

④ ***More ascites with higher CT value.***

⑤ The tumor can transfer to multiple organs and tissues, such as implantation metastasis, greater omentum metastasis, liver metastasis, and peritoneal metastasis of lymph nodes.

(3) MRI

① Tumor margin is irregular with no clear boundary.

② T1WI presents equal or low signal, while T2WI has slightly high signal.

③ Enhanced scan shows obvious enhancement.

④ Pelvic and omental fat infiltrates, with even signal on T1WI and T2WI.

⑤ Peripheral organ metastasis, with high signal on T2WI.

⑥ Abdominal lymph node metastasis; lymph nodes show even signal on T1 and T2.

⑦ Ascites shows long T1 and long T2 signal.

⑧ MRS shows the tumor is significantly high in Cho peak (Fig 7-3-3-A/B/C/D).

[**Diagnosis**]

Based on the CT or MRI examination, diagnosis can be made directly; also, the extent of tumor invasion, or peritoneal metastasis and lymph node metastasis can be displayed.

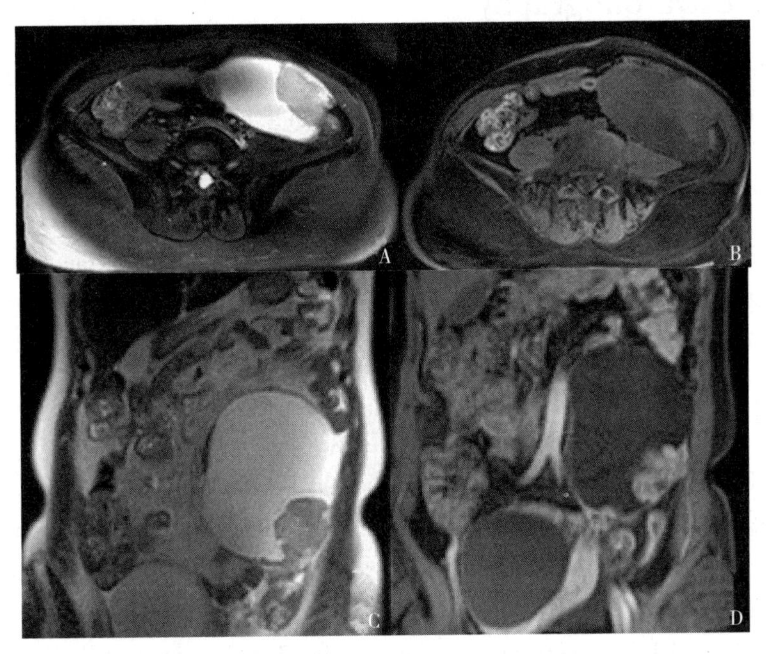

Fig 7-3-3-A/B/C/D MR: Ovarian serous cyst adenocarcinoma Large pelvic mass is composed of cystic and solid components; enhanced scan shows the solid part is significantly enhanced.

Lesson 4 Male Genital System

Section 1 Imaging methods

1 Radiography

Examination: due to the lack of natural contrast, radiography of the male genital system provides limited information, and is now rarely used.

2 Ultrasonography

It is usually used as a preliminary investigation method to detect the disease of male genital system, and especially it can guide biopsy.

3 CT

Examination: CT is not commonly used in the examination of the male genital system. If used, the examination should be carried out in fasting and bladder filling condition.

4 MRI

MRI is the most valuable imaging method for the detection of male genital system diseases. MRI can show the anatomical structure of each zone of prostate clearly, and is helpful in detecting the prostate diseases and determining the scope and staging clearly.

MRS and DWI functional imaging has significantly improved the sensitivity and specificity for the diagnosis of prostate cancer.

(1) Plain MRI

Routine axial T1WI and axial sagittal coronal T2WI sequences are conventionally used, and if necessary, fat suppression T2WI sequence is added.

(2) Enhanced MRI

After intravenous injection of contrast agent Gd-DTPA, usually dynamic enhanced MRI is used for dynamic analysis of the lesions' enhancement characteristics.

(3) MRS

Analysis of prostate lesions in citrate (Cit), choline (Cho) and creatine (Cr) concentration of metabolites are made to reflect the metabolic characteristics of the lesion.

(4) Functional magnetic resonance imaging

Currently functional magnetic resonance imaging (fMRI) clinically used in diagnosis of prostate disease includes diffusion weighted imaging (DWI) and perfusion weighted imaging (PWI).

Section 2 Normal imaging findings of male genital system

1 Ultrasonography

The prostate appears as oval shape in longitudinal section and chestnut shape in transverse section. Its internal echo is homogeneous and medium-level echogenicity with clear and smooth capsule.

2 CT

Normal prostate shows soft tissue density, and its size increases with age. Dynamic enhancement: in arterial phase, the density of center land increases, and then in advanced phase the densities of central gland and peripheral zone become consistent. (Fig 7-4-1-A/B)

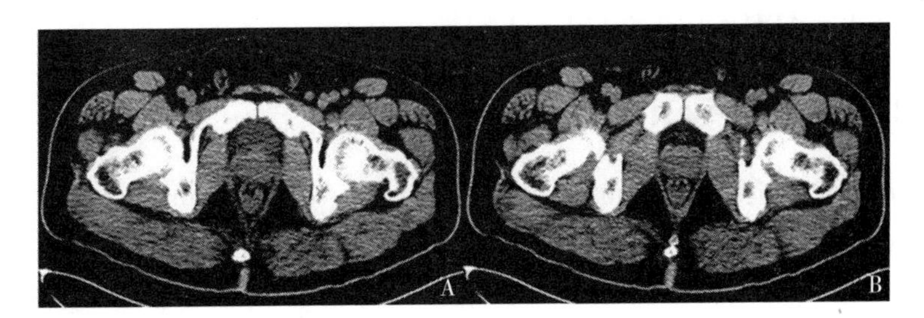

Fig 7-4-1-A/B Normal prostate of a young male has chestnut shape and soft density.

3 MRI

Normal prostate shows homogeneously low signal on T1WI, so it cannot identify each zone of prostate. Low T1WI signal venous plexus is located at the adipose tissues around prostate

T2WI can better show each zone of prostate: Central glade shows low signal, representing the transitional zone and the central zone; peripheral area shows crescent shaped high signal, representing the surrounding belt; it is coated with a thin ring of low signal.

Section 3 Imaging signs of male genital system diseases

1 Enlargement of the prostate gland

The symmetrical prostate enlargement often occurs in benign prostatic hyperplasia and inflammation, and it can also be found in prostate cancer occasionally. The internal density or signal of prostate is often not uniform. If the prostate has a higher Cit peak, lower Cho peak on ^{1}H-MRS, and higher ADC value, it tends to be benign. Asymmetry prostatic enlargement is common in prostate cancer, and shows localized nodular bulge or lobulated change. If rich in blood supply, it is prompt to prostate cancer; if the Cit and Cho peaks on ^{1}H-MRS are inverted and with low ADC value, it also indicates prostate cancer.

2 Seminal vesicle mass

Seminal vesicle cyst, abscess and primary or secondary tumor all appear as seminal vesicle masses. Malignant tumor often has complex echo, density, and signal and has rich blood supply. Malignant tumor can also invade its adjacent structures. Cyst has clear boundary, homogeneous internal echo, density and signal. However, hematoma and abscess seminal vesicle have relative characteristics of echo, density and signal.

3 Testicular mass

Testicular mass appears as testicular increase, and it is common in testicular tumors. Different types of tumors have different echoes and signals.

Section 4 Diagnosis of diseases

1 Benign prostatic hyperplasia

Benign prostatic hyperplasia is a common disease in men aged 60 years and above, with an incidence rate of up to 75%.

[**Clinical and pathological**]

Prostate hyperplasia occurs mainly in the transitional zone, shown as its glands and stroma with different degrees of hyperplasia. When the hyperplasia presses against the urethra and bladder hyperplasia adjacent to it, there may be different degrees of bladder obstruction. The clinical expression is unusual micturition.

(1) Ultrasonography

The prostate is enlarged and the shape changes into roundness. Nevertheless, the prostate still has well-defined border. The proportion between inner gland and outer gland is abnormal (the normal proportion is 1 : 1). Hyperplastic nodules and sometimes stone are present.

(2) CT

① Prostate volume increases but the edge is smooth and clear.

② Transitional zone and central zone increase, and peripheral zone becomes narrowed.

③ Enhanced CT scan shows obviously uneven enhancement, and delayed enhancement is uniform.

(3) MRI

① ***T1WI***: enlarged prostate shows homogeneous low T1WI signal.

② ***T2WI***: enlarged prostate glands mainly show high T2WI signal, and often can be seen with false capsule, while the interstitial hyperplasia mainly shows low T2WI signal.

[**Diagnosis**]

CT and MRI can detect the prostate enlargement uniformly and symmetrically. MRI has higher diagnostic value than CT.

The main basis of the diagnosis of benign prostatic hyperplasia is T2WI: the peripheral zone of increased prostate is squeezed but its signal is normal.

2 Prostate carcinoma

Prostate carcinoma has a high incidence in Europe and America, and occurs more often in the elderly men. It is the second male malignant tumor in the USA.

[**Clinical and pathological**]

Prostate carcinomas occur mainly in peripheral zone of the prostate (70%), and more than 95% are adenocarcinomas. The clinical manifestations are oliguria, anuria, and even incontinence. Bone metastasis is common and the majority of which are osteoblastic metastasis.

(1) Ultrasonography

Most prostate carcinomas occur in the outer gland. The prostate is often enlarged, the shape becomes asymmetrical and the capsule becomes discontinuous. The hypoechogenic area is present within the homogeneous gland. Blood flow is present on CDFI in the hypoechogenic area.

(2) CT

① Most prostate carcinomas increase irregularly, especially in the peripheral zone.

② Prostate tumors show equal density, but sometimes calcification can be found in them.

③Enhanced CT scanning can detect the limitations or multiple abnormal enhancement focusing on peripheral zone with low density.

④ Advanced prostate carcinoma has obvious space occupying effect and metastasis features.

(3) MRI

① ***T2WI***: The normal prostate peripheral zone shows high T2WI signal. When prostate lesions appear, single or multiple patchy with low signal or mixed signal can be found in the high signal.

② ***Enhanced MRI***: The lesions are early enhanced, then in delayed phase the enhancement degree of lesions decreases and the lesions show low signal.

③ ***MRS***: Prostate nodules' choline and inositol levels increase; citric acid levels decrease significantly.

④ ***Low ADC, high signal on DWI.*** (Fig 7-4-2-A/B/C/D)

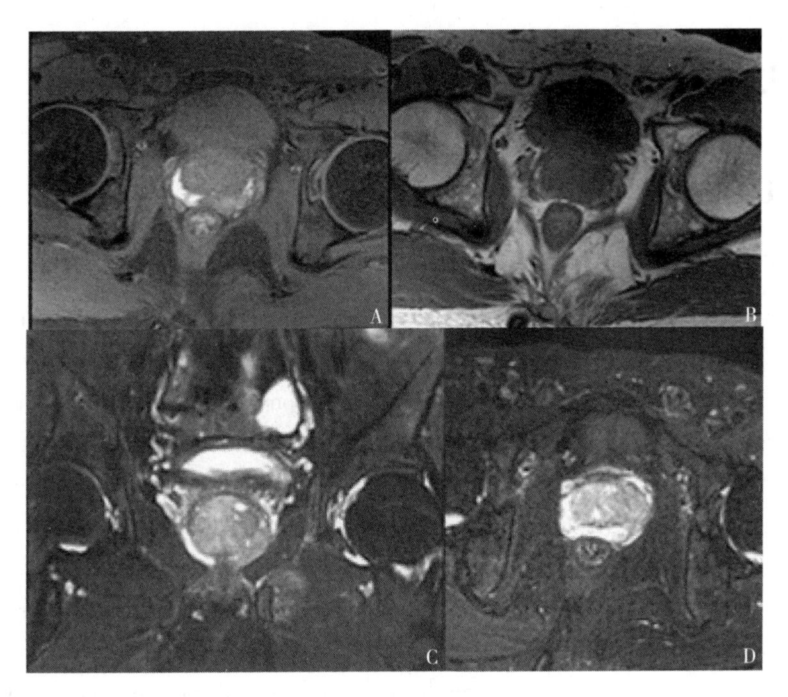

Fig 7-4-2-A/B/C/D

MRI of prostate carcinoma: the prostate is enlarged and the peripheral zone of the right prostate shows normal high TWI2 signal, but the signal of the left prostate is declined.

[**Diagnosis**]

Early prostate carcinoma is confined to the prostate membrane. MRI should be used as the preferred imaging method. The main basis for the diagnosis is that among high T2WI signal there are one or multiple low signal nodules in the peripheral zone of prostate.

Chapter 8

Imaging of the Mammary Glands

Lesson 1 Imaging Methods

1 Radiography

(1) Mammography

As US, it is the most common approach to detecting and screening the breast diseases. Conventional mammography is called screen-film or analog mammography (SFM): Radiography photons are converted to light by phosphor screens, and exposed films are chemically processed to create visible images. In recent years, full field digital mammography (FFDM) is widely used in clinical setting, which uses a flat panel detector to convert X-ray photons to digital signals and create an image. The superiority of the FFDM is: a) improving image contrast, tissue equalization and penetration, especially in dense breasts; b) more consistent than SFM; c) lower image noise; d) comparable or lower dose; e) enabling electronic image display, storage and transmission, telemammography.

Mammography is best performed in midcycle of the menses (week 2; between days 7 and 14). Imaging protocols include: bilateral (or unilateral) craniocaudal view (CC), bilateral (or unilateral) mediolateral oblique view (MLO), mediolateral view (ML), lateromedial view (LM), inframammary fold (IMF) and focal or full breast exaggerated craniocaudal view (XCC). CC view and MLO view are the routine imaging protocols.

(2) Galactography

Galactography is an optimal application for pathologic nipple discharge with the contrast injected into the ducts from the discharged duct orifices. This method can display the dilatation/filling-defect or cut off of the ducts.

2 Ultrasonography

Breast ultrasound can clearly show each zone from superficial zone to deep zone. The initial role of diagnostic breast sonography was to distinguish between cysts and solid nodules, and observe real-time dynamic active lesions. A good general rule for breast ultrasound is that lesions that appear to be just under the skin on the mammogram or that are palpable and pea-sized or smaller are most prone to volume averaging and should routinely be imaged through an acoustic standoff. Specific goals of targeted diagnostic sonography are to prevent biopsies and short interval follow-up mammography of benign lesions, to guide interventions of all types, to give feedback that improves clinical and mammographic skills, and to find malignancies that are missed by mammography. The breast neoplasm biopsy pathology distinguishes benign and malignant tumors through puncture guided by high frequency ultrasound. Ultrasonography plays a very significant role in pregnant and lactating women. Ultrasound evaluates the lesions after breast prosthesis implantation. Transducers with frequency of more than 10MHz can find calcifications, which are suspicious mammographic findings that have been applied directly to sonography. The disadvantages of sonography are: the accuracy of ultrasonic diagnosis depends largely on the equipment used and the doctor's personal experience; also, it is difficult to detect the small lesions and decide if they are benign or malignant.

(1) 2D

Sonography and mammography have the same indication, and complementary advantage.

(2) D-mode and CDFI

D-mode and CDFI characteristics of breast masses are important factors of diagnosis, and are valuable in the differentiation of benign and malignant breast tumors,

(3) Ultrasonic elastography

It can objectively evaluate the relative elastic hardness of breast tumors, and identify whether the breast lumps are benign or malignant with high diagnostic value.

(4) Ultrasound-guided core needle biopsy in diagnosis of breast lesions

Ultrasound-guided core needle biopsy, as a preoperative diagnosis modality for breast lesions, is safe, effective, and accurate. Any unsatisfactory, suspicious, or atypical change on ultrasound-guided core needle biopsy should be followed by an open biopsy.

3 MRI

Magnetic resonance imaging (MRI) of the breast is widely used as an adjunct diagnostic procedure to mammography and ultrasound. Because of its high sensitivity and effectiveness in detecting dense breast tissue, there are a number of clinical indications for the application of breast MRI: a) evaluation of women with questionable mammographic or ultrasonic findings; b) evaluation of patients with axillary carcinoma and negative mammographic and clinical findings; c) pre-operative staging of the known cancer diagnosed by percutaneous needle biopsy; d) distinguishing postsurgical or post-radiational scar from recurrent carcinoma; e) screening in high-risk populations; f) assessing tumor response to neoadjuvant chemotherapy; and g) evaluating silicone breast implant integrity.

The major limitation of breast MRI is the low-to-moderate specificity and insensitivity to microcalcifications.

Occasionally, the normal hormonally-sensitive breast parenchyma may be enhanced intensely and in a mass-like distribution. For this reason, breast MRI examination is best performed in midcycle of the menses (week 2; between days 7 and 14) with patients lying in the prone position, with both breasts hanging freely in the bilateral openings of the breast coil support. MRI is by nature a very multiparametric technique involving trade-offs between image characteristics such as contrast, signal-to-noise ratio, resolution, field of view, and scan time. Other parameters can also be varied, including orientation (transaxial, sagittal, or coronal), format (unilateral or bilateral), and use of fat suppression (FS). Commonly the contrast is gadolinium-DTPA. Typical imaging protocols include:

transaxial and (or) sagittal non-fat suppression TlWI; transaxial and (or) sagittal T2WI FS (or STIR); 3D SPGR FS pre-and post-contrast T1WI; special imaging protocols include: DWI (diffusion weighted imaging) and MRS (spectrum), which in some distance can differentiate benign lesions from malignant ones.

4 CT

CT is not used to detect breast diseases, but it is useful in pre-operative stages and post-therapeutic assessment of the breast cancer.

Lesson 2 Normal Imaging of Breast

Section 1 Anatomy

Breast projects at midclavicular line of the front chest wall, extending from 2nd intercostal space to 5th intercostal space and overlying pectoralis major muscle with round or hemispherical shape (adult). Nipple everts from the center of the non-pendulous breast, and there are 8 ~ 12 duct orifices at bases of crevices on nipple surface. Areola is circular and pigmented, measuring 3~4 cm in diameter around the nipple. Breast is comprised of ducts, lobes, lobules, acini and stromata (fat, fiber tissue, nerves, blood vessels and lymphatics). There are 15~20 lobes in each breast. Each lobe is composed of many lobules, and each lobule is composed of many intralobular terminal ducts and acini. Most lobes drain to corresponding ducts. Ductal system is composed of duct orifices, lactiferous sinus, major ducts and terminal ducts (extralobular terminal ducts and intralobular terminal ducts). Lactiferous sinus is the widened duct segment just deep to nipple orifice, 4~5mm in diameter. Major duct drains 20~40 lobules, usually 1mm in diameter. Premammary (subcutaneous) zone contains subcutaneous fat, blood vessels, anterior suspensory (Cooper) ligaments. Retromammary zone contains fat and posterior suspensory ligaments which attach postmammary fat to chest wall.

Section 2 Mammography

1 Nipple

Nipple lies in the center of the areola, usually everted, and should be seen in profile on at least one of two standard mammographic views. Nipple is high in density, symmetric in size bilaterally, but different in size individually.

2 Areola

Areola is discoid around the nipple, thicker than other regions of breast skin, usually 1 ~ 5mm thick.

3 Skin

Normal skin appears linear, smooth and measures usually 0.5 ~ 3.0 mm thick, except caudally where it may be slightly thicker due to its usual dependency.

4 Subcutaneous fat

Subcutaneous fat is low dense region beneath the skin, 5 ~ 25mm thick. There are fibrous intervals, vessels, suspensory ligaments, or Cooper ligaments.

5 Fibroglandular tissue

Fibroglandular tissue is the dense region on mammogram. The quantity of the fibroglandular tissue in breast is changing with age. For young women, the breast is rich of fibroglandular tissues and less of fat tissues, so parenchyma is dense on mammogram; For middle-aged women, fibroglandular tissues are atrophying and fat tissues increase, so the density decreases. For old women, the whole breast is composed of almost entirely fat and ducts, residual fiberous tissues, and vessels, so the density is very low on mammogram. According to breast imaging reporting and data system (BI-RADS), breast parenchyma is classified as four types: a) Almost entirely fat: Mostly fatty replaced, mammographic sensitivity 97%~98%; b) Scattered fibroglandular densities, which can be further described as minimal or moderate; c) Heterogeneously dense: 51%~75% glandular, mammographic sensitivity reduced: 64%~70%; d) Extremely dense: > 75% glandular, mammographic sensitivity reduced: 30% ~ 48%. (Fig 8-2-1-A/B)

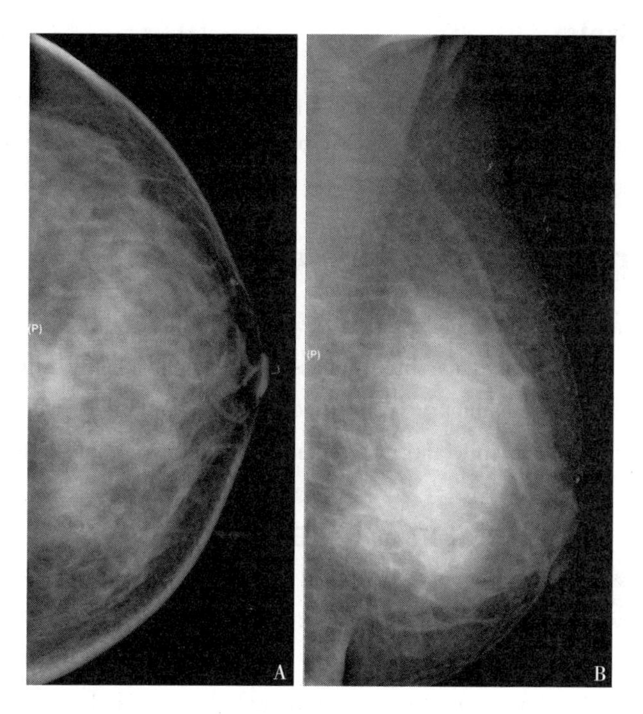

Fig 8-2-1-A/B

A: normal breast on mammogram in craniocaudal view

B: normal breast on mammogram in mediolateral oblique view

6 Duct

On mammogram, it is difficult to distinguish linear isodense ducts from fibrous tissues, so they are together called breast trabeculae. Galactography can demonstrate ducts and their branches. Occasionally, the major duct is shown as linear isodensity beneath nipple and is in radial distribution in parenchyma.

7 Post mammary fat

Post mammary fat is low density region between mammary gland and pectoralis major muscle, 0.5~2mm thick.

8 Vessels

Vessels are linear isodense to breast parenchyma. Vessels located in subcutaneous fat or in the fatty type of breast parenchyma are easily seen, especially calcified ones.

9 Intramammary lymph node

Intramammary lymph node is mall, oval, reniform or lobulated smoothly-marginated, intraparenchymal breast mass with eccentric fatty hilum or notch, typically<1 cm. Intramammary lymph node may be anywhere within the breast and may be multiple, while the most common location is upper outer quadrant.

Section 3 Ultrasonography

The breast is a modified sweat gland that is composed of 15 to 20 lobes that are not well delineated from each other, overlap, and vary greatly in size and distribution. Each has many separate terminal ductal lobular units (TDLUs) which contain the terminal ducts. The TDLUs are surrounded by loose and dense connective tissues. The Cooper's ligaments surround and suspend each of the TDLUs within surrounding fatty tissues.

1 Normal Breast (Fig 8-2-2)

(1) Nipple

It is located in the center of surface in front of breast. Its size and character of the echo depend on age, developmental stage and the production. Usually hypoechogenic type circular nodules with clear boundary can be seen.

(2) Skin

It is hyperechogenic smooth band, 0.5 ~ 3mm in thickness, with smooth and well-defined edge.

(3) Subcutaneous fat and the suspensory ligament

The echo of subcutaneous fat is hypoechoic. Inside there scatter funicular hyperechoic bands or triangles, which are called suspensory ligaments.

(4) Fibroglandular tissue and duct

Fibroglandular tissue presents moderate echoes with scattered hypoechoic fat in it. Duct is anechoic fluid area.

(5) Post mammary fat

It is hypoechoic and lies between fiber layer glands and chest muscle, parallel to the chest wall.

(6) Vessels

In two-dimensional ultrasonographic images, the vessels of glands are in the tubular anechoic area, and veins are superficial compared with arteries. Doppler spectrum and CDFI can show blood flow signals, and can measure values.

(7) Intramammary lymph nodes

Normal intramammary lymph nodes in two-dimensional ultrasonographic images are circular or ovoid. The shapes are regular. The boundaries are clear, and the surfaces are smooth. The hillus is echogenic.

2 Foreign language books on US of normal breast

In foreign language ultrasonic books, the breast can be divided into three zones from superficial to deep—the premammary zone, the mammary zone, and the retromammary zone.

(1) The premammary zone

The most superficial zone is the premammary or subcutaneous zone that lies between the skin and the anterior mammary fascia. The premammary zone is really part of the integument, and processes that arise primarily within the pre-

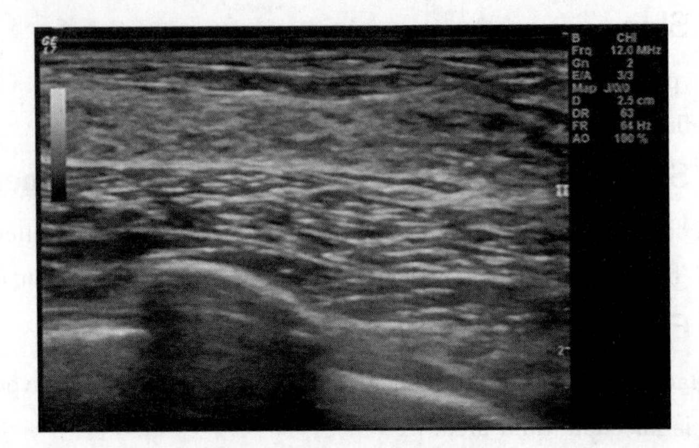

Fig 8-2-2 Normal breast

mammary zone are usually not true breast lesions. Rather, they are lesions of the skin and/or subcutaneous tissues that are identical to those that arise from skin and subcutaneous tissues that cover any other part of the body. Subcutaneous zone is hypoechogenic.

(2) The mammary zone

It is the middle zone and lies between the anterior mammary fascia and the posterior mammary fascia. It contains the lobar ducts, their branches, most of TDLUs, and most of the fibrous stromal elements of the breast. This zone varies greatly in thickness and echoes, depending on the patient age, and hormonal status. For instance, in pubertal women, the mammary layer is thick and the internal echoes are hypoechogenic. In pregnant and lactating women, the mammary layer is thick and ductal dilation can be seen. In women after lactation, the internal echoes of mammary layer are homogeneous hypoechogenic and hyperechogenic mixtures. In postmenopausal women, the mammary layer is thin and the internal echoes are hyperechogenic.

(3) The retromammary zone

The deepest zone is the retromammary zone. It contains mainly fat, blood vessels, and lymphatics and is usually much less apparent on sonograms than on mammograms because sonographic compression compresses it against the chest wall. This differs greatly from mammography, where mammographic compression pulls the retromammary fat away from the chest wall and expands it in the antero-posterior direction.

Conclusion: the mammary zone is where most of ducts and lobules of the breast that give rise to breast pathology lie. The retromammary zone is compressed during real-time sonography in the recumbent position and is relatively small and unapparent in comparison to its appearance on mammography. The mammary zone is enveloped in thick, tough fascia. Anteriorly it is delineated from the subcutaneous fat by the premammary or anterior mammary fascia and posteriorly from the retromammary fat by the posterior or retromammary fascia. The anterior mammary fascia is continuous with Cooper's ligaments, with each ligament being formed by two apposed layers of anterior mammary fascia.

3 BIRADS Nomenclature and Lexicon

An official breast imaging reporting and data system (BIRADS) ultrasound lexicon has been developed by the American College of Radiology (ACR) in an attempt to standardize the reporting and data. In general, BIRADS categories are 1, 2, 3, 4a, 4b, and 5.

The sonographic BIRADS 1 category corresponds to sonographically normal tissues that cause mammographic or clinical abnormalities. The sonographic BI-RADS 2 category corresponds to benign entities and includes intramammary lymph nodes, ecstatic ducts, simple cysts, and definitively benign solid nodules, such as lipomas. sonographic BIRADS 3 category corresponds to probably benign lesions that have a 2% or less chance of being malignant and includes some complex cysts, small intraductal papillomas, and a subset of fibroadenomas. We simply divide the BIRADS 4 category that is termed suspicious into two subcategories because it is so large, extending from>2% risk to<90% risk of malignancy. We simply divide the BIRADS 4 category at 50% or greater risk into 4a and 4b subcategories. We term the BIRADS 4a category mildly suspicious. It carries a risk between 3% and 49%. We term the BIRADS

4b category moderately suspicious. It carries a risk of 50% to 89%. These categories include lesions that do not meet strict criteria for BIRADS 3 or lower characterization. The BIRADS 5 category is termed malignant and indicates a risk of malignancy of 90% or greater. The management rules for each category have already been developed for mammography and are quite simple. BIRADS 1 and 2 characterizations enable the patient to return to routine screening follow-up. BI-RADS 3 characterization presents the patient with three choices—surgical biopsy, image-guided needle biopsy, or short interval sonographic follow-up. BIRADS 4a, 4b and 5 lesions require biopsy.

Section 4 MRI

1 Fat

On non-fat-suppressed T1-weighted and T2-weighted precontrast images, fat is high in signal intensity and low signal after fat suppression. Fat does not enhance.

2 Fibroglandular tissue

Fibroglandular tissue is low or intermediate in signal intensity in T1-weighted images, similar to the muscles, and intermediate in signal intensity in non-fat-suppressed T2-weighted images, higher than muscles while lower than liquid and fat. In fat-suppressed T2-weighted images, fibroglandular tissue is intermediate or slightly higher in signal intensity. In fat-suppressed T1-weighted images, normal breast parenchyma mildly, persistently enhances after contrast administration. During menstruation or before menstruation, breast parenchyma moderately or obviously enhances. Breast density, which is a representation in mammography of the amount of breast parenchyma present in the breast, can be assessed on MRI in both T2-and T1-weighted images. Breasts are characterized using BI-RADS (Breast Imaging Reporting and Data System) criteria: a) almost entirely fatty; b) scattered fibroglandular densities; c) heterogeneously dense; and d) extremely dense as with mammography.

3 Skin and Nipple

Normal skin appears smooth and measures usually 0.5~2.0 mm thick, except caudally where it may be slightly thicker due to its usual dependency. The skin routinely enhances. Skin scars demonstrate focal skin thickening that does not enhance if mature. The nipple-areolar complex enhances intensely on MRI following contrast administration due to the presence of numerous vessels. Differentiation of normal from abnormal patterns is facilitated by use of the opposite breast for comparison. (Fig 8-2-3-A/B/C)

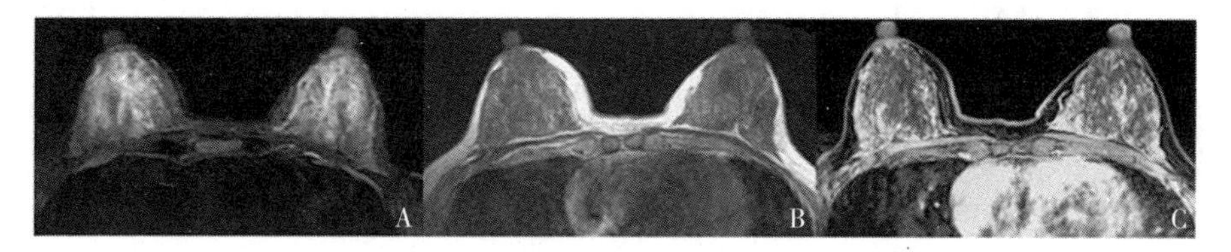

Fig 8-2-3-A/B/C

A: normal breast on fat-suppressed T2WI; B: normal breast on non-fat-suppressed T1WI; C: normal breast on fat-suppressed T1WI

Section 5 CT

The normal breast manifestation on CT is similar to that on mammogram. The superiority of CT is the evaluation of CT values (Housfield Unit) and obtainment of enhanced images. Normal breast parenchyma is mildly enhanced, with an increase of 10~20 Hu.

Lesson 3 Imaging Signs of Breast

Section 1 Mammography

1 Mass

Masses can be seen in both benign and malignant diseases. Mass shape, margin, and density should be described.

(1) Mass shape

Mass shape can be described as round, oval, lobular, and irregular; in this order, the possibility of malignant increases.

(2) Mass margin

Mass margin can be described as circumscribed, obscured, microlobulated, indistinct, and spiculated. Most of masses with circumscribed, smooth margins are benign, while masses with microlobulated, indistinct, or spiculated margins are suggestive of malignant lesions. For the obscured margins, spot compression views should be added to identify whether the margin is hidden by overlying tissue or not.

(3) Mass density

Compared to equal volume of fibroglandular tissue, the mass density can be described as high, equal, low, and fat-containing. Generally, benign lesions are in low or equal density, while malignant lesions are more in high density though a small part of cancers are in low or equal density. Fat-containing masses are likely benign, such as lipoma, fibroadenolipoma, galactocele, etc.

2 Calcification

Calcification can be seen in both benign and malignant diseases. Calcification morphology and distribution should be described. Generally, coarse, punctate, "popcorn" like, "egg-shell" like, rod-like, round, and circular calcifications with high density, following a scattered distribution, are likely benign. Fine sand-like, fine linear or branching calcifications, variable in sizes and density, following a clustered, linear, segmental distribution, are likely malignant. Calcification morphology and distribution are important in differentiating benign lesions from malignant ones. Calcifications can be a primary finding or associated with a mass. For most of clinically insidious breast cancers, calcifications on mammogram may be the only signs to diagnosis.

3 Architectural distortion

Architectural distortion is defined as alteration of the normal breast architecture with thin spiculations radiating from a point without a definite mass or focal retraction or distortion at the parenchymal margin. Architectural distortion can be seen in breast cancers and some benign diseases such as chronic inflammation, fat necrosis, radial scar, and post-surgical scar. It is manifested as straightening, angulation of the fibroglandular tissue on mammogram. This sign should be seen at least in two position views to exclude the possibility of overlapping of normal tissues.

4 Focal asymmetrical density

New focal asymmetry, especially with density increasing by follow-up, is highly suggestive of invasive carcinoma.

5 Skin thickening and dimpling

Skin thickening and dimpling are more likely seen in breast carcinomas. With progressive enlargement, carcinomas can become adherent to the deep fascia of the chest wall and so become fixed in position. Extension to the skin or fibrosis associated with the tumor can also cause dimpling sign. Peaud' orange or skin thickening with an orange skin pattern occurs secondary to a local blockage of lymphatic drainage. Dimpling sign can also be seen in benign diseases, such as post-surgical scar.

6 Nipple retraction (inversion)

Nipple retraction (inversion) can be caused by both infiltration of the malignant lesions under the nipple and congenital displasia of the nipple. The detection of nipple inversion can be impossible if breast positioning does not place the nipple in profile, so the positioning is very important. New developing nipple inversion requires diligent search for subareolar pathology, especially if nipple inversion is unilateral.

7 Lymphadenopathy

Pathologic enlargement of lymph nodes are usually round or irregular in shape with indistinct margins, high in density, and absent of central fat. Lymphadenopathy may be caused by metastasis of carcinomas or inflammatory response.

8 Increased vascularity

Increased vascularity is manifested as increased, thickened, or tortuous vessels in breast. This sign is usually seen in malignant tumors.

9 Ductal change

Galactography is useful to demonstrate abnormal ductal changes, such as ductal ectasia, filling defect, shut-off, shift, destruction, or arrangement disorder.

Section 2 Ultrasonography

1 Lesion

All lesions should be scanned in their entirety in two orthogonal planes to assess the surface and internal characteristics and shape. Hard copy images should be obtained in a minimum of two orthogonal planes. These can be longitudinal and transverse, but radial and antiradial planes are preferred. It is important to document the maximum diameter of the lesion, an important prognostic indicator. Breast sonographic evaluation depends heavily on special dynamic maneuvers performed during the examination.

The goals of sonographic evaluation of lesion correspond to size, shape, edge, echogenicity, margin features, orientation, attenuation (e. g. shadowing or enhancement), longitudinal-transverse ratio, and CDFI.

(1) Benign lesion

Benign lesions are usually round or oval in shape, with circumscribed and smooth margins. The transverse diameters of benign lesions are often greater than the vertical diameters. The internal echoes are uniformly hypoechoic and there are no or low flow signals within lesions on CDFI. Simple cysts are anechoic fluid areas.

(2) Malignant lesion

Most of the malignant lesions are shown irregular in shape, with no or incomplete capsule. The vertical diameter is greater than the transverse diameter, and internal echoes are usually hypoechogenic and heterogeneous.

2 Calcification

Calcifications are suspicious mammographic findings that have been applied directly to sonography. Most benign calcifications lie within a fairly echogenic background, so when volume is averaged with the surrounding tissues, they are no longer bright enough to be identified sonographically. Malignant calcifications lie within rather homogeneous hypoechoic tumor substance and remain visible even though they are subject to volume averaging with surrounding tissues. Sonography can generally demonstrate a higher percentage of malignant calcifications than benign ones.

3 Architectural disorder

The breast is thickened, and internal echo is either grid-like or hypoechogenic. It can be seen in benign or malignant lesions.

4 Duct change

Duct ectasia: echogenic duct walls are separated by secretions within the duct lumen and the isoechoic periductal loose stromal tissue becomes thinner, either by compression or because of atrophy. Intraductal lesions may be benign or malignant.

5 Lymph nodes enlargement

The location, size, internal echo, lymph hilum, corticomedullary structure and flow pattern of lymph nodes are explored. The round or fused shape, internal hypoechcocity, hilar disappearance, vague corticomedullary structure and abundant flow are mainly observed in metastatic lymph nodes.

Section 3 MRI

Generally, the imaging analysis of breast MRI should include morphology, signal intensity and internal architecture of the lesions, especially the dynamic enhancement characteristics, such as early phase enhancement rate and type of time-signal intensity curve. DWI and ^{1}H-MRS in some distance can contribute to differentiating benign and malignant lesions.

1 Morphologic analysis

The morphologic parameters include lesion type (focus, mass or nonmass), mass shape and margins, and internal enhancement.

(1) Focus

A focus is a single tiny punctate enhancement that is nonspecific and too small to be characterized. A focus is not a space-occupying lesion or mass, usually less than 5mm. If there are multiple foci in a breast, the term stippled can be applied. Stippled refers to multiple, often innumerable punctate foci that are approximately 1 to 2mm in size and appear scattered throughout an area of the breast that does not conform usually to a duct system. Stippled enhancement is more characteristic of benign normal variant parenchymal enhancement or fibrocystic changes.

(2) Mass

Mass shape can be described as round (spherical), oval (elliptical), lobulated or irregular. Margins of masses are smooth, irregular or spiculated. Spiculated and irregular masses are suspicious for carcinoma, whereas a smooth margin is more suggestive of a benign lesion. Internal enhancement of masses can be described as homogeneous, heterogeneous or rim enhancement. Rim enhancement can be seen in invasive carcinoma, ruptured or inflamed cyst, abscess, fat necrosis. Thick, irregular rim, rapid enhancement and washout kinetics are usually malignant signs. Homogeneous enhancement is suggestive of a benign process. Heterogeneous enhancement is more characteristic of malignant lesions, especially if rim enhancement is present. Dark internal septations are classic for fibroadenomas. Similarly, nonenhanced masses are also likely benign fibroadenomas that have a high hyaline content.

(3) Non-mass-like distribution

It includes focal area (<25% of quadrant in confined area and contains interspersed fat or normal glandular tissue), linear (in a line, not definitely a duct, may be sheet-like), ductal (in a line, pointing to nipple, can branch, conforming to a duct), segmental (triangular region or cone with apex pointing to nipple), regional (geographic, ≥ 25% of quadrant), multiple regions (≥2 regions, patchy) or diffuse distribution (uniform, even throughout breast). Ductal or segmental enhancement is generally suggestive of malignance, especially ductal carcinoma in situ (DCIS). Regional enhancement and diffuse enhancement are more characteristic of benign diseases such as proliferative changes.

2 Signal intensity and internal architecture

Signal intensity can be described as homogeneous or heterogeneous. Benign lesions are generally homogeneous in signal, whereas malignant lesions are heterogeneous. On noncontrast T1WI, breast lesions, benign or malignant, are generally low or moderate signals similar to the surrounding parenchyma; on T2WI, the signal intensity is variable depending on different contents of cells, collagen and liquad in lesions, so the lesions demonstrate complexity of high, moderate, low, or mixed signals. Cysts, lymph nodes, and certain types of fibroadenomas (myxomatous) are high in signal on T2WI. Breast carcinomas are generally not high in signal on T2WI, but carcinomas with necrosis, liquefaction, and cystic degeneration can exhibit high signal.

3 Kinetics of enhancement

The type of time-signal intensity curve should be evaluated after contrast injection. There are two phases: Initial phase: change in signal intensity (SI) within first 2 minutes of injection, which can be described as slow (<60% increase in SI within 2 minutes), medium (60%~100% increase in SI within 2 minutes), rapid (> 100% increase in SI within 2 minutes); Delayed phase: change in signal intensity (SI) after 2 minutes of injection, which most contributes to the curve types. There are three types: persistent (Type Ⅰ): progressive, continued increase in signal over time; plateau (Type Ⅱ): SI does not change over time after initial rise; washout (Type Ⅲ): SI decreases after peaking. Generally, persistent pattern is suggestive of benign lesions (83%~94% positive predictive value, PPV), while washout pattern is suggestive of malignant lesions (87% PPV), and plateau pattern can be seen in both benign and malignant lesions (64% PPV for malignance).

4 DWI (diffusion weighted imaging) and MRS (MR spectrum)

DWI and ^{1}H-MRS are used to differentiate benign lesions from malignant ones. Generally, malignant tumors are high signal on DWI with decreased ADC values, while benign tumors are low signal on DWI with increased ADC values. Most breast carcinomas demonstrate choline peak on ^{1}H-MRS, while only a small part of benign lesions demonstrate choline peak on ^{1}H-MRS.

Section 4 CT

The abnormal signs on CT of breast diseases, including mass, calcification, nipple retraction, skin thickening and dimpling, lymphadenopathy, are similar to those on mammogram. But fine calcifications are not well demonstrated on CT compared with mammogram.

Lesson 4 Diagnosis of Diseases

Section 1 Fibroadenoma

[**Pathology and clinical manifestations**]

Fibroadenomas are the most common benign neoplasms of the breast. They may occur in all age groups, but are most common in young women with peak incidence in the 30s. Usually a highly mobile palpable painless firm mass can be touched in the breast by physical examination. They may be solitary or multiple. Histologically, fibroadenomas are most often smooth, occasionally lobulated, circumscribed, round, or oval masses. They are comprised of epithelial and stromal elements surrounded by a pseudocapsule. The epithelial component is composed of gland-like, duct-like spaces containing terminal duct and lobular tissues. The stromal elements consist of surrounding connective tissue containing varying amounts of collagen and acid mucopolysaccharides. The predominance of epithelial versus stromal components varies with age. The epithelial elements usually predominate in younger women. In older postmenopausal women, the stromal component dominates and may hyalinize or calcify.

[**Imaging appearances**]

(1) Mammography

On mammogram, fibroadenomas are usually round, oval, or lobulated masses with low density or isodense to breast parenchyma. Often most parts of margins are smooth and circumscribed and are partly obscured. Calcifications always can be seen, which are clustered coarse heterogeneous or "popcorn" shaped. (Fig 8-4-1-A/B)

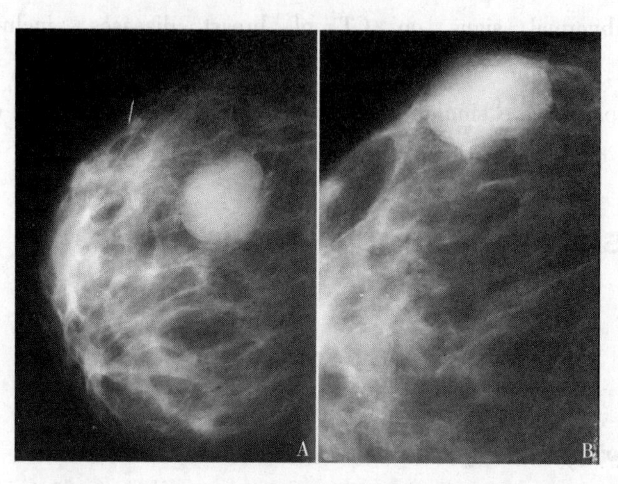

Fig 8-4-1-A/B An oval isodense mass on mammogram in MLO and CC views

(2) Ultrasonography

It is the most common cause of a breast lump in women under 30 years of age. It is characterized by a firm, painless, smooth, often highly mobile lump in the breast. Ultrasound finding is as Fig 8-4-2-A/B.

①The classic shape of benign fibroadenomas is elliptical. The second most common shape is gently lobulated. Classic lobulated fibrodenomas have three or fewer lobulations.

②The width of such lesions is larger than their length. They are completely encompassed by a complete thin, echogenic capsule, and can be characterized as BIRADS 3.

③The internal echoes are uniformly hypoechogenic.

④Most show posterior acoustic enhancement.

⑤ In some lesions, CDFI may show blood flow.

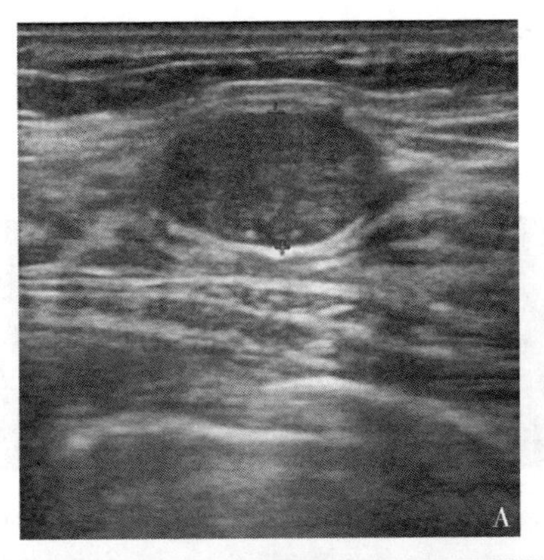

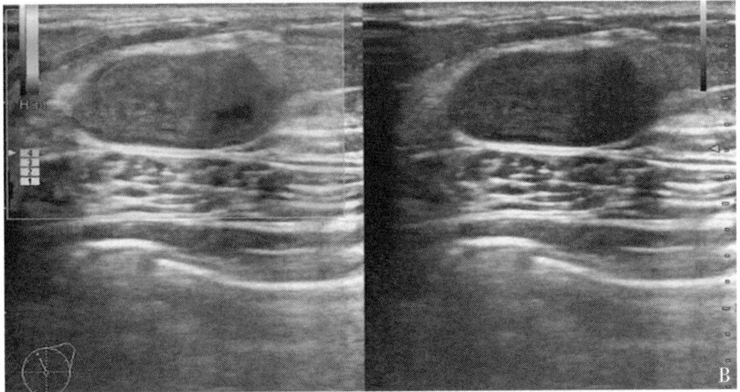

Fig 8-4-2-A/B Fibroadenoma in 2D and ultrasonic elasticity imagings

(3) MRI

Fibroadenomas are of low signal in T1W non-contrast images and most often cannot be distinguished from adjacent glandular tissues. In non-contrast enhanced T2WI images, signal intensity varies depending on the fluid content of the lesion. Cellular, myxomatous lesions, often seen in younger patients, are high in signal. Less cellular and sclerotic lesions, seen in older patients, vary from intermediate to low signal intensity. In T1WI contrast-enhanced images, cellular, myxomatous fibroadenoma lesions demonstrate uniform and homogeneous enhancement. If the lesions contain non-enhancing internal septations, they are highly suggestive of the diagnosis. Less cellular fibroadenomas enhance less or not at all. The enhancement kinetic curves generally are continuous or plateau. (Fig 8-4-3-A/B/C)

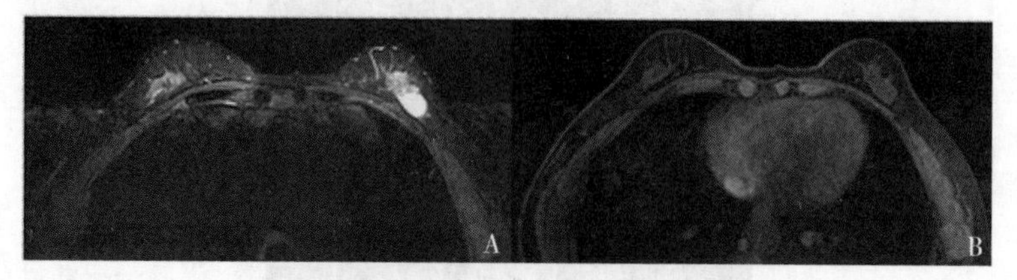

Fig 8-4-3-A A high signal lesion onT2WI in left breast; B the same lesion on T1WI

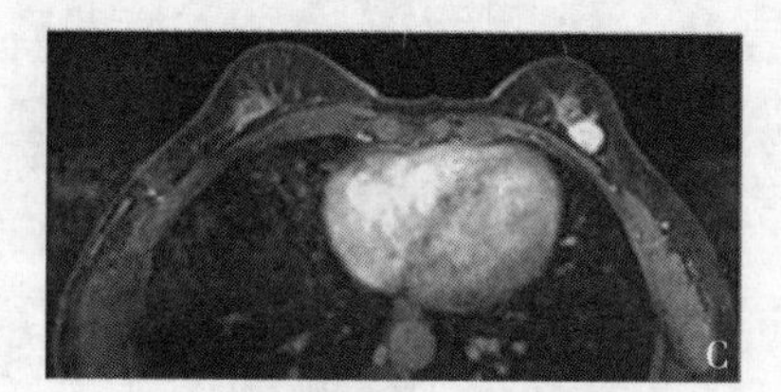

Fig 8-4-3-C The same lesion enhanced homogeneously in a T1WI contrast-enhanced image

(4) CT

The morphologic characteristics of fibroadenomas on CT are similar to those on mammogram. Fibroadenomas are usually homogeneously enhanced, with CT value increases of 30~40 HU.

[**Diagnosis**]

Best diagnostic clue: Most common solid mass in women of all ages; Mammogram: oval or lobulated circumscribed mass with dense coarse calcifications; Ultrasound: hypoechoic circumscribed oval mass with homogeneous internal echoes; MRI: smooth, moderately enhanced lobulated mass with nonenhanced internal septations.

Section 2 Fibrocystic disease

[**Pathology and clinical manifestations**]

Fibrocystic disease, also called chronic cystic mastitis or mammary dysplasia, is the most common, most often bilateral, disorder of the breast. It is the result of distortion and exaggeration of normal menstrual cyclic changes of ductal epithelium and stroma. Histopathologically, non-proliferative fibrocystic changes, which are not associated with an increased risk of breast cancer, consist of cysts of varying sizes, stromal fibrosis, and apocrine metaplasia. Proliferative fibrocystic changes include hyperplasia without atypia, papillomas, and sclerosing adenosis. Atypical hyperplasias, such as atypical lobular hyperplasia and atypical ductal hyperplasia, included in the spectrum of fibrocystic disease, may be associated with a slight increased risk of cancer. It happens bilaterally in 30~40 years old women. The clinical symptoms are distending pain, multiple "clumps" in breast, especially during premenstrual cycle.

[**Imaging appearances**]

(1) Mammography

It shows focal or diffused nodules or thickened dense parenchyma with vague margins. Calcifications can be seen, which are punctate in scattered or clustered, diffused distribution, 2~4mm in diameter. If calcifications are scattered, it suggests benign disease; if calcifications are clustered or diffused, it is difficult to distinguish benign diseases from malignant ones. Small cysts are round, or oval in shape with low or isodense to breast parenchyma. Linear calcification can be seen in cystic wall.

(2) Ultrasonography

① Most appear as thickening of mammary gland structure disorder, and the internal echo is uniform.

② If there are ectatic ducts, they present as anechoic areas in different sizes. (Fig 8-4-4)

(3) MRI

Fibrocystic parenchyma is most often difficult to distinguish from normal breast parenchyma on both T2WI and T1WI non-contrast imaging series. This is because fibrocystic parenchyma, like normal parenchyma, has a variable appearance dependent on the water and collagen content of the tissues. The pattern may be similar to that seen on the mammogram. One may identify clusters of small cysts, less than 3mm. In T1W contrast-enhanced images, there may be a prominent presence of stippled regional enhancement. Occasionally, this pattern may seem to coalesce and appear as a region of clumped enhancement or even as a heterogeneous large mass. Proliferative changes, such as sclerosing adenosis, may appear as mass-like lesions due to the compression of stroma with distortion or the glandular elements. These patterns are difficult to distinguish from carcinoma. Generally, if these patterns vary with the menstrual cycle, least conspicuous in mid-cycle, the diagnosis of fibrocystic disease is more likely. Evaluation of enhancement kinetics can be helpful if continuous or plateau kinetic patterns are observed.

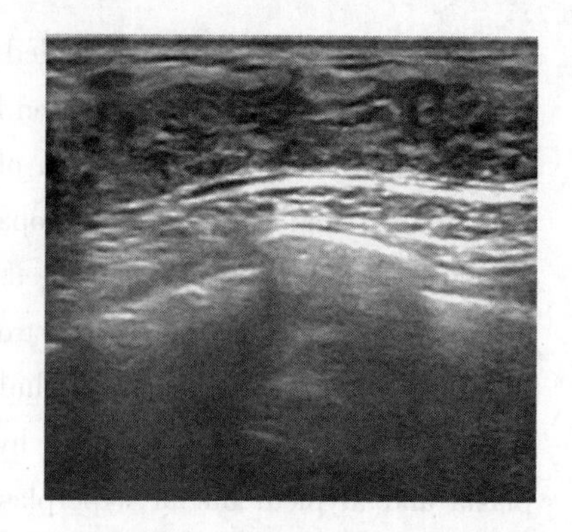

Fig 8-4-4 Fibrocystic disease

(4) CT

CT can demonstrate thickened, dense breast parenchyma with scattered low density. If there are cysts, they are round, or oval in shape with low density like water.

[**Diagnosis**]

Best diagnostic clue: bilaterally, most in women of 30~40 years old, with associated clinical symptoms changed in menstrual cycle; Mammogram: nodular or diffused densities in breast. MRI: chronic and continuous enhancement with persistent dynamic curve type.

Section 3 Breast cancer

[**Pathology and clinical manifestations**]

The prevalence of breast carcinoma in China is increasing. It can be unilateral or bilateral. Approximately 80% of breast cancers arise in the ducts, with the most common histology of invasive cancer being invasive ductal carcinoma not otherwise specified (NOS). Specialized subtypes of invasive ductal carcinoma also occur, including mucinous, tubular, medullary, and papillary carcinomas. Less than 10% of breast cancers arise in the lobules of the breast and are invasive lobular carcinomas. Other unusual primary malignant lesions that arise in the breast include lymphoid and hematopoietic malignancies and mesenchymal stromal neoplasms, such as malignant phyllodes tumors and sarcomas. Metastatic lesions can also involve the breast. Breast carcinoma is most often seen in women of 40~60 years, but also can be seen in men. Most common symptoms are palpable thickening or firm lump with or without nipple and/or skin retraction. Some others have no symptoms and cancers are detected on screening mammogram.

[**Imaging appearances**]

(1) Mammography

The mammographic findings of breast carcinomas include mass, calcification, mass associated calcification, focal asymmetric density, distortion, distortion associated calcification, etc. Mass is the most common sign, which is usually irregular or lobulated in shape with spiculated margins. The density of mass is often higher than that of benign tumor of the same size. Calcification is the second most common sign, which is fine sand-like, linear, or linear-branching in shape and is clustered, linear, or segmental in distribution. Calcification can be the only sign or associated with mass. The shape and distribution of calcification are very important in differentiating benign lesions from malignant ones. Most ductal carcinomas in situ (DCIS) are detected by characteristic calcification on mammogram with no mass at all. Other associated signs include ductal sign, vascularity increasing, skin thickening and dimpling, nipple retraction, or lymphadenopathy. (Fig 8-4-5-A/B)

(2) Ultrasonography

1) Most invasive duct carcinoma components may extend away from the invasive tumor within surrounding lobar ducts and grow toward the nipple to create duct extensions. The microlobulations are pointed or angular and associated with speculations or thick, echogenic halo. The border is indistinct and irregular without intact capsule.

2) As malignant solid modules enlarge, invasive ductal carcinoma components are taller than wide.

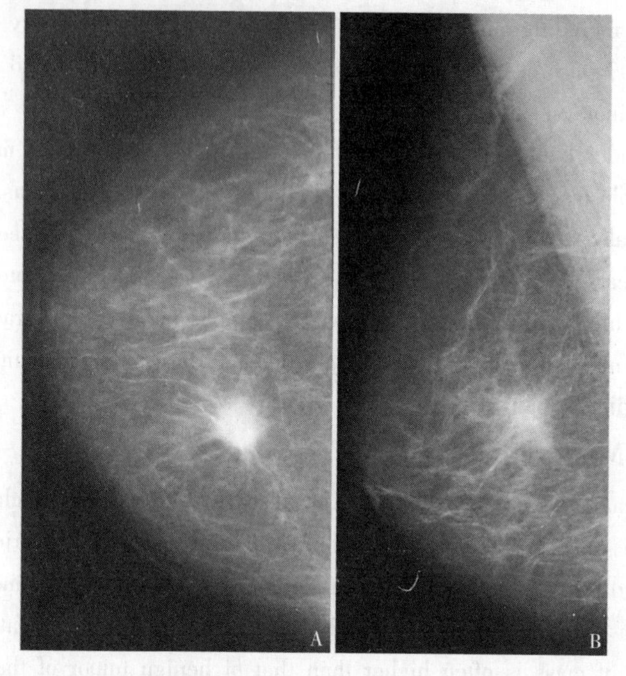

Fig 8-4-5-A/B A spiculated isodense mass on mammogram in MLO and CC views

3) The internal echoes usually is hypoechogenic and heterogeneous.

4) In some lesions, the microcalcifications can be seen. In some degree, it is regarded as a specific sign in diagnosing carcinomas of breast.

5) Posterior acoustic attenuation can be seen.

6) In most lesions, CDFI can show blood flow. (Fig 8-4-6-A/B)

(3) MRI

MRI is highly sensitive in the detection of breast cancer. Most carcinomas present as irregular or spiculated masses. This spiculated lesion is characterized by extensive fibrosis and consists of a central mass that radiates into the surrounding breast tissues. Less frequently, carcinomas are well defined with lobulated shape and circumscribed margins. The mass lesions are lower or isointense to surrounding breast parenchyma in T1W non-contrast images, heterogeneous higher or isointense in fat-suppressed T2-weighted images. In T1-weighted contrast-enhanced images, the mass lesions usually have peripheral or rim enhancement.

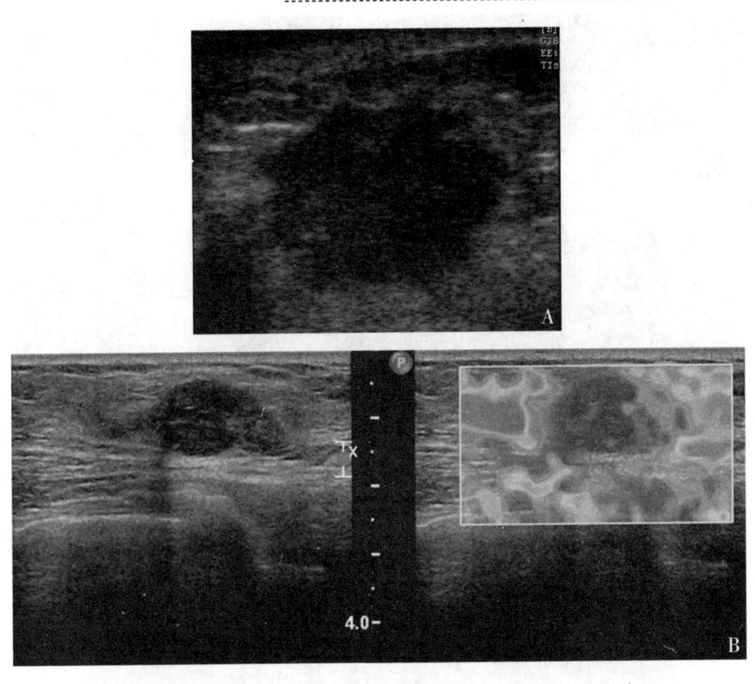

Fig 8-4-6-A/B Breast cancer in 2D and ultrasonic elasticity imagings

Irregular enhancement within the mass is frequently seen. The enhancement kinetic curves generally are washout or plateau. Nonmass-like enhancement also can be seen. For example, ductal enhancement should be viewed with suspicion as possibly representing in situ carcinoma. Regional or diffuse enhancement is rare but can be seen in multicentric DCIS. Most carcinomas are high signal on DWI with decreased ADC values. For some breast carcinomas, choline peak lying in 3.2 ppm can be detected on ^{1}H-MRS. (Fig 8-4-7-A/B/C/D/E/FG)

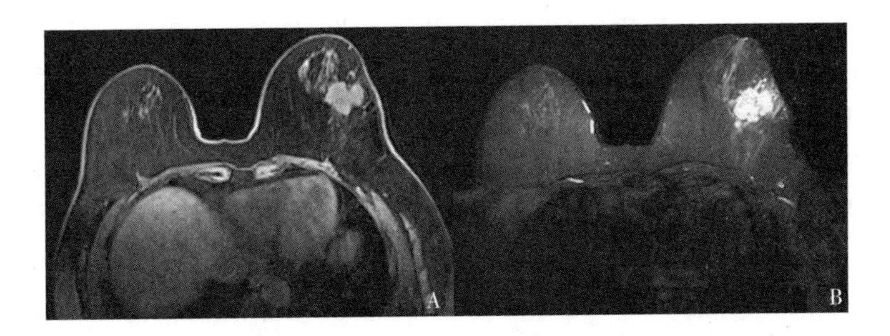

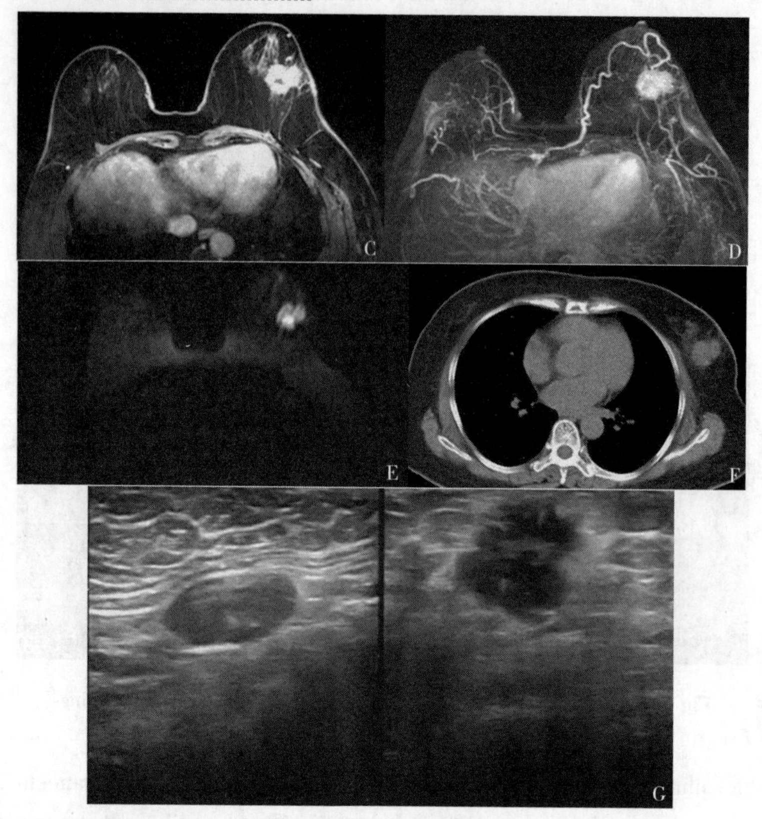

Fig 8-4-7-A/B/C/D/E/F/G

A：A high signal lesion onT2WI in left breast；B：the same lesion on T1WI
C：The lesion is enhanced heterogeneously in T1WI contrast-enhanced images；
D：MR angiography shows thickened arteries to the lesion.
E：The lesion is high signal on DWI；F：the same lesion on CT
G：The same lesion on US

(4) CT

The morphologic characteristics of breast carcinoma on CT are similar to those on mammogram. Breast carcinomas usually heterogeneously enhance in "rapid in and rapid out" pattern, with CT values increasing by more than 50HU.

[**Diagnosis**]

Best diagnostic clue：Most in women aged 40～60 years，with associated clinical symptoms. Mammogram：irregular，spiculated mass with fine sand-like，linear，or linear-branching calcifications in clustered，linear，or segmental distribution. MRI：rapid enhancement and rapid washout pattern of dynamic curve.

Chapter 9

Imaging of the osteoarticular and muscular systems

Lesson 1 Skeleton

Section 1 Imaging Methods

1 Radiography

The radiography the preferred method in the diagnosis of bone diseases. However, the appearances in many bone diseases such as inflammation and early stage of tumors can be negative for the first time to check, which appear later than the pathological changes and clinical symptoms, and need periodic review or further CT and MRI. The following rules in radiography should be noted: a) multiple position: antero-posterior, lateral position should be taken for limbs, joints, and spine. b) Special position, such as oblique position for rib fracture, axial position for patellar fracture and calcaneus fracture, which will help to avoid missing of indistinctive lesions. c) The surrounding soft tissue should be included in the radiography. d) For limbs, spine examination, adjacent joint or vertebra should be included in the radiography. e) For comparison, in the identical position and photographic parameter, the bone or joint on the other side need to be examined usually.

2 CT

CT is used as a further examination when clinical observasions and radiography fail to prompt a diagnosis. It is also the first choice for some complex anatomic sites like pelvis, shoulder, knees etc., because it can not only provide more details about the anatomy of lesion, but also easily distinguish between destruction, sequestrum, calcification and ossification etc.

(1) Plain CT scanning

Both sides including the lesion part should be scanned at the same time as far as possible, for comparison. Transect scanning is often used. According to the quality and scope, the thickness may be 2 to 5mm, with L60, W300 to observe soft tissues, and L400, W1500 to observe bones, owing to the great difference of CT values between bone and soft tissue. When necessary, a variety of image post-processing techniques are needed.

(2) Enhanced CT scanning

Convenient for qualitative diagnosis, contrast-enhanced scanning is often used to show the blood supply of lesions, and to determine the scope of the disease or whether there is necrosis.

3 MRI

MRI is the newest and most sophisticated imaging technique as a further examination. Especially for the early stage of bone destruction and occult fracture, MRI is better than radiography and CT. MRI also has advantages in revealing the anatomy and lesions of spine. But it is inferior to radiography and CT in showing calcification and tiny ossification.

(1) Plain MRI scanning

Spin echo T1-weighted imaging (T1WI) and T2-weighted imaging (T2WI) are the basic scanning sequences, and stir sequence is often used for bone examination. As the high signal of adipose tissue in the bone marrow is restrained, differences between lesions and normal tissues can be more obvious. Generally, two different ranges of levels including T1WI and T2WI should be checked.

(2) Enhanced MRI scanning

The purpose and significance of contrast-enhanced MRI scanning are the same as enhanced CT.

Section 2 Normal imaging findings of bones

1 The structure and growth of bones

(1) Structure

The bones of human body can be divided into 4 types: long, short, flat and irregular bones. According to its structure, the skeleton is made up of compact and spongy bones. Compact bone contains cortex of long bone and internal and external plates of flat bone, mainly formed by Haversian system. While spongy bone is composed of bone trabeculae, and the spaces between them are occupied by fat or hemopoietic marrow.

(2) Growth

The ossification of bones, including membrane bones and endochondral bones, begins from the fetal period. The mesenchymal cells change into fibroblasts, form the connective tissue, and turn into the ossification center, and then gradually expand, to complete the development of bone. Another way is that the mesenchymal cells change into cartilage primordial, and form the primary ossification center by osteogenesis. After birth, the secondary ossification center appears, and continues to expand. The primary and secondary ossification centers completely heal mutually, to complete the development of bone.

During the process of bone growth, the bones remodel through the absorption of bones by activity of osteoclast. The formation of medullary cavity is mainly due to the absorption of the internal surface of the cortex.

(3) Factors affecting the development of bones

There must be two conditions in the growth of bones: osteoblast cells make formation of osteoid tissues, and then sediment of minerals on osteoid tissues. At the same time, the absorption of bones by osteoclast cells can help to maintain the balance of the metabolism of bones. Any change of the above processes may affect the development of bones.

2 Long bones

(1) Pediatric bones

The pediatric long bone generally has more than 3 ossification centers. After birth, most of the diaphysis ossifies, and there are epiphyseal cartilages at both ends. The characteristics of pediatric long bones are the epiphyseal cartilage and incomplete ossification. Pediatric long bone can be divided into diaphysis, metaphysis, epiphysis and epiphyseal plate (Fig 9-1-1-A/B).

1) Diaphysis:

① ***radiography***: cortical bone is high density and uniform density, with well-defined edge. It is thicker in the middle of diaphysis while thinner at the ends. The surface and inner face of cortical bone are covered with periosteum. The medullary cavity which contains fat and hemopoietic tissues is like an increased translucency.

② ***CT image***: the cortical bone is like a linear or ribbon shadow, the bone trabecula can be seen as a reticular shadow, while the medullary cavity is low density.

③ ***MRI***: On T1WI and T2WI of MRI, the cortex appears as a line or girdle-shaped low-signal shadow, and the marrow cavity may be high signal similar to fat. The periosteum is not shown in a normal image of radiography, CT, nor MRI.

2) Metaphysis

It is made up of spongy bones, and lies at the ends of the diaphysis.

① ***Radiography***: The compact bone trabeculae are crossing each other, and on the top there is a transverse thin shadow called provisional calcification zone. The demarcation between diaphysis and metaphysis is not clear.

② ***CT***: The bone trabeculae of metaphysis can be seen as a reticular shadow, and the provisional calcification zone is high density.

③ ***MRI***: The marrow of metaphysis can be seen as lower signal on T1WI and T2WI, while the provisional calcification zone shows hypointensity, too.

3) Epiphysis

It is made up of varying amounts of cartilages and spongy bones.

① ***Radiography***: The epiphyseal cartilage is invisible on radiography. When the secondary ossification center appears, the epiphyseal cartilage enlarges, and forms the spongy bone.

② ***CT***: The epiphyseal cartilage shows soft tissue density, and the density of ossification center is similar to metaphysis.

③ ***MRI***: The epiphyseal cartilage shows isointensity, and the signal of ossification center is similar to metaphysis.

4) Epiphyseal plate

It is situated between the epiphysis and diaphysis, which is a cartilaginous plate remaining for a long while as a suturing or connecting cartilage during the period of growth.

① ***Radiography***: The epiphyseal plate shows a transverse transparent strip shadow. It becomes thinner and linear, and is called epiphyseal line. Finally it disappears, and completes the growth of bone. Instead, it may appear as a translucent line situated between epiphysis and metaphysis on X-ray radiograph.

② ***CT and MRI***: The appearance is similar to epiphysis in CT and MRI images.

(2) Bone age

The appearance and fusion of the secondary ossification will take place at certain time and with certain regularity, and this is referred to as bone age. To know the order of the appearance of the ossification centers in different regions of the body is of importance.

(3) Adult bones

The shape of adult bones is similar to those of children. But they develop fully and there is bony fusion of the epiphysis with the shaft, and the epiphyseal line disappears. The cortical bone is thicker, and with higher density. The signal of bone marrow is also higher in MRI images.

3 Spine

Spine consists of vertebra and intervertebral disc. Except C1, every vertebra consists of two parts, body and arch. Vertebral arch is composed of pedicle, plate, spinous process, transverse process and articulating process.

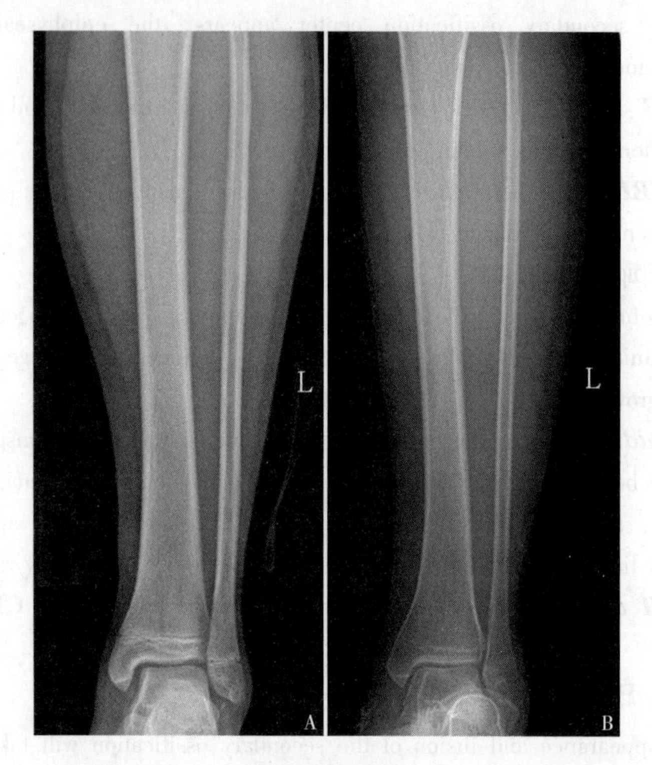

Fig 9-1-1-A/B

A: long bone of child: diaphysis, metaphysis, epiphysis, epiphysis line of tibia and fibular.

B: long bone of adult: only diaphysis and end of bone, with no metaphysis and epiphyseal plate.

(Fig 9-1-2-A/B)

1) Radiography

On AP view each vertebra appears rectangle and it enlarges gradually downwards. It is composed of spongy bones, with uniform density, well-defined edge. The upper and lower edges are called end plates. Transverse process can be seen on both sides as a transverse outward-extending shadow, and in the inner side there is an oval ring shadow called vertebral arch ring. Spinous process is a pointed triangular shadow partial below the middle of the vertebral body. On lat-

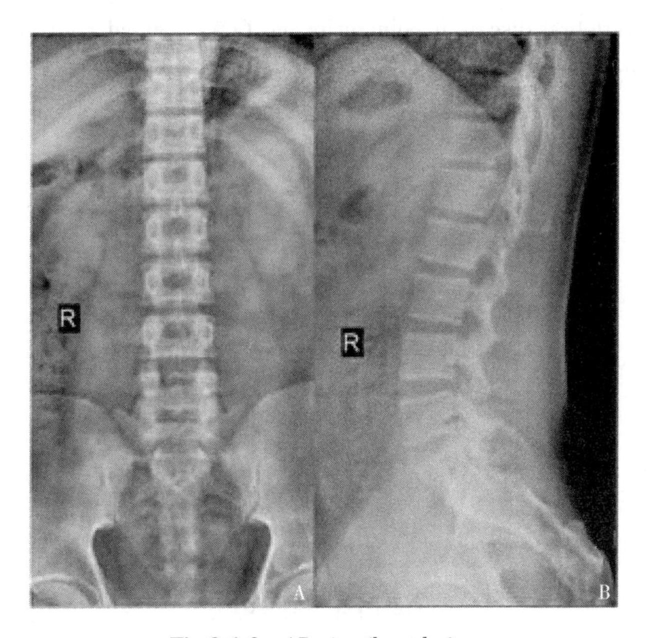

Fig 9-1-2 AP view/lateral view

eral view the intervertebral space and intervertebral foramen can be easily seen.

2) CT image

On axial view, the trailing edge of vertebrae concaves forward. The spinal bone ring is enclosed by vertebrae, vertebral pedicle and laminae of vertebral arches. Spinal dural sac is a low density shadow living in the middle of spinal bone ring. Ligamenta flava is usually 2~4mm thick, attached to the inside of laminae of vertebral arches. Lumbar nerve roots are located in the anterolateral dural sac symmetrically and bilaterally, which is a round isodensity shadow. Lateral recess is like funnel-shaped, and its anteroposterior diameter is no less than 3mm. Intervertebral disc is composed of nucleus pulposus, annulus and cartilage plate, and its density is lower than vertebrae. The CT value is 50~110 HU. (Fig 9-1-3)

3) MRI image

Cortical bone and ligaments are hypointensity on both T1WI and T2WI.

Bone marrow is high signal on T1WI, isointensity or slightly higher signal on T2WI. Intervertebral disc is hypointensity on T1WI. Spinal cord is isointensity on T1WI, higher than the signal of cerebrospinal fluid; while on T2WI it is lower. (Fig 9-1-4)

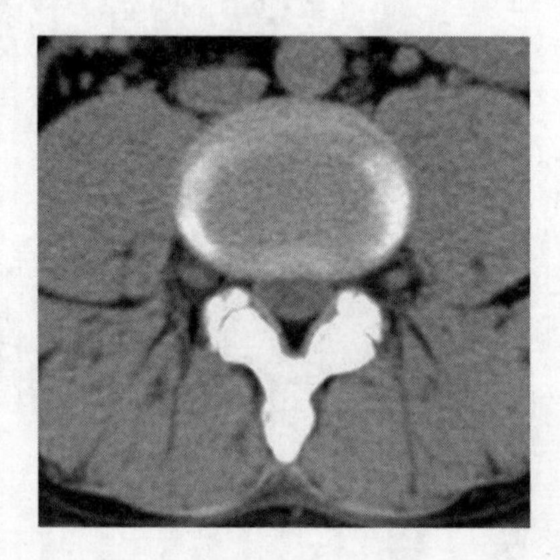

Fig 9-1-3 Plain CT

Intervertebral disc shows soft tissue density, and endplates of adjacent vertebra appear as new moon high density shadow.

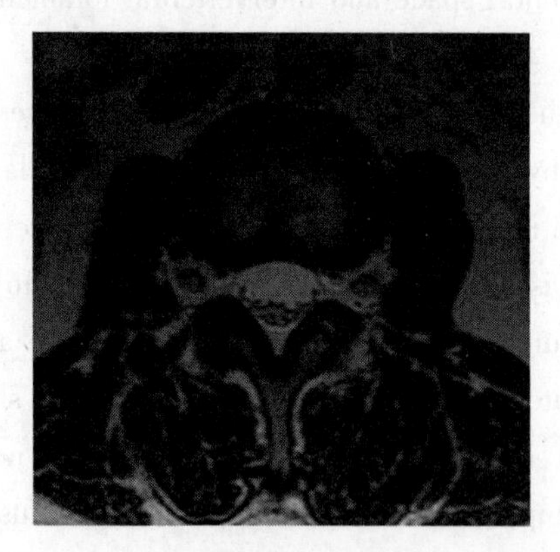

Fig 9-1-4 MRI T2WI

Intervertebral disc, dural sac, cauda equian, intervertebral foramen and spinous process are seen.

Section 3 Imaging signs of bone diseases

The imaging signs of bone diseases are varied. Different diseases may have identical basic features. It is an important approach to diagnose bone diseases by mastering of the basic signs.

1 Osteoporosis

In a certain unit volume of bone, the organics and calcium are decreased, but the ratio of them is still normal. Histological changes include thin of the cortex, enlargement of Harson system, and decrease of trabecula. (Fig 9-1-5-A)

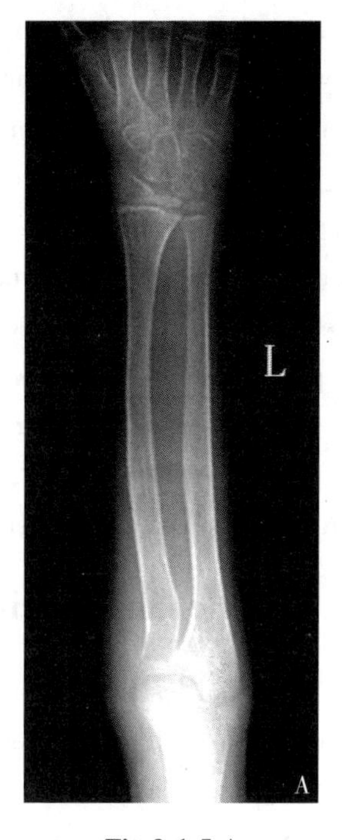

Fig 9-1-5-A

Density of bone decreases, the cortex becomes thinner, and bone trabecula decreases.

(1) Radiography

The main sign is decreased density of bone. In a long bone, the cortex becomes thinner and layered, the bone trabecula decreases, with the gap widened, and the marrow cavity becomes enlarged. In spine, the cortical bone of vertebrae becomes thinner. In serious cases, the normal vertebral structure disappears, vertebrae become flat, and its upper and lower edges become concaved, with the fusiform intervertebral gap widened. Osteoporosis is prone to fracture.

(2) CT

The appearance is similar to that of radiography.

(3) MRI

In addition to the bone shape changes, signal increases on T1WI and T2WI.

Generalized osteoporosis is mainly seen in old people, postmenopausal women, hyperparathyroidism, hypovitaminosis C, alcoholism, etc. Localized osteoporosis is more common in fracture, infection, and tumors.

2 Osteomalacia

In a certain unit volume of bone, the organic ingredients are normal, but mineral content is decreased. The osteoid tissue is short of calcification in histology. There is a central part of the trabecular bone with calcification, and usually a layer of non-calcified bone-like tissue appears around it. The bones thus become softened and bend or even break.

Radiography appearance: the main sign is decreased density of bones, especially in spine and pelvis. In contrast to osteoporosis, the edges of trabecular and cortical bones are "ground glass" like. Because of osteomalacia, a variety of skeletal deformation often occurs, and pseudo-fracture lines are seen, which are transparent lines 1-2mm in width that are perpendicular to the cortical bone.

Many diseases affecting calcification in the osteoid can cause osteomalacia, such as vitamin-Ddeficiency, kidney diseases, and disturbance of calcium-phosphorus metabolism. It is seen in osteomalacia in adults and rickets in children.

3 Bone destruction

Abnormal lesion or tissue replaces normal bone structure, which is caused by the lesion itself or more active osteoclast movement. (Fig 9-1-5-B/C)

Imaging appearances:

(1) Radiography

it appears as a localized area of decreased bone density and rarefaction of trabecular bone, erosion of the cortex or loss of a part of bone, and normal bone structure disappears. In early stage, spongy bone destruction appears as patchy trabecular bone defect, and cortical bone destruction appears as erossion-like change in margin. In advanced stage, there may be great loss of cortical bones and spongy bones.

(2) CT

it is useful for differentiation of destruction of position and range. Spongy

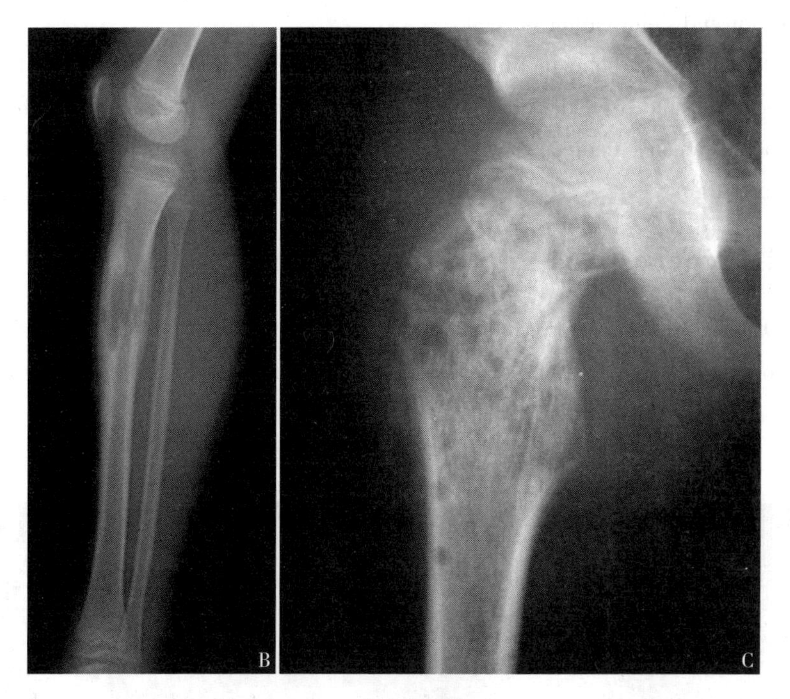

Fig 9-1-5-B/C

bone destruction appears as patchy loss areas, cortical bone destruction appears as erossion-like and cribriform change, and cortical bone becomes thinner.

(3) MRI

it appears as a hypointensity bone replaced by different signal intensity lesions. Cortical bone destruction appears similar to CT, and spongy bone destruction appears as a high signal marrow change into hypointensity or heterogeneous signal.

Destruction of bone is a common change in inflammation, tumor and tumor-like lesion. Different diseases have different destruction appearances. Acute inflammation and malignant tumor may cause an osteolytic bone destruction, which is quickly developed with irregular ill-defined margin. Chronic inflammation and benign lesion may cause expansive bone destruction, with regular well-defined margin. Sometimes hyperostosis surrounding the destruction area, bone expansion and deformation is seen.

Destruction of bone in tibia, with bone density decreased, bone trabecula disappeared, and well-defined margin. Osteolytic bone destruction in femur: with bone density decreased, bone trabecula in disorder, and irregular ill-defined margin.

4 Hyperostosis and osteosclerosis

Osteosclerosis is referred to as an increase of amount of bone matrix in a certain volume of bone. Various diseases involving activities of osteoblast cells cause hyperostosis and osteosclerosis. (Fig 9-1-6-A/B)

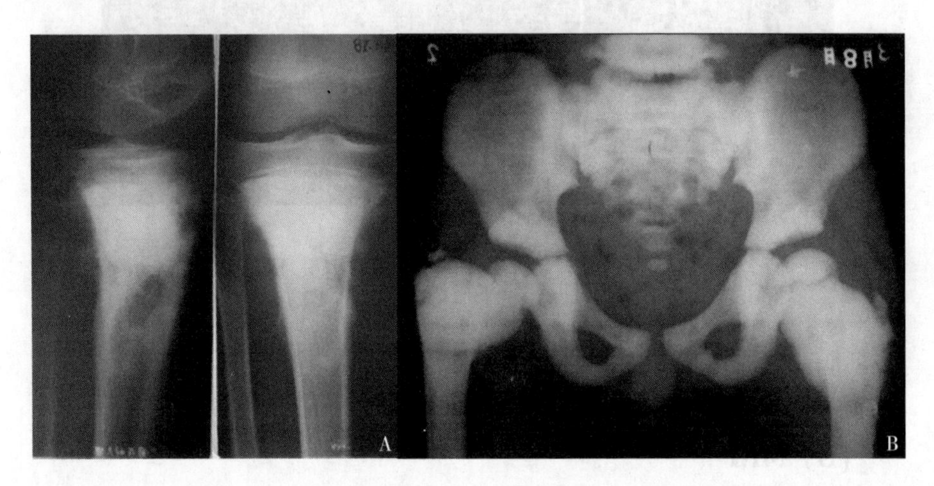

Fig 9-1-6-A/B proximal tibia:

Bone density increases, and cortical bone is thickened. It is osteosclerosis.

(1) Radiography

It appears as bone density increased, with or without bone enlarged. Trabecular bone and cortical bone are thickened. Bone marrow cavity may be narrowed or disappear in long bones.

(2) CT

The appearance is similar to radiography.

(3) MRI

It appears as hypointensity on both T1WI and T2WI.

Local osteosclerosis is commonly seen in chronic inflammation, degeneration, repair after injury, and osteogenic tumor. General osteosclerosis occurs in metabolic bone disease, toxic bone disease and hereditary dysostosis.

5 Periosteal proliferation (periosteal reaction)

Due to the edematous thickening periosteum and increased osteoblast activity, sub-periosteal new bone is formed eventually. It's pathological in general. (Fig 9-1-7)

(1) Radiography and CT

In the early stage, it appears as a variable length linear shadow, which is parallel to the cortical bone, with a 1~2mm wide translucent gap. Later the sub-periosteal new bone is thickening, with linear, layered and lacy change. Usually, it is widely seen in inflammation and is localized in tumors. With the improvement of lesions, sub-periosteal new bone may become compacted and gradually fuse with the cortical bone. Sub-periosteal new bone may also be destructed and the bilateral vestigial triangular structure is called "Codman triangle", which is a sign of malignant tumor.

(2) MRI

Periosteal proliferation in MRI image is earlier than radiography and CT. In early stage, periosteal edema is isointensity on T1WI, and high signal on T2WI, and sub-periosteal new bone is hypointensity on both T1WI and T2WI.

Periosteal proliferation is commonly seen in inflammation, tumor, injury, subperiosteum bleeding.

6 Calcification within bone or cartilage

Calcification within bone or cartilage can be physiologic (calcification of costal cartilage), or pathologic (calcification of tumor cartilage).

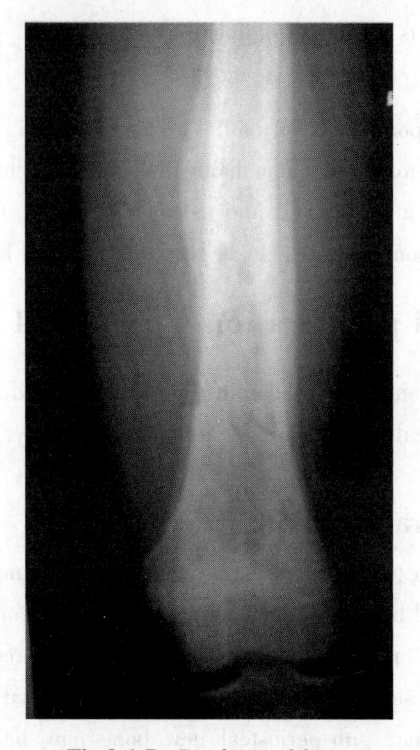

Fig 9-1-7 Diaphysis of femur
Long linear and triangular shadow, which is parallel to the cortical bone.

(1) Radiography

It appears as granular, ringlike, semi-circular ringlike high density shadows, widely distributed or restricted to a particular area in tumors.

(2) CT

It is more sensitive in finding small calcification than plain film, but on the contrary, MRI has less sensitivity. Calcification is hypointensity on both T1WI and T2WI.

7 Bone necrosis

Bone necrosis is defined as the death of bone tissue caused by gradual vascular impairment or cessation of metabolism of local bone tissue. A fragment of necrotic bone that becomes separated from healthy bone is called sequestrum. Histological changes include bone cell death and loss, bone marrow liquefaction and atrophy. In early stage, there is no change about bone structure and calcium content of bone. The sequestrum lies in a space surrounded by granulation tissue, then it is absorbed and new bone appears.

(1) Radiography and CT

In early stage, it's normal on radiography and CT image; the sequestrum appears as a localized high density shadow.

(2) MRI

The sequestrum is isointensity or hypointensity on T1WI, and isointensity to high signal on T2WI. The granulation tissue around is hypointensity on T1WI, and high signal on T2WI. New bone is hypointensity on both T1WI and T2WI. Bone necrosis may occur in inflammation, injury, etc.

8 Mineral sedimentation

Minerals such as lead, phosphorus, bismuth get into human body, and are mainly deposited in the metaphyseal bone in children.

Radiography

It appears that a few compact bands are parallel to epiphyseal line in the metaphyseal bone, which seldom appears in adults.

Fluorine is not a kind of mineral, but if fluorine intake is excessive, it stimulates endosteal and periosteal osteoblastic activity and bone formation, but the resulting bone is morphologically abnormal and mechanically inferior, because fluorine in high concentrations has a toxic effect on the osteoblasts and osteocytes. The skeletal changes consist of increased density of the bones, particularly the cancellous bone, which remodels more rapidly than the cortex.

9 Deformity of bone

Deformity of bone may be localized or generalized, and it usually occurs with the size change of bone. Bone tumor and growth malformation can cause local bone enlargement and deformity. Osteomalacia and osteogenesis imperfecta can lead to bone deformity throughout the body.

Section 4 Diagnosis of bone diseases

1 Injury of bone

The purposes of taking radiological examinations are as follows: a) to ensure whether fracture exists; b) to determine whether it is pathologic fracture; c) to know displacement of fracture; d) to decide effect of treatment after reposition, to observe healing and complications, and to remove pathological fracture. Radiography is the primary method for diagnosis of fracture, while CT is better for complex structure. MRI is prior to injury of cartilage and soft tissue.

(1) Fracture

Fracture is a complete or incomplete break in the continuity of bone or cartilage, which usually occurs in long bones and spine.

[**Pathology and clinical manifestations**]

After fracture, hemorrhage around fracture is fundamental for healing. Patients generally have obvious traumatic history, local continuous pain, swelling, dysfunction, and sometimes deformity may be present.

[**Imaging appearances**]

1) Radiography

It is the first choice to examine bone fracture. (Fig 9-1-8-A/B)

①***Appearance and classification***: The break or incontinuity of a bone often shows as an irregular translucent line, called fracture line, which is usually clear in cortex and shows interruption, distortion, and displacement of trabecular bone in spongy bone.

Depending on whether the fracture line is complete or not, bone fractures can be divided into complete and incomplete fracture; according to the direction of fracture line, they can be divided into transverse fractures, oblique fractures, spiral fractures, etc.; according to fracture line shape, complex fractures can be divided into T-shape, Y-shape, etc.; according to bone chips and the relationships between fracture fragments, they can be divided into avulsed fractures, embedded fractures, compressed fractures, and comminuted fractures. Embedded fractures appear that the fracture fragments are embedded into each other, which occur more often in femoral neck. They appear as irregular high density bands, and may be misdiagnosed.

While in radiography, the x-ray should be perpendicular to the wound site and parallel to the fracture fragments, so that the fracture line is clear.

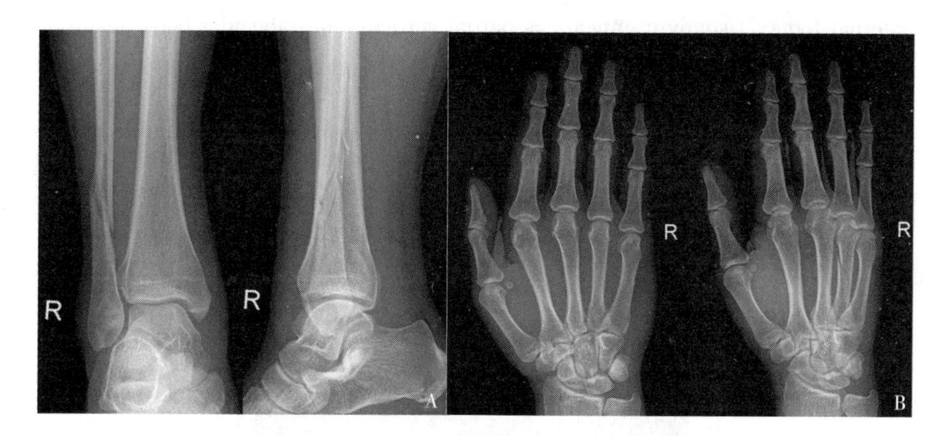

Fig 9-1-8-A/B

Oblique fracture in tibia, with good fracture alignment and contraposition

angulated fracture in the fifth metacarpal bone

② ***Fracture displacement***: proximal fracture fragment is used to determine the shifting of the distal fracture displacement, such as inward or outward, forward or backward. Fracture sites may be overlapped or separated from each other. Sometimes the two fracture fragments can form an angulation, which is called angulated displacement. In addition, fractures can also appear as rotating displacement: the distal fragment rotates inward or outward around the longitudinal axis of bone.

Fracture alignment and contraposition: poor alignment and contraposition appear when there is inward, outward, forward or backward fracture displacement or angulated displacement. The frontal view and lateral view should be taken at least in radiography. Observing alignment and contraposition of fractures is very important for diagnosis and prognosis.

③***Fractures in children***: epiphyseal fracture often occurs in long bones of children. Epiphyseal cartilage does not develop on radiography. When there is epiphyseal injury, the epiphysis displaces with metaphysis as the distance increases, and it is called epiphyseal separations. (Fig 9-1-9) In a bigger child the failure pattern resulting from this type of stress is more likely to create a metaphyseal fragment. Children's skeleton is flexible; therefore it is not easy to break by external force. Usually it appears as partial cortical and trabecular bone distortion only, without fracture line but sunken or bulged cortical bone, and it is called Greenstick fracture. (Fig 9-1-10-A/B)

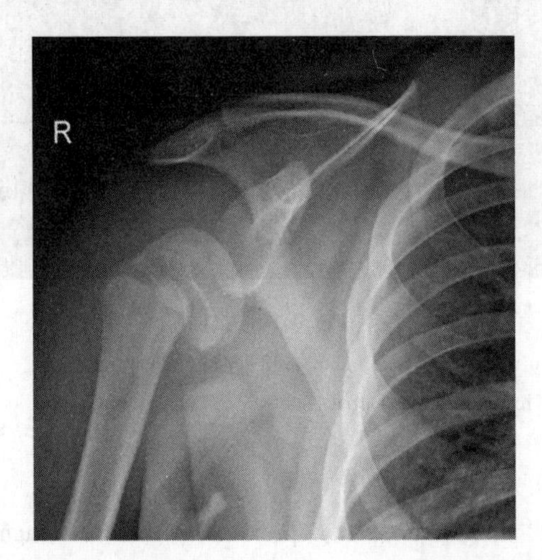

Fig 9-1-9 Epiphyseal fracture of humeral head with dislocation of shoulder joint at the same time.

④***Healing of fracture***: After fracture, hemorrhage is formed around

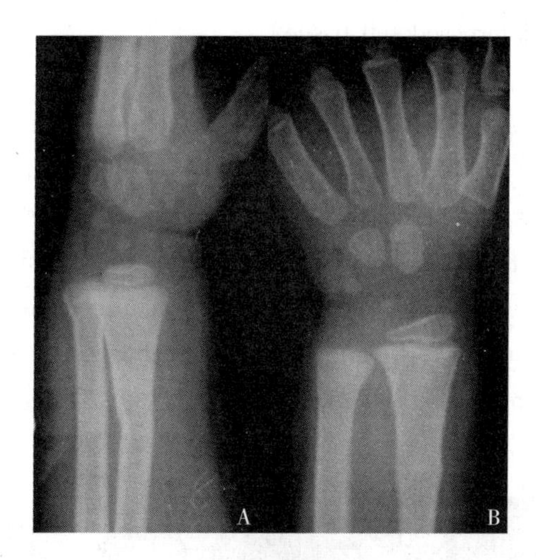

Fig 9-1-10-A/B

Greenstick fracture in radius.

fracture fragments and in bone marrow cavity. Two or three days later, hemorrhage organizes and forms fibrous callus, and then changes into osseous callus. Fracture line is blurred and indistinct on radiography, and osseous callus is seen.

With the formation and growth of callus, the fracture line disappears and fracture healing is finished. Fracture healing rate is related to many factors, like age, fracture type, fracture position, nutritional status and treatment, etc. Normally, the fracture fragments unite more rapidly in children fractures, muscle-rich region fractures, and embedded fractures; while slowly in elderly fractures, intra-articular fractures, serious fracture displacement, poor nutritional status or concurrent infection.

⑤***Common complications of fractures***: Complications of fractures include un-union or delayed union; deformity of union; osteoporosis after trauma; infection of bone and joint; hemorrhagic necrosis of bone; degeneration of joint; ossifying myositis, etc. Faulty healing of fractures results in non-union, which is more common in the femoral neck and the shaft of humerus. The non-united fragments soon become atrophic and osteoporotic owing to disuse and there is usually a point of false motion at the junction of the fragments, which may be separated by a wide mass of interposed soft tissue.

2) CT

It is not used as a routine examination for fractures, but it's preferred for the spine, facial bone and pelvis, as well as joints like hip, shoulder, knee, wrist, etc. in order to facilitate the display of complex or overlapping bone structures, and ensure the number and location of fracture fragments. Three-dimensional reconstruction technique can display the fracture stereoscopically. In addition, CPR reconstruction technique is helpful in diagnosing occult fractures and costobrachial fractures. (Fig 9-1-11-A/B)

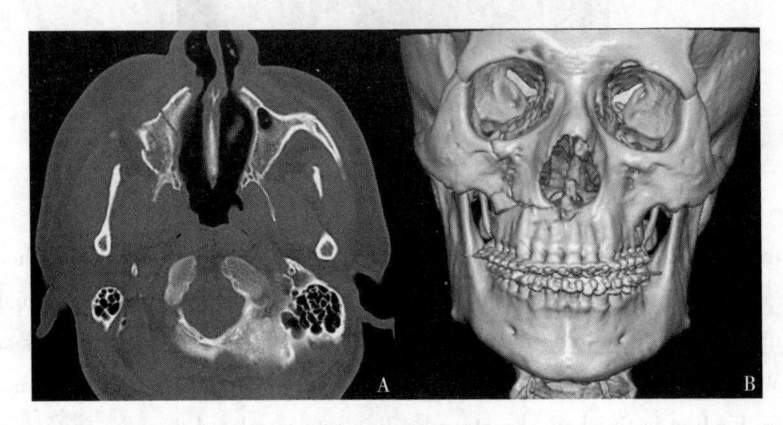

Fig 9-1-11-A/B

A: CT axial view: upper maxillary fracture.

B: SSD reconstruction: more intuitive to show the fracture line.

3) MRI

Fracture line is hypointensity in MRI image, and MRI image shows clearly hemorrhage, edema and soft tissue injury around the fracture fragment, as well as the damage of organs and tissues nearby. Bone marrow edema can be seen as long T1 and long T2 echo time. The value of MRI for bone trauma mainly lies in showing bone bruise, occult fracture, cartilage fracture, and determining whether it is a pathologic fracture. (Fig 9-1-12-A/B)

Bone bruise includes trabecular bone fracture, bone marrow edema, hemorrhage caused by external force, and often shows no abnormal findings on radiography and CT images. It appears blurred hypointensity in T1-weighted images and high signal in fat-suppression T2-weighted imaging, and is generally confined to the area of action of external force.

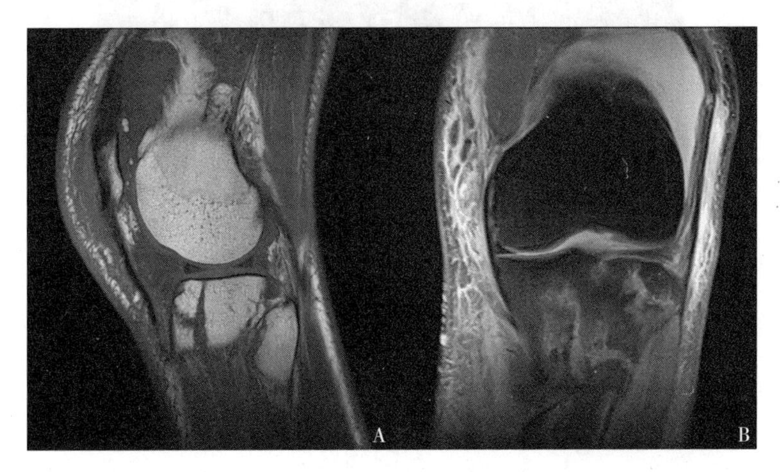

Fig 9-1-12-A/B

A: T1WI: fracture line in tibia is hypointensity.

B: T2WI: bone marrow edema is high signal.

[**Diagnosis**]

When the fracture line appears, combined with the history of injury, fracture can be diagnosed. In addition, the adjacent bone should be taken notice that whether there is destruction to exclude pathological fractures. Sometimes bone fractures overlap or have no displacement, so that radiography is useless to display them. CT and (or) MRI can be chosen to show the occult fractures and bone bruise. When the fracture is indeterminate on radiography for the first time, review is needed after 1 week.

(2) Common long bone fractures

①***Colles fracture***: A transverse or comminuted fracture occurs in 2~3cm distal radius, with dorsal displacement and angulation of the distal radial fragment. The malalignment is classically described as a "silver fork" deformity. (Fig 9-1-13)

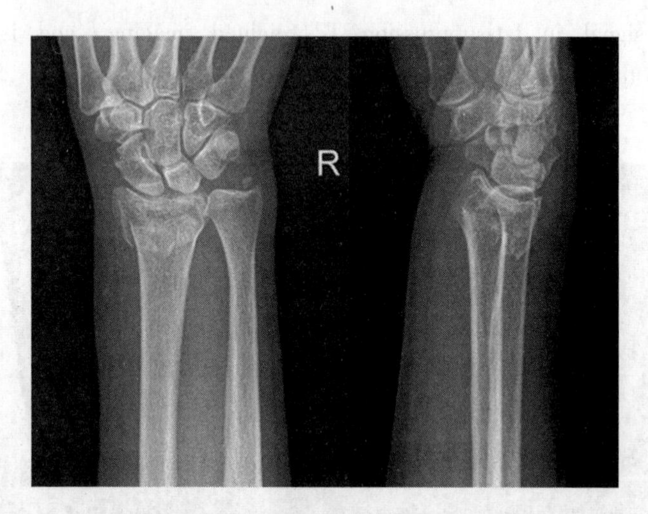

Fig 9-1-13 Colles fracture

②***Epicondylar fracture of humerus***: It occurs more often in children. Fracture line appears across the coronoid fossa and olecranon fossa of humerus, with dorsal displacement of the distal fragment.

③***Femur neck fracture***: It occurs in the collum femoris of old women, usually with displacement and bone fragment embedded. The fracture fragments unite slowly because of the poor blood supply, and ischemic necrosis of femoral head may occur in serious cases.

[**Imaging appearances**]

Radiography

Fracture line is easily seen in Colles fracture and epicondylar fracture of humerus. Fracture displacement and angulated change are also clear on radiography. But 10% of femur neck fractures are indeterminate because of the bone fragments embedded. In this case, a further CT or MRI examination is needed.

(3) Facture of vertebrae

[Pathology and clinical manifestations]

The patient always has a traumatic history of falling down from high place. The most common sites are lower (C5~C6) cervical spines and the thoracolumbar junctions (T11~L2), with single vertebrae fracture usually. The patient may has swelling, pain, dysfunction and some symptoms due to injury of nerve or spinal cord.

[Imaging appearances]

1) Radiography

There are three types of vertebrae fractures as follows:

①***Simple compression fracture***: the vertebrae is wedge-shaped without fracture line; the front edge of vertebrae is shortened; it appears as irregular transverse band shadow. The upper and lower intervertebral spaces generally remain normal.

②***Burst fracture of spine***: a comminuted fracture caused by compression from the vertical; the vertebrae is flattened. CT is the preferred examination.

③***Fracture and dislocation***: there is vertebral dislocation besides fracture, with zygapophysial joints displaced. Sometimes free fracture fragments can be seen in vertebral canal. (Fig 9-1-14-A/B)

2) CT

MSCT and post-processing techniques are helpful in determining the classification of vertebrae fracture and displacement of fracture fragments; showing the deformation, stricture of vertebral canal, and bone fragments inside; and diagnosing spinal injury. Fractures of appendix of vertebra and dislocation of articulations are also easily displayed in CT images.

3) MRI

MRI is better than radiography and CT in displaying bone bruise, intervertebral disc injury, ligamentous injury and spinal cord compression, etc., and is of great help for the operation treatment and prognosis.

①***Intervertebral disc injury***: acute injury appears hypointensity on T1WI and high signal on T2WI.

②***Ligamentous injury***: normal spinal ligaments appear hypointensity,

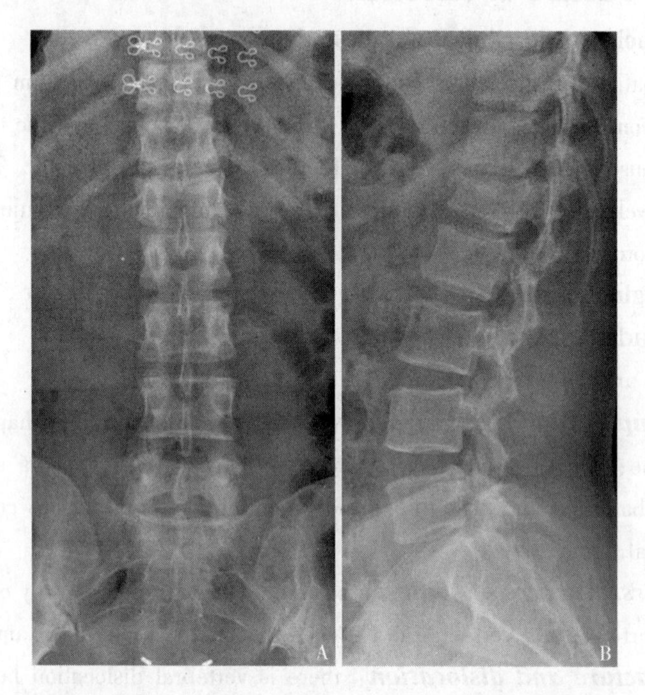

Fig 9-1-14-A/B Simple compression fracture: L1 is wedge-shaped

including anterior longitudinal ligament, posterior longitudinal ligament, interspinal ligament and interspinous ligament, etc. After injury, the hypointensity shadow is discontinuous and appears high signal in T2WI fat-suppression images.

[**Diagnosis**]

Based on the history of injury and appearance of deformation, it is not difficult to diagnose bone fractures and vertebrae fractures. Spinal traumatic fractures should be differentiated from fractures caused by osteoporosis, vertebral tuberculosis and metastasis. These lesions may have vertebral osteoporosis, intervertebral space narrowing or disappearance, paravertebral abscess or soft tissue mass. Combined with the clinical history, it is usually not difficult to identify them.

(4) Protrusion of Intervertebral Disc (Discal Herniation)

[**Pathology and clinical manifestations**]

Discal herniation often occurs in middle-aged people, and mainly in males, with traumatic or chronic injury history. The intervertebral disc consists of annulus fibrosis, nucleus pulposus, and vertebral end plates. The most common site is lower lumbar intervertebral disc. The anulus fibrosus is thinnest at the posterior part, so the nucleus pulposus always protrudes backward. The protruded nucleus pulposus can oppress the adjacent tissue and nerve root, causing the clinical symptoms. Traumatic disc injuries which produce annular tears or vertebral end plate damage may cause painful symptoms.

[**Imaging appearances**]

1) Radiography

Plain film is limited in the diagnosis of discal herniation. However, some special signs on plain film may suggest of probable diagnosis:

Intervertebral space is asymmetrically narrowed, especially the anterior part. Posterior and lateral marginal vertebral body osteophytes are often present due to degenerative changes. Displacement or herniation of portions of a degenerating intervertebral disc into the spinal canal can be associated with gas formation in both the disc and the canal (vacuum phenomenon). Protrusion of intervertebral disc material through a break in the subchondral bone plate, with displacement of this material into the vertebral body, leading to an abnormal contour of the spine on radiographs, is referred to as Schmorl's nodes. Radiographically, Schmorl's nodes appear as a radiolucent lesion within the vertebral body surrounded by helmet-shaped sclerosis that borders on the intervertebral disc.

2) CT

On CT, density of intevertebral disc is lower than that of vertebral body and higher than that of spinal capsule. According to deformation degree of intevertebral disc, discal bulge, extrusion and sequestration are all forms of herniation.

CT scan can be used to identify symmetric uniform degenerative changes of the disc that result in a diffuse annular disc bulge, seen as diffuse peripheral extension of disc material. The margin of the annular bulge usually is uniform and smooth in contour but may be asymmetric, whereas a disk protrusion is a posterior circumscribed bulge of the disk, central or eccentrical. Calcification of intervertebral discs may occur in many discal herniations. (Fig 9-1-15)

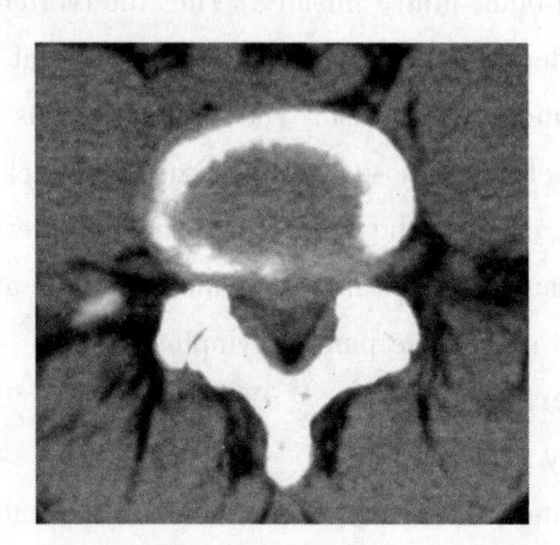

Fig 9-1-15 Plain CT

A distinct protrusion on the posterior part with dural sac and spinal cord Compressed.

In addition, indirect signs sometimes may suggest of diagnosis, for example, epidural layer of fatty tissue may be compressed, deformed, or even disappear; dural sac or ipsilateral sheath of nerve root may be compressed, and so on. But CT has less value in diagnosing cervical discal herniation than diagnosing lumber discal herniation.

3) MRI

MRI currently is the criterion standard imaging modality for detection of disc pathology. (Fig 9-1-16)

The annulus fibrosis contains 75% water in the first decade of life and 70%~80% water in adults. Degeneration of the intervertebral disc results in diminished signal intensity on T1WI and T2WI of MRI. These signal intensity changes result from diminished water and glycosaminoglycan content and increased collagen content of the intervertebral disc. Sagittal images provide the best visualization of loss in intervertebral disc height. Bulging or protruding of the disc annulus appears as a hemicycle or triangle hypointensity signal shadow ante-

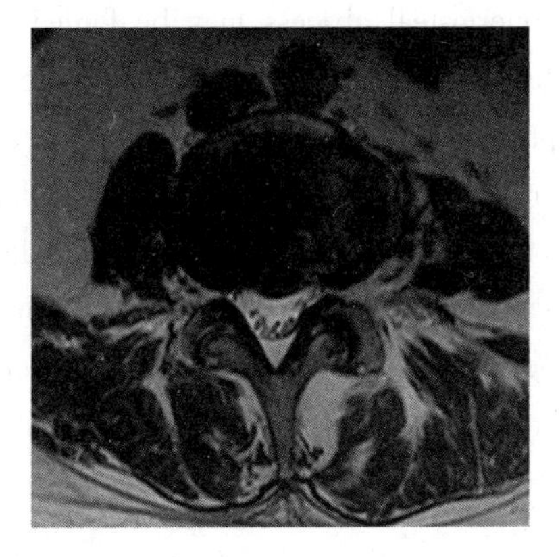

Fig 9-1-16 T2WI

The appearance is similar to CT, but the protrusion is not serious.

rior of dura mater in both axial and sagittal images. MRI has an advantage in showing compressed spinal nerve and spinal cord.

2 Infectious diseases of bones

(1) Pyogenic Osteomyelitis

Pyogenic osteomyelitis is caused by *Staphylococcus aureus* entering bone marrow. Three main routes of infection include hematogenous metastasis, directly spreading from a primary staphylococcal lesion around bone, and open fracture or firearm injury.

Acute Pyogenic Osteomyelitis

[**Pathology and clinical manifestations**]

Typical clinical signs are as follows: acute high-fever and conspicuous toxic symptom, motion disorder and deeper pain, local red swelling and tenderness.

The commonest route of spread is by direct extension through the haversian canals of the overlying cortex to the subperiosteal space, where the periosteum is lifted off the cortex by the formation of a subperiosteal abscess. The periosteum itself then may rupture, with extrusion of the infection into the overlying soft tissues. Pus from the subperiosteal abscess may be forced back into the medulla and set up secondary foci of infection in the marrow tissues. The articular tissues may be infected by rupture of the periosteum when the metaphysis is intracapsular or by extension through the epiphyseal plate into the cartilage and hence onto the synovial. The metaphysis, the medullary canal in the middle of the shaft, the epiphysis and the cortex may be infected singly or in combination, concurrently or at intervals. Repair begins with localization of the infection and the reduction of intra-osseous and subperiosteal tension. The dead segment or sequestrum may be completely detached and discharged. Large sequestrums may persist until removed surgically.

[**Imaging appearances**]

1) Radiography

Plain radiographs should always be the first step in the imaging assessment of osteomyelitis, because they may provide clues for other pathologic conditions. The earliest sign is the deep soft tissue swelling. Further swelling involves the muscles and the superficial subcutaneous soft tissues. Regional soft tissue swelling near the site of bone tenderness and pain is the only evidence of infection of the underlying bone within 2 weeks.

Bone destruction and periosteal reaction may be obvious but only 10 to 21 days after the onset of the disease. The first roentgen signs in the bone are local osteoporosis and one or more small shadows of diminished density at or near the end of the shaft caused by foci of bone necrosis. Pathologic fracture may occur because of the osteopenic early bone.

After the 2nd or 3rd week periosteal reaction shows a strip of increased density outside and parallel to the shaft.

Sequestrum usually casts a denser shadow compared to the diminished density of the surrounding bones.

2) CT

CT is better than radiography in showing the infection of soft tissue, subperiosteal abscess, inflammation of marrow cavity, as well as destruction of bone and sequestrums, particularly a small lesion.

3) MRI

Findings by MRI truly reflect the pathologic process. In early osteomyelitis the edema and exudate of the medullary space account for the ill-defined low signal intensity in T1-weighted images and the high signal in T2-weighted images. Poorly defined soft tissue planes, lack of cortex thickening, and poor interface between normal and abnormal marrows are good predictors of early osteomyelitis. MRI is the best in assurance of invasion of marrow cavity and infection of soft tissue.

Chronic Pyogenic Osteomyelitis

[**Pathology and clinical manifestations**]

After acute phase, the fistula may always discharge pus due to the existence of pus cavity or sequestrum.

It has a more insidious presentation, with on and off mild fever and some focal pain. This may be related to prior antibiotic therapy or to a less virulent pathogen.

[**Imaging appearance**]

1) Radiography

There is a predominant bone sclerosis, with periosteal apposition. Sinus tracts may be present. There is destruction as well as new bone formation. As a result of periosteal new bone formation, the bone is deformed and increased in density.

2) CT and MRI

CT is best in assessing bone details (e. g., cavity and sequestrum).

MRI shows any soft tissue abnormality, thickened cortex, and focally diseased marrow. Differential diagnosis of chronic osteomyelitis includes mainly bone neoplasms.

2 Tuberculosis of bone

Tuberculosis of bone is a chronic secondary TB characteristic for destruction of bone and osteoporosis, more common in children and adolescents. Hematogenous spread of tubercle bacilli to the skeleton may take place early during the active phase of the primary complex in the thorax or later from post-primary tuberculous foci. Tuberculosis of bone prefers to involving cartilage and causing local bone destruction, sometimes a cold abscess.

[**Pathology and clinical manifestations**]

Lesions may be present for a number of years without showing progression until trauma occurs to produce recrudescence. The presenting symptoms and signs usually depend on the stage of the disease. Acute symptoms are rare. Swelling, mild pain, weakness, and dysfunction are some clinical manifestations.

TB pathological changes include three components, one is a kind of exudative lesion, having large macrophage and neutrophil, another one is hypertrophic lesion, having many tuberculous granulomas, and the last one is caseating necrotic lesion, having large caseating necrosis areas. Healing occurs by fibrosis, calcification, and even ossification. Clinical symptoms and imaging features are compacted with pathological features.

[**Imaging appearance**]

1) Radiography

①***The tuberculosis of tubulous bone***: The initial focus of infection is generally the epiphysis and/or metaphysic (Fig 9-1-17). A small focal area of osteolysis located eccentrically in the metaphysis with little or no surrounding os-

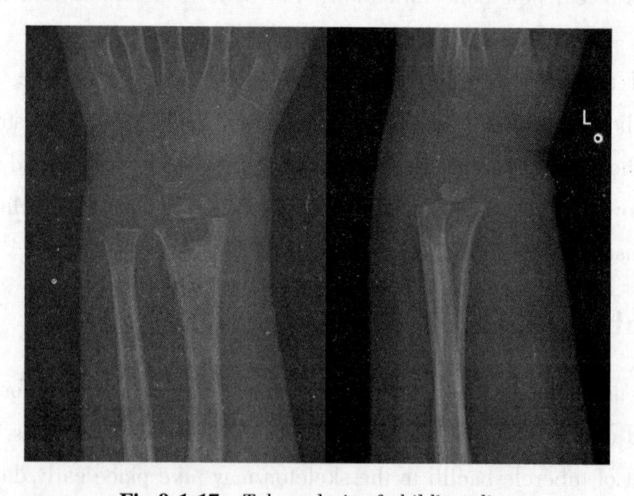

Fig 9-1-17 Tuberculosis of child's radius

teosclerosis and periosteal reaction is characteristic, and the margins of lesion usually are defined but not very clear-cut. The presence of osteopenia helps to diagnose tuberculosis and to differentiate it from infection by pyogenic organisms. Sequestration is less common in tuberculosis than in pyogenic infection. Sequestra if present are tiny irregular structureless particles only slightly more dense than the surrounding bones. Chronically draining sinuses are common. On occasion, a large soft tissue mass is present out of proportion to the depth of bone destruction with extensive periosteal reaction.

Extension of focal area of osteolysis to the epiphysis is present with the development of the lesion, then causing articular TB, but seldom metaphyseal focus extending into diaphysis.

TB is seldom in the diaphysis, and a lytic area often occurs in the mid-shaft of a short tubular bone of the hands and feet, particularly children younger than 5. It may produce fusiform enlargement of the entire diaphysis. The shaft of the involved phalanges may be broader than normal, giving rise to an expanded new bony shell (spina ventosa-swelling of the shaft).

②***Tuberculosis of spine***: Lesions in the axial skeleton are more common than lesions of the peripheral skeleton. Involvement of the vertebral body is more common than that of the posterior appendages, such as spinous and transverse processes, and more lesions may be seen on the lumbar vertebrae.

More often the infection originates at the articular margin and involves the intervertebral disc, often spreading through one disc to adjacent vertebrae. Therefore, it commences with erosion of the disc surfaces; usually two adjacent vertebra show equal changes. The normal disc surface of a vertebral body appears as a hard white line. The erosive change removes this line.

Narrowing of the disc constitutes one of the most important and early diagnostic features. It serves to differentiate the condition from fracture, malignant disease, osteomyelitis and osteoporotic collapse of the vertebral body.

Paravertebral abscess occurs in about 95% of cases. It may be unilateral or bilateral and may assume any shape. Cold abscess formation in the cervical region appears as widening of the retropharyngeal soft tissue shadow, in the thoracic region as spindle-shaped paravertebral soft tissue shadow, and in the lumbar region as widened shadow of psoas muscle.

2) CT

CT has been of great value in the early detection of soft tissue masses and calcifications, which are not easily identified in routine radiographs. CT can show the narrowing of vertebral canal due to the backward protrusion of vertebral body and may have ring-shaped intensification after contrast, yet CT helps finding epidural abscess. (Fig 9-1-18-A/B)

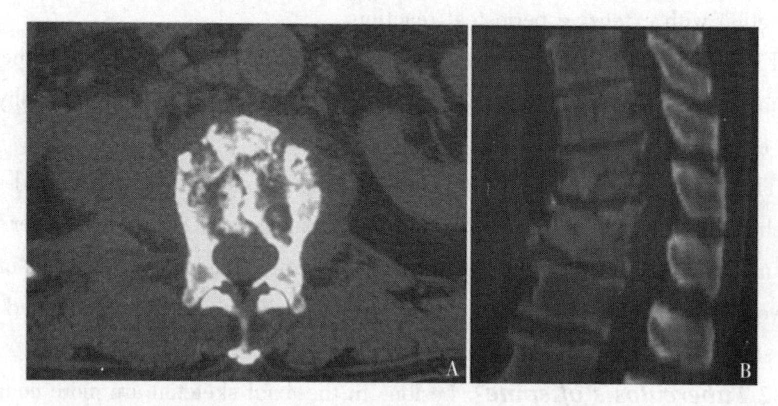

Fig 9-1-18-A/B Axial view and sagittal MPR:
Soft tissue masses surrounding the destructed vertebra

3) MRI

The destructive area shows low signal on T1WI and high signal on T2WI, and the same as the adjacent marrow due to edema. (Fig 9-1-19-A/B)

Narrowing of the disc and destructive spinal margin. Destructive area shows hypointensity on T1WI, and the same as paravertebral abscess.

3 Tumor and tumor-like diseases

The diagnosis of bone tumors is an important issue as it is mainly seen in young males, although unusual, representing 1% of all body malignant tumors.

Radiology is an essential tool to diagnose bone tumors, which can show their location, sizes, changes of adjacent bones and soft tissues as well as their fea-

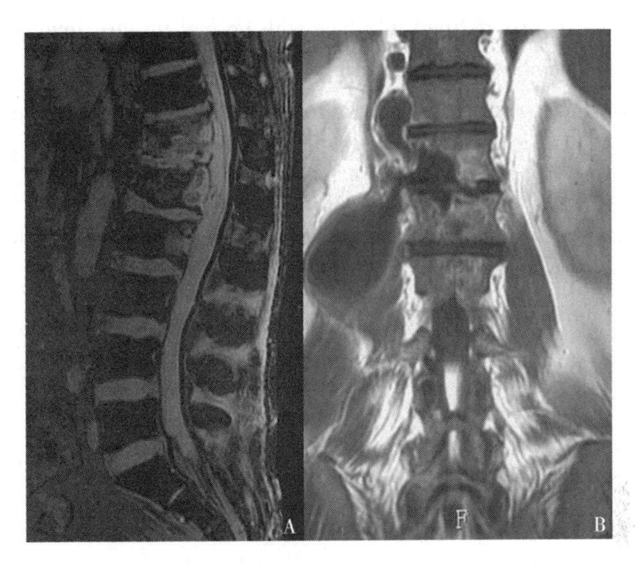

Fig 9-1-19-A/B Sagittal and coronal T2WI

tures. Due to its variety of imaging characteristics, accurate diagnosis is based on clinical, radiographic identification and experimental information, combined with pathology.

The requirements of bone tumor imaging diagnosis are as follows:

a) Tumor or not? b) If a tumor, benign or malignant, primary or metastatic? c) Histological type; and d) Invasive areas.

In the imaging evaluation of a suspected bone lesion, information about lesion location, number, osseous change, periosteal reaction and soft tissue changes should be provided.

(1) Differentiation between benign and malignant tumors

①***Biological behavior***: Benign tumor usually grows slowly; results in no invasion to surrounding structures but dislocation; no metastases may present. Malignant tumor is usually with rapid growth; invasion to surrounding structures with metastases.

②***Bone changes***: Benign tumor may appear as bulky destruction with clear margin to normal structure; thinning cortex usually is preserved but contiguous with surrounding normal tissue. Malignant tumor usually appears as infiltrative destruction; poorly defined interface with normal tissue; involvement of cortex is sometimes combined with a variety of new bone formation.

③ ***Periosteal reaction***: Benign tumor is usually with no periosteal reaction or a little after pathological fracture; no interruption to periosteal reaction is present. Malignant tumor is usually associated with different kinds of periosteal reactions and may be interrupted to form "Codman triangle".

④***Soft tissue***: No soft tissue swelling; no mass or mass with clear margin is present in benign tumor. While invading soft tissue and forming mass within the soft tissue, its interface with surrounding tissues is poorly defined, and it is usually present in malignant tumor.

(2) Benign bone tumors

Giant Cell Tumors of Bone

[**Pathology and clinical manifestations**]

The tumor is usually found in the ends of long bones and particularly at the knee joint and lower end of the radius. The usual age of onset is 20 to 40.

[**Imaging appearance**]

1) Radiography

Tumor is usually eccentric and destructive (osteolytic). The rarefaction produced by the tumor is due to the destruction of the cancellous network. The tumor is expansive and radiolucent and extends to the articular end of a long bone. The edge is poorly defined without a margin of sclerosis demarcating the tumor. Within the area of rarefaction there may be septa. The trabeculated, soap-bubble-like appearance may be present within the area of rarefaction, whereas absence indicates rapid growth. Despite tumoral extension, the periosteal new bone reaction is limited or absent. (Fig 9-1-20)

Anteroposterior and lateral positions of the knee: an osteolytic eccentric lesion extending to the articular end of femur with lower density; the edge is poorly defined without a margin of sclerosis.

Pathologic fractures may develop in large lesions, particularly those in weight-bearing bones.

2) CT

The destructive area appears as density of soft tissue, or even lower density

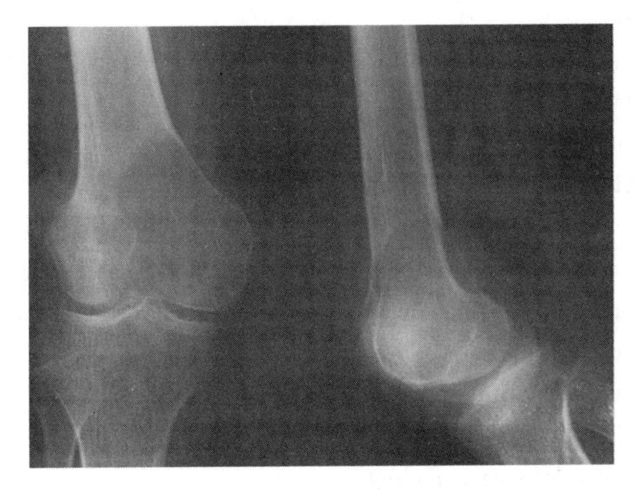

Fig 9-1-20 Giant cell tumor

due to necrosis, without calcification and ossification. Obvious intensification is seen after contrast administration.

3) MRI

The tumor shows hypointense or isointense signal on T1WI and usually hyperintense on T2WI.

Bone cysts

[**Pathology and clinical manifestations**]

The tumor is usually found in the metaphysis of long bones and particularly at the proximal ends of femur and humerus. It often occurs in adolescents without symptoms.

[**Imaging appearance**]

1) Radiography

It appears as round or oval translucent area, and may develop along the longitudinal axis of original bone; the bone cortex is thinner with regular border without any periosteal reaction.

2) CT

The destructed area appears as density of water, without intensification after contrast administration.

3) MRI

The tumor shows hypointensity on T1WI and hyperintensity on T2WI.

(3) Malignant bone tumors

Osteosarcoma

[**Pathology and clinical manifestations**]

This occurs mainly in children and adolescents. The prognosis is not good. The term "osteogenic" indicates an origin from tissues capable of forming bones. The site of predilection is the metaphysis of a long bone. The commonest region locates near the knee joint.

[**Imaging appearance**]

1) Radiography

A mass in soft tissue is present.

Periosteal reaction: parallel layers: the formation of a layer or layers of periosteal reaction may be an early indication of neoplasm. A characteristic of many tumors is the reactive triangle or periosteal cuff near the edge of the mass (Codman's triangle). This is due to the absorption of periosteal bone at the center of the tumor. Sunray spicules: this kind of periosteal reaction is often regarded as a characteristic of osteosarcoma.

For easy description, it is divided into osteolytic and osteoblastic forms artificially.

①***Osteolysis***: The early osteolytic tumor presents a difficult problem as the sclerotic form is easier to recognize.

②***Osteosclerosis***: Sclerosis of bone may be central or unilateral, and patchy or diffuse. And the patchy one is usually situated in the medulla. Some sclerotic lesions involve the whole medulla and cortex. They obliterate all bone structures and cause increase in density (Fig 9-1-21).

Pathological fracture may occur in osteolytic type of osteogenic sarcoma.

2) CT

CT can be helpful locally when the radiographic appearances are confusing, particularly in areas of anatomy complex. Clearer bone destruction and extent of any soft-tissue mass is obtained in cross-sectional images than radiographs. CT can depict small amounts of mineralized osseous matrix not seen on radiographs.

It is particularly helpful in flat bones in which periosteal changes can be more difficult to indicate.

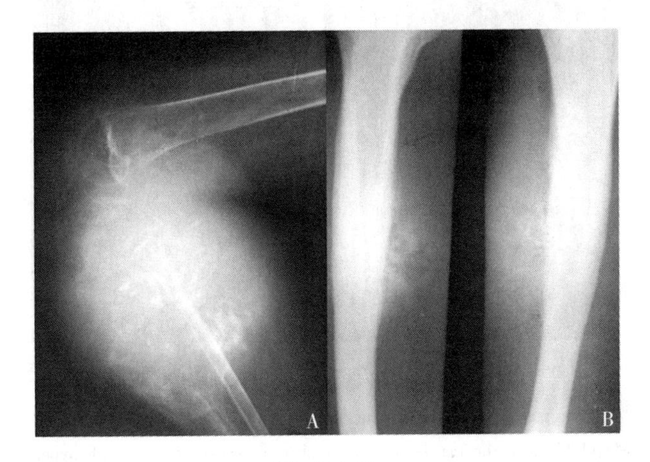

Fig 9-1-21

A patchy destructive area with irregular osteoblast formation; periosteal reaction as sunray spicules; soft tissue mass.

3) MRI

MRI is a suitable choice in staging of musculoskeletal lesions. Its multiplanar capability and soft tissue contrast allows accurate determination of the intraosseous extent of tumor, cortical disruption, adjacent soft tissue mass, or articular invasion.

MRI is the most important imaging technique for accurately evaluating local stage of osteosarcoma and assisting in determining the most appropriate surgical management. For the purposes of staging, assessment of the relationship of a tumor to the anatomic compartment in which it originated is of vital importance.

Most osteosarcomas indicate irregular inhomogeneous iso-intensity on T1WI and hyper-intensity on T1WI with ill-defined margin. (Fig 9-1-22-A/B)

Bone metastasis

Metastatic tumor of bone is the most common of all malignant bone tumors, which is transmitted from distant primary cancer or sarcoma by way of the blood vessels.

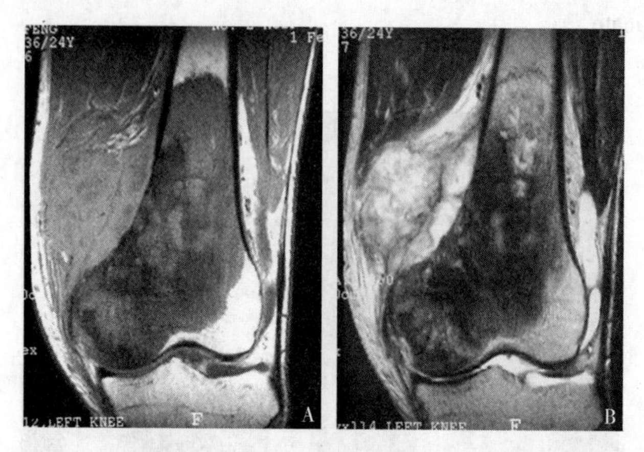

Fig 9-1-22-A/B Coronal T1WI and T2WI

A large patchy irregular destruction with nonuniform hypointense signal on T1WI and T2WI in the marrow cavity, and a circumjacent mass with hypointense signal on T1WI and hyperintense signal on T2WI.

[**Pathology and clinical manifestations**]

In skeletal metastasis, the malignant neoplasm spreads to osseous structures. The skeleton is a frequent site of metastasis, while the most common sites are the spine, bones of the pelvis, ribs, sternum, femoral and humeral shafts, and skull. The primary lesions involved most frequently are carcinoma of the breast, lung, thyroid gland, prostate and kidney. Patients often have bone tenderness, a soft tissue mass, and deformity.

[**Imaging appearance**]

1) Radiography

Bone response to metastasis can be classified broadly as bone resorption or bone formation, with the radiographic patterns described as purely osteolytic, purely osteosclerotic, and mixed osteolytic and osteosclerotic, with purely osteolytic being the most common.

Long bone osteolytic lesions are often located in backbone or metaphysis nearby, manifesting with worm eclipse-like defection in cancellous bone. When the lesions develop, the range of destruction is enlarging, the cortex is also invaded from the medulla. The involved bone may undergo pathological fracture, but frequently may be not associated with periosteal thickening. Involvement of the spine may show destruction of pedicle and vertebral body. Metastasis to the body will cause compression of the body to form a wedge-shaped deformity but the intervertebral disc is intact.

Osteosclerotic lesions are less common. It usually comes from carcinoma of prostate, breast, lung or bladder. It is located in cancellous bone with patches or nodules, appearing with high and homogeneous density. It has intact cortex but poorly defined interface with normal tissue. The lesions are frequently multiple, and the spine and bones of the pelvis are the common sites. It is without vertebral body deformity (Fig 9-1-23). Mixed osteolytic and osteosclerotic lesions often cause the above two bone changes.

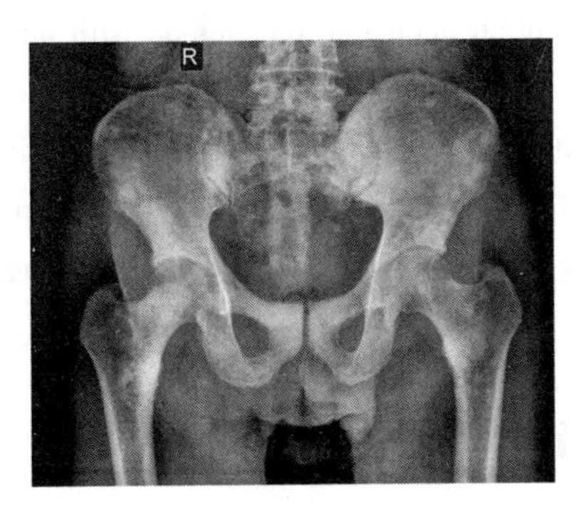

Fig 9-1-23

Prostate carcinomawith bone metastasis

2) CT

CT is more sensitive than radiography in showing the skeletal metastasis. It can also show more details such as range, size and relationship with adjacent organs, especially on the peripheral soft tissue. Osteolytic metastasis shows decreased density defection area in cancellous and (or) cortex bone on CT. Its margin is clear and without sclerosis. It is frequently with small soft tissue masses. Osteosclerotic metastasis shows increased density lesion in cancellous bone, with patchy, lamellar cotton-ball like or nodose shape. It is frequently without soft tissue masses, rarely with periosteal reaction. Mixed osteolytic and osteosclerotic lesions often cause the above two bone changes.

3) MRI

MRI is very sensitive in showing tumor tissues in marrow with fat compositions and adjacent edema. So it can detect lesions, while radiography, CT or radionuclide imaging can not. Furthermore, it can detect skeletal metastasis without obvious destruction of bone. It can also determine the amount, size, and distribution of tumors and whether adjacent tissues are involved. It can provide reliable information for prompt clinical diagnosis or prognosis appraisal. On T1WI, metastasis lesions are of low signal intensity, obviously with high signal intensity of the marrow; on T2WI, they are of inviable high signal intensity; in fat-suppression sequences, lesions are accurately depicted.

[**Diagnosis**]

Skeletal metastasis often occurs in old person with multiple lesions. It is not common with periosteal thickening or soft tissue mass when long bone is invaded. It rarely invades bone below knee or elbow joints. According to these characters, primary tumors and metastasis can be differentiated. When lesions are not typical or tumors are in earlier period, MRI or radionuclide imaging should be considered.

Lesson 2 Joints

Section 1 Imaging methods

The joints of body can be classified as three types: fibrous joints or synarthroses, cartilaginous joints or amphiarthroses, and synovial joints. The synovial joint is a movable articulation, such as the articulation of arms and legs. This kind of articulation includes three parts: capitulum, articular cartilage, and joint capsule. The bony articular surface of the capitulum is covered with hyaline cartilage. The hyaline cartilage can protect the bony articular surface, but it cannot regenerate when the hyaline cartilage has been destructed. There are various radiographic examinations to evaluate the joint diseases. The essential and most common method is radiography. Computed tomography, magnetic resonance imaging and digital subtraction angiography are widely used. The purposes of radiographic examinations of joints are detecting the joint disease, determining the extent and severity of the lesions, assessing the activity of joint disease, choosing the appropriate methods of treatments, evaluating the therapeutic efficacy, and finding the complications. Establishing the etiology diagnosis of joint diseases must take clinical manifestations and laboratory parameters into consideration.

1 Radiography

Radiography is the first choice to evaluate the joint diseases in routine work. It is the foundation of other imaging examinations. Bone substance, because of its calcium content and its high density, differs from the surrounding soft tissues and thus its image on a film is full of contrast and detail. This is the advantage of radiography. The joint capsule, the ligament and the articular cartilage, because of the lack of natural contrast, are invisible on radiography, and this is the disadvantage of it. The basic principle for radiography of joint is the same as skeletal system examination.

2 Digital subtraxtion angiography (DSA)

DSA is applied to diagnose the tumors and vascular abnormalities. It is an invasive examination. Its use is uncommon.

3 Arthrography

Arthrography is an examination by injecting some negative or positive media into the articular cavity to display the intra-articular structures. It is an invasive examination, too. It is often used to evaluate the joint diseases. CT and MRI are applied to study the joint disorders widely, and have replaced it gradually.

4 CT

CT is an essential tool to diagnose the joint diseases. It is a quick, accurate, and un-invasive method. The important characteristics of CT, such as cross-sectional display, excellent density resolution, and the ability to allow the measurement of specific attenuation values, enable CT to gain the obvious advantage over plain film. Therefore, CT is used widely when the lesions are located in complex anatomy regions, where the lesions are more difficult to be detected by conventional radiographs. The scan method includes plain scanning, enhanced scanning, and CT arthrography. Plain CT means scanning without intravenous contrast medium. Enhanced CT indicates scanning with intravenous injection of iodinated contrast medium. There are two main purposes of enhanced CT. One is elevating density difference between the lesion and normal tissue in order to discover the lesion. The other is showing the characteristics of enhancement in order to diagnose accurately. CT arthrography implies the scanning after arthrography. The transaxial scanning and reformation are used commonly. Usually 2 ~ 5mm collimation is adequate after locating on the lateral or coronal scout image. All images should be reviewed at window and center settings appropriate for visualization of both bone and soft tissues.

5 MRI

MRI can reveal the normal structure of joint, such as capitulum, bony articular surface, articular cartilage, joint capsule, tendon, ligament, and fat tissue and soft tissue around the joint. It also can detect the pathologic tissues, such as masses, edema, joint effusion, hemorrhage, and traumatic and degenerative tissues. It is able to show the early changes of lesions. So MRI plays an important and unique role in diagnosis of joint diseases. Using surface coils can increase the signal-noise ratio. MRI is a multi-parameter imaging examination. Spin echo or fast spin echo sequences with T1 and T2 weighting and fat-suppressed sequences are common sequences. MRI is a multi-plane imaging examination. According to the diagnostic requirement, the transaxial, coronal, sagittal and oblique scanning may be selected. The use of intravenous injection of gadolinium-enhanced MRI for the joint lesions can increase the accuracy of diagnosis, and know the characteristics of blood supply of the lesions.

Section 2 Normal imaging findings of joint

1 The articular capitulum and articular cartilage

The cortex of the articular capitulum forms the bony articular surface. It is affluent in calcium content. So it reveals as smooth and regular linear high-density shadow on radiology (Fig 9-2-1-A/B) and CT imaging, and presents low signal zone on all sequences in MRI (Fig 9-2-2-A/B). The medulla of the articular capitulum abounds with fat tissue. It reveals as high signal intensity on both T1WI and T2WI. The articular cartilage that covers the bony articular surface is invisible on radiography and CT. It shows as 1 ~ 6mm middle signal arc on both T1WI and T2WI, and high signal arc on fat suppression sequence. The epiphysis is a mass of chondral bone. It consists of varying amount of ossified and non-ossified cartilage. The proportion is depending on the size of the ossified center. The imaging appearances of non-ossified epiphysis are the same as the articular cartilage.

2 The joint capsule and the ligament

The joint capsule and the ligament are the main structures to maintain the stability and integrality of joint. They consist of fibrous tissues. The joint capsule and the ligament are invisible on radiography. They reveal as soft tissue density on CT imaging, and low signal on all sequences of MRI.

3 The joint space

The joint space reveals as low density space between the opposite capitulum on radiography and CT imaging. It includes the veritable anatomical cavity, the articular-cartilage and a little synovia. So the joint space of a child seems wider than that of an adult. MRI can distinguish the veritable anatomical cavity, the articular cartilage and a little synovia. The synovia displays as thin low signal area on T1WI, and thin high signal area on T2WI.

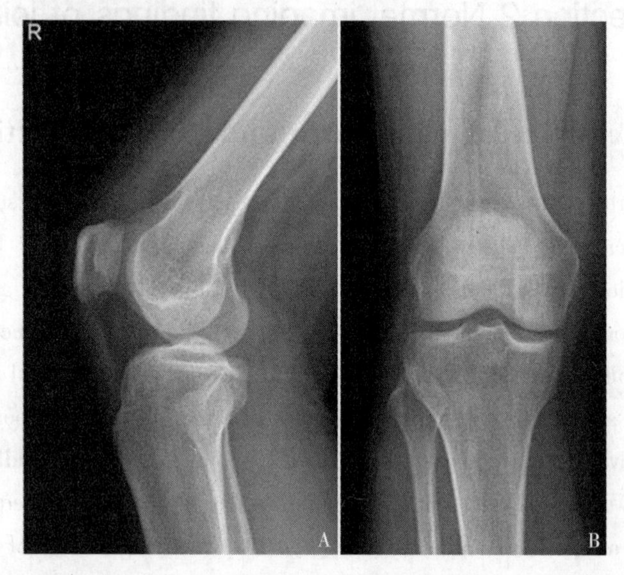

Fig 9-2-1-A/B Radiography of adult joint shows the bony articular surface, joint space, and surrounding soft tissue.

Section 3 Imaging signs of joint diseases

There are several common radiologic signs in joint diseases. We can gain a lot of diagnostic information by analyzing these radiologic signs. These radiologic signs include destruction of joint, changes of joint space, swelling of the joint, ankylosis of joint, and dislocation. They may occur alone or in combination when joint disorders occur.

1 Destruction of joint

It indicates the articular cartilage and the sub-chondral bone have been invaded or replaced by pathologic tissue. When the articular cartilage is involved, the joint space will be narrowed. When the bony articular surface and the sub-bony articular surface are involved, there will be defect or destruction of the bony

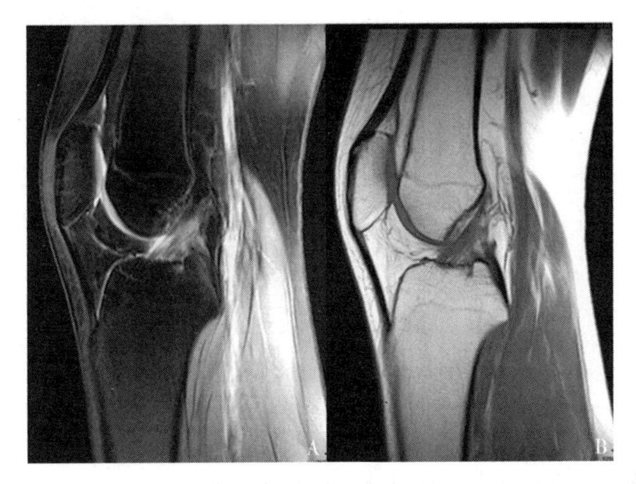

Fig 9-2-2-A/B

MRI T1-weighted image and fat-suppressed T2-weighted image of joint: showing the bony articular surface, subarticular bone, articular cartilage, meniscus, ligaments and the fat pads.

articular surface and sub-bony articular surface. It shows low-density areas of lose bone structure on radiography and CT (Fig 9-2-3, 9-2-4). In MRI image the destruction of spongy bone revealed as the high signal of marrow has been replaced by low signal or mixed signal of pathological tissue; and the destruction of cortex revealed as the low signal of the normal cortex has been replaced by high or mixed signal of pathological tissue. Destruction of joint is the important evidence to diagnose joint diseases. The involved sites may be different according to different etiology. CT can reveal the occult or minute bone destruction more sensitively than plain film; and MRI is superior to CT.

2 Changes of joint space

The large intra-articular effusion may lead to an increase in the width of the joint space. The narrowed joint space indicates the destruction of articular cartilage. It allows considerable accuracy in radiologic diagnosis, according to its location, distribution, and pattern of erosion. It may occur in pyogenic arthritis,

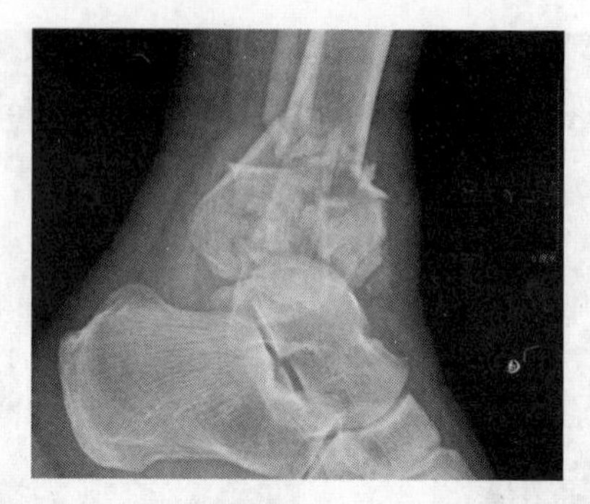

Fig 9-2-3 Radiography of joint destruction shows. the deficiency of os at the site of bony articular surface, and subarticular bone; and the joint, in right tibia and fibula. Space is narrowing, and surrounding soft tissue is tissue.

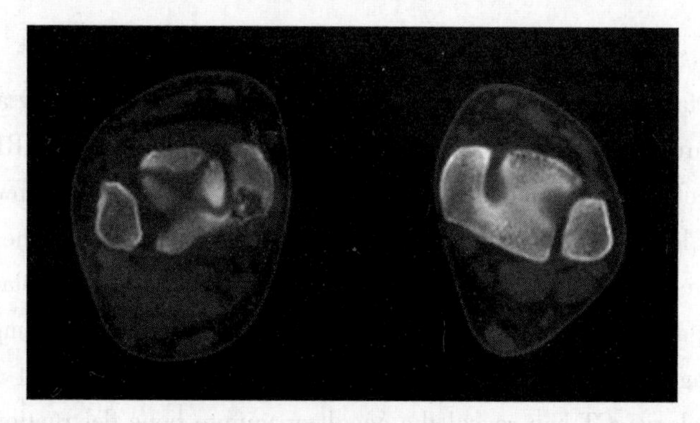

Fig 9-2-4 CT of joint destruction shows the bony destruction and swelling of surrounding soft swelling.

tuberculosis arthritis, degenerative arthritis, and rheumatoid arthritis. The slight change of joint space is difficult to be found, unless compared with the normal joint on the other side.

3 Swelling of the joint

It may be caused by inflammation, trauma, and hemorrhage of the joint. The hyperaemia of synovial membrane, the swelling of the periarticular soft tissues and joint capsule, and the intra-articular effusion and hemorrhage are the pathologic foundation of the sign. A good radiography of joint may reveal the increased density of the surrounding soft tissue of the joint, the loss of definition or displacement of the fat line in the soft tissue (Fig 9-2-5-A). CT and MRI are more sensitive in showing this sign than radiography. The swelling of the periarticular soft tissues and joint capsule shows the enlargement of the contour, decrease of the density, and displacement of the fat line in the soft tissue on CT (Fig 9-2-5-B). The intra-articular effusion reveals as hydro-density imaging in the intra-articular on CT (Fig 9-2-6). When it is accompanied by hemorrhage or pus collection, the density of the lesion will be heightened, and the CT attenuation values may range between 60HU and 80HU. MRI can show not only the thickness of the joint capsule, but also the abnormal signal; swelling of the joint reveals as low signal lesion on T1WI and high signal lesion on T2WI with no en-

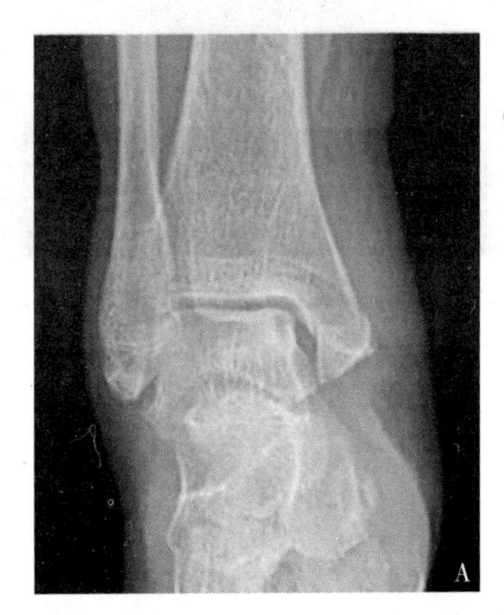

Fig 9-2-5-A Radiography of joint swelling shows enlargement and increased density of the soft tissue surrounding the right ankle.

hancement after enhanced MRI; joint effusion reveals as low signal lesion on T1WI and high signal lesion on T2WI (Fig 9-2-7) with no enhancement after enhanced MRI. The acute hematoma shows low signal on both T1WI and T2WI; sub-acute hematoma shows high signal on both T1WI and T2WI; chronic hematoma shows low signal on T1WI and high signal on T2WI. Sometimes a fluid level is noted between two components of the bloody joint effusion. The upper component is serum and the lower component relates to the cellular components of blood, and each of the two has different CT and MRI findings. The abscess reveals as low-density area with rim enhancement after enhanced CT; low signal lesion on T1WI, and high signal lesion on T2WI with rim enhancement after intravenous administration of a gadolinium contrast agent. The rim of enhancement about abscesses relates to a peripheral, cellular inflammatory zone, and the central non-enhancing region indicates necrotic tissue.

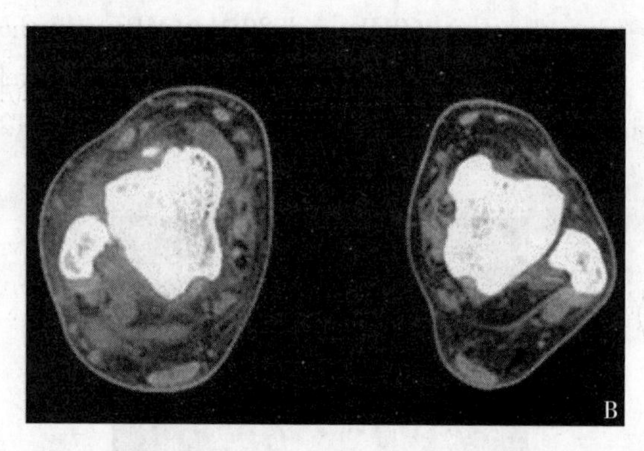

Fig 9-2-5-B CT of joint swelling shows the bony destruction of the soft tissue surrounding the right ankle

4 Ankylosis of joint

Ankylosis of join is the consequence of destruction of joint. It may be classified as bony ankylosis and fibrous ankylosis. The former means the total obliteration of joint space, and the articular capitulums are crossed by bony trabecula-

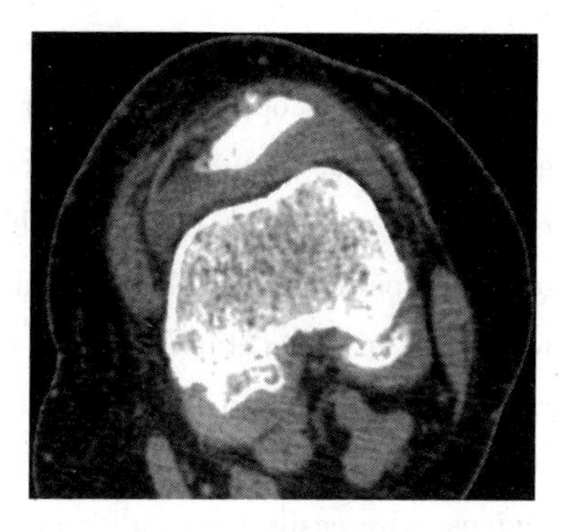

Fig 9-2-6 CT of joint effusion: A fluid density signal can be seen in the articular capsule.

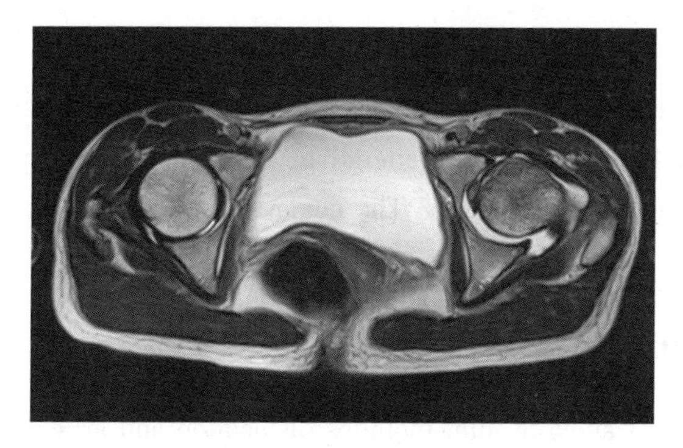

Fig 9-2-7 MRI T2WI of joint effusion shows the high area in the articular capsule.

tions. It can be seen commonly in pyogenic arthritis. The bony ankylosis can be discovered by radiography easily. The fibrous ankylosis indicates that the joint space is crossed by fibrous tissue. It can be seen commonly in tuberculosis arthritis. Fibrous ankylosis cannot be detected by radiography alone. Clinic information must be combined to obtain the right diagnosis.

5 Dislocation

The changes of the location of the opposite articular capitulum of joints are called dislocation. It means the loss of continuity at the joint. It may be complete or incomplete, the later being named as sub-luxation. The causes of dislocations may be traumatic, congenital or pathological. Any joint disease that can bring on destruction of the joint will result in dislocation. We can diagnose the dislocation according to the radiography generally, but some occult dislocations cannot be found unless compared with the healthy joint. CT may detect some dislocations of more complex anatomy regions more easily than radiography. MRI can display not only the dislocation, but also the complications of dislocation, such as intra-articular hemorrhage, ligament injury, and tendon tear.

Section 4 Diagnosis of diseases

There are great amounts of joint diseases and there is no uniform classification of them. According to the etiology classification, arthropathy may be classified as infectious, degenerative, immune, traumatic, congenital, metabolic, and tumorous diseases. The common joint diseases are introduced as follows.

1 Trauma of joint

The common trauma of joint includes dislocation and articular cartilage injury.

(1) Dislocation of joint

Traumatic dislocation mostly occurs in large-range moving, slack joint capsule and ligaments, and unstable joints. As for limbs, it is more commonly seen in the shoulders and elbows, while rarely seen in the knees.

[**Pathology and clinical manifestations**]

After trauma, the patients will feel swelling, pain, dysfunction, and even deformity of traumatic joints, Dislocation is often accompanied by tearing of the capsule, and sometimes by fractures.

[**Imaging appearances**]

Radiography

The common dislocations of joint are introduced as follows.

① ***Dislocation of shoulder***: The shoulder joint has the greatest range of motion of any joint in the body and as a result the ability to move makes the joint inherently unstable and also makes the shoulder the most often dislocated joint in the body. Dislocation of the shoulder is divided into anterior and posterior types: a) Anterior dislocation: over 95% of shoulder dislocation cases are anterior (Fig 9-2-8). Most anterior dislocations are sub-coracoid, sub-glenoid and sub-clavicular. A fracture of the humeral head, neck or greater tuberosity can occur at the same time. b) Posterior dislocation: this type is rare. It can only be diagnosed correctly on radiography lateral position, showing the humeral head has moved backward toward the shoulder blade, while it is easily missed on antero-posterior position.

② ***Dislocation of elbow***: Elbow dislocation is the second most common major joint dislocation, usually resulting from fall onto elbow with hyperextension. a) Posterior dislocation: Posterior elbow dislocation (both ulna and radius) is the more common type and the mechanism of injury is typically a

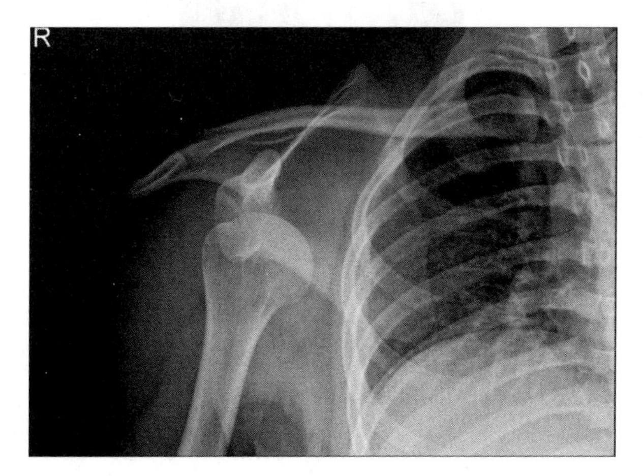

Fig 9-2-8 Radiography of shoulder joint, shows dislocation of the shoulder anteriorly.

fall onto an outstretched hand. Associated fractures are not infrequent (Fig 9-2-9). b) Lateral dislocation: This type is less. This type of dislocation is often accompanied by fracture, by joint capsule and ligament injury in severe cases, and by vascular and nerve damages. Anteroposterior and lateral plain-film radiographs of the elbow should be obtained to both confirm the diagnosis and detect fractures. CT is useful in evaluating intraarticular fractures (such as radial head, capitellum, coronoid process), which is important for deciding the appropriate treatment of the injury. MRI is indicated to assess bone marrow, capsule ligament, and soft-tissue injuries. The medial collateral ligament and lateral collateral ligament are responsible for the ligamentous stability of the elbow.

(2) Injury of articular cartilage

The fracture of the end of bones often causes articular cartilage injury or breakage.

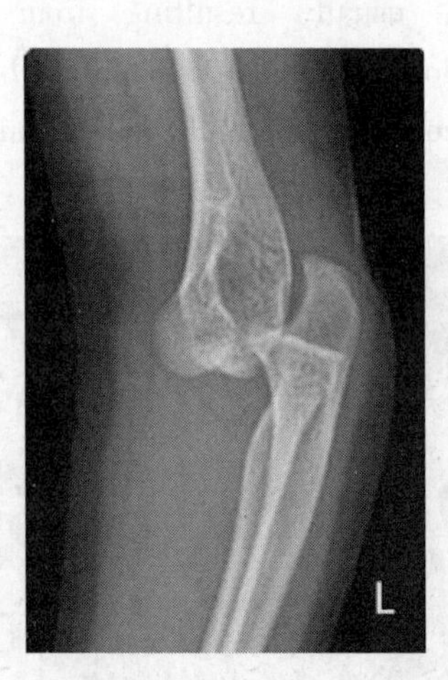

Fig 9-2-9 Radiography of elbow joint, shows dislocation of the elbow posteriorly.

[**Imaging appearances**]

1) Radiography and CT

Radiography and CT cannot find direct signs of chondral injury, but if the fracture line involves the joint surface, it can provide a clue to chondral injury. If the fracture line involves the bony joint surface, especially when the bony joint surfaces are staggered, chondral fracture should be considered.

2) MRI

MRI can find the following signs of damaged articular cartilage directly: the chondral defect, the chondral intra-articular bodies, high signal areas in the normal low signal articular cartilage on T2-weighted sequences and fat suppression sequences. Sometimes the marrow edema may be complicated, and MRI can detect it easily. It can reveal as low signal lesion on T1WI, high signal lesion on fat-suppression T2-weighted sequence with no enhancement after enhanced MRI.

2 Pyogenic arthritis

The pyogenic arthritis is a severe acute joint disorder. The staphylococcus aureus, alpha and beta hemolytic streptococci, gonococci, and pneumococci are the most common infecting organisms. The weight bearing joints, such as the hip or the knee joints are often affected. Mono-articular involvement is the major pattern.

[**Pathology and clinical manifestations**]

Although the pyogenic arthritis predominates in the youth, it affects people of all ages. With acute pyogenic arthritis, fever and chills are the common systemic symptoms. Pain, tenderness, redness, heat, and soft tissue swelling of the involved joint are typical local clinical manifestations. Pathological changes include the synovial membrane hyperaemia, edema, and thickness. The increased amounts of intra-articular extravasate are produced. The fluid contains large numbers of leukocytes, fibrin, and proteolytic ferment, surrounding soft tissue edema is evident, and osseous erosions ensue. Bony ankylosis can eventually occur.

[**Imaging appearances**]

1) Radiography

Radiographic abnormalities are in accordance with the pathologic changes in pyogenic arthritis. In the early stage, radiological changes may be minimal and escape from detection even there are marked symptoms and signs clinically. By careful observation some changes may be discovered within the first several days, such as the soft tissue density around the joint increases, the fascial planes or bursal fat pads are displaced, especially in the knee or ankle. The inflammatory effusion may lead to an increase in the width of the joint space. Later the destruction of articular cartilage and narrowing of the joint space occur first at points of maximum weight bearing or stress. Bone changes become evident two weeks later after the onset of the disease. The sites of the bone destruction locate at maximum weight bearing areas, too. A sequestrum may occasionally develop. Infrequently, gas formation may occur within a joint and surrounding soft tissue. Dislocation and sub-luxation result from the destruction of the joint capsule. The periarticular calcification sometimes appears several weeks after onset of the infection. Bony ankylosis ensues if the articular cartilage is entirely destroyed. Vigorous antibiotic therapy modifies the course of disease.

2) CT

The advantages of CT in evaluating the pyogenic arthritis are as follows: 1) In the early stage, CT can find the changes of soft tissue more sensitively. 2) Joint effusions may be detected by CT when routine radiographs are normal. 3) CT can delineate the osseous and soft tissue extent of the disease process. 4) CT can reveal the slight bone destructions, sequestrum, and the lesions located in the complex anatomy site that may not be evident on radiography. 5) The detection of gas is a reliable diagnostic sign of pyogenic arthritis. 6) CT scanning allows the detection of intra-articular fragments complicating septic arthritis.

3) MRI

MRI is the most sensitive imaging diagnostic method to evaluate the pyogenic arthritis. MRI is superior to CT in revealing the changes of soft tissue and the lesions of the joint capsule, the articular cartilage, and the ligament. It is possible to diagnose the pyogenic arthritis in early stage by MRI. It can accurately describe the range of inflammation involved. The specificity of the MRI findings in cases of pyogenic arthritis is limited. The edema of soft tissue and medulla presents low signal intensity lesions on T1WI, high signal intensity lesions on T2WI and fat-suppression sequence and with no enhancement after enhanced MRI. The bone destruction demonstrates hypo-intensity focus on T1WI, hyper-intensity focus on T2WI and fat-suppression sequence, and with enhancement after enhanced MRI. The signal intensity of focus is not uniform. The border is not clear. MRI is capable of noting the abscess and sequestrum, too. The abscess reveals as low signal lesion on T1WI, and high signal lesion on T2WI with rim enhancement after enhanced MRI. Sequestra appear as regions of low to intermediate signal intensity on both T1WI and T2WI, and do not show enhancement of signal intensity after enhanced MRI.

[**Diagnosis**]

In the presence of a hot, painful and swollen joint, pyogenic arthritis must be considered. Early radiographs may be normal. MRI is better at demonstrating bone involvement.

3 Tuberculosis arthritis

In the majority of cases of joint tuberculosis, pulmonary lesions are also present. Tuberculous arthritis most typically affects large joints such as the hip, the knee and the spine, although any joint may be involved. It is generally mono-articular involvement. But poly-articular tuberculosis has also been reported.

[**Pathology and clinical manifestations**]

Tuberculous arthritis can affect people of all ages, although it is usually encountered in children and young adults. Clinically, it often runs a chronic course as compared with that of pyogenic arthritis. The patient often complains of chronic pain and swelling of the joint with minimal signs of inflammation. Delay in diagnosis is frequent. Pathological changes include the synovial membrane hyperaemia, edema, and thickness, cartilaginous destruction, and osseous erosion.

[**Imaging appearances**]

1) Radiography

Radiologically, tuberculosis of joint may be classified according to their primary site of infection as osseous type and synovial type. The osseous type: the primary focus lies in the metaphysis or epiphysis or it may be a secondary extension of tuberculous infection from the adjacent metaphysis or epiphysis. It more commonly occurs in adults. The synovial type: due to hematogenous infection and the initial focus, it appears in the synovial membrane. This type occurs often in children and affects the knee or ankle joint frequently. Despite the types, the end results are the same: in the later type, bone is always almost involved later on. In the early stage, there often shows little change on radiography except for some soft tissue swelling around the affected joint and progressive osteoporosis, which makes the early diagnosis more difficult. The infectious nature of the process may be obscured until osseous and cartilaginous destruction becomes evident. Marginal erosions are especially characteristic of tuberculosis in weight-bearing articulations, such as the hip and knee. They produce Comer defects simulating the erosions of other synovial processes, such as rheumatoid arthritis. Sub-chondral osseous erosions are also encountered in tuberculosis arthritis. They appear as poorly defined gaps in the sub-chondral bone plate and subjacent trabeculae that may be apparent at a stage when the articular space is well preserved. Narrowing of the joint space duo to extensive destruction of cartilage always occurs. In some patients, diminution in this space is a late finding that occurs after marginal and central erosions of large size have appeared. In other patients, loss of the space can be appreciated at a time when only small marginal osseous defects are apparent. Bony proliferation is not general unless a secondary pyogenic infection. Dislocation may occur duo to the destruction of joint. The eventual result in tuberculous arthritis is usually fibrous ankylosis of the joint. Bony ankylosis is occasionally seen.

2) CT

CT can detect these abnormalities too. Furthermore, CT can detect the swellings of the joint capsule, the soft tissue surrounding the joint, the intra-articular effusion, the occult destruction, small "kissing sequestrum", and the cold abscess. The cold abscess reveals as low-density area with rim enhancement after enhanced CT.

3) MRI

MRI is more sensitive than CT in evaluating abnormalities of tuberculosis arthritis. In the early stage, MRI can find the swelling of the joint easily, including the thickness of synovial membrane, the swelling of the periarticular soft tissues and joint capsule, and the tiny intra-articular effusion. MRI can find the destruction of articular cartilage, the osseous erosions, and the cold abscess. Main radiological features of tuberculosis arthritis may be summarized as following: a) Monoarticular involvement. b) Soft tissue swelling and slight but progressive osteoporosis. c) Marginal, mouse-eaten like subarticular bone erosion occurs in the non weight-bearing articular surface. d) Uneven narrowing of joint space, late appearance, and unparallel to the degree of the bone destruction. e) Absence of bone sclerosis and periosteal reaction, unless secondary infection supervenes. f) Small "kissing sequestrum" may present. g) Cold abscess formation with discharging sinus and calcified debris. h) Pathologic dislocation occurs when there is extensive destruction of the joint. i) Fibrous ankylosis.

[**Diagnosis**]

It is easy to diagnose typical tuberculosis arthritis by its performances on radiography, CT or MRI.

4 Rheumatoid arthritis

The rheumatoid arthritis (RA) is a systemic non-pyogenic inflammatory disease of connective tissue which locally involves the synovial membrane. The epidemiological data shows that the incidence of the disease is approximately 0.3%~1.5%.

[**Pathology and clinical manifestations**]

Young women are more commonly affected. The rheumatoid arthritis most typically affect the small joint of the hand and foot; the proximal inter-phalangeal joints, the metacarpophalangeal joints, and the wrists are the favorite sites, but practically any joint may be affected. The systemic symptom includes fatigue, anorexia, weight loss, and malaise; the local manifestations include pain, morning stiffness, swelling, and dislocation or subluxation. Rheumatoid factor, elevated erythrocyte sedimentation rates and C-reactive protein levels are important laboratory parameters of rheumatoid arthritis. The pathologic abnormalities of rheumatoid arthritis are synovial inflammation, intra-articular effusion, pannus formation, destructions of cartilage and subchondral bone, and ankylosis.

[**Imaging appearances**]

1) Radiography

Radiographic findings may lag considerably behind the clinical symptoms, and a long interval between the onset of symptoms and the appearance of radiographic changes is not unusual. In general there is multiple and symmetric joint involvement. The earliest radiographic change is periarticular soft tissue swelling due to joint effusion and synovitis; although usually fusiform, the swelling may occasionally appear lobulated. Regional osteoporosis is characteristic and initially juxta-articular. As the disease progresses, irreversible erosion of the articular cartilage results in uniform joint space narrowing (Fig 9-2-10). The subarticular bony cortex losses its sharp outline and disappears, either focally or diffusely. Erosion of bone tends to occur, especially at the edges of the joint, where articular cartilage is absent. The erosion has poorly defined edges without a sclerotic rim. Mechanical stress may play a role in the location and development of the erosion. Periosteal reaction is very infrequent. With progression, diffuse osteoporosis becomes apparent, and eventually subluxation, contractures, and bony ankylosis may develop. Bony ankylosis is most frequent in the wrist and carpal bones. It is uncommon in the metacarpophalangeal and interphalangeal joints. Secondary changes of osteoarthritis with spurring and sclerosis may develop because of altered joint mechanics. Synovial cysts often develop in an affected joint, causing disproportionate soft tissue swelling. Around the knee, the cysts may become huge, extending into the soft tissue well beyond the joint boundaries. Synovial cysts are best demonstrated by arthrography. Cervical spine involvement occurs in over 80 percent of well-advanced cases. Occasionally this may be the only area affected. Both the disc space and the apophyseal joints may be involved. Osteoporosis, eroded or blurred facets, and disc space narrowing are the most common findings. Subluxation of one or more joints is not an uncommon complication. The odontoid process may show erosive changes, volume decrease, and pointing of its normally rounded upper border. The space between the odontoid and anterior arch of the atlas may be widened. Cervical spine involvement in the rheumatoid patient should not be confused with progressive ascending spondylitis of the entire spine, which may sometimes be of rheumatoid origin but is a separate entity. It is considered under ankylosing spondylitis. The most significant and frequent findings in a rheumatoid joint are uniform narrowing of the joint space, marginal erosions, and periarticular osteoporosis. Prolonged corticosteroid therapy may result in a number of complications, some of which can be detected radiographically. Among these is peptic ulcer. A Cushing syndrome can also develop with resultant osteoporosis and pathologic fracture, the latter occurring most frequently in the spine.

2) CT

CT plays an important role in diagnosis of rheumatoid arthritis. When the radiography shows no positive findings, CT can demonstrate the bone erosions (Fig 9-2-11), especially when the lesion is located in complex anatomy regions, such as sacroiliac joint and spine, swelling of soft tissue, the articular effusion, the para-articular masses, such as rheumatoid nodes and synovial cysts. Rheumatoid nodes vary in size from a few millimeters to over 5 cm. CT reveals as a soft density mass, which is enhanced after intravenous administration of iodinated contrast medium. Synovial cyst reveals as a hydro-density lesion with no enhancement after intravenous administration of iodinated contrast medium.

3) MRI

MRI is superior to radiography in showing the abnormities of rheumatoid arthritis. It may permit an earlier diagnosis of RA, though MRI findings of rheumatoid arthritis are diagnostically nonspecific. MRI can demonstrate bone erosions, the intra-articular structure abnormities (cartilage injury, articular effusion, tendon, and ligament), the activity of rheumatoid arthritis and therapeutic effect, the extent of inflammatory synovial membrane and synovial cyst, and rheumatoid nodes. Enhanced MRI can make difference between synovial fluid and pannus. After the intravenous injection of a gadolinium-containing agent, the effusion remains of low signal intensity in T1WI images, and the pannus demonstrates enhancement with increased signal intensity. Rheumatoid nodes show low signal intensity on T1WI and high signal intensity on T2WI, and the nodes may show enhancement of signal intensity after the intravenous administration of a gadolinium-containing agent. The appearance of a rheumatoid node may resemble that of a soft tissue tumor. Furthermore, the complication of rheumatoid arthritis, such as ischemic necrosis of bone, can be detected far more easily by MRI than by radiology.

[**Diagnosis**]

Bilateral symmetrical erosive arthropathy predominantly involves proximal small joints of hand and wrist. Diagnosis of rheumatoid arthritis is based on a combination of clinical, laboratory and radiological investigations.

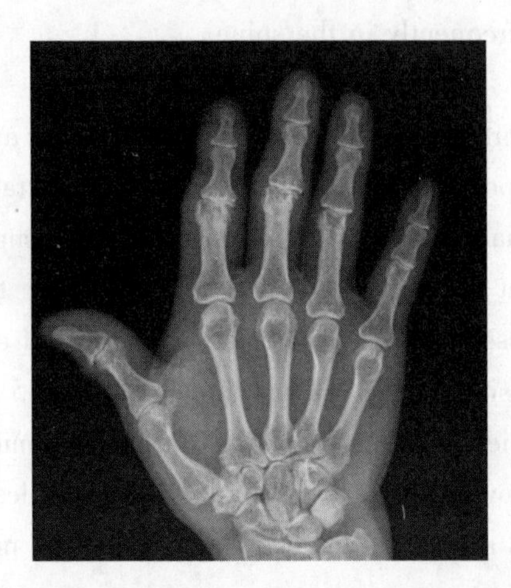

Fig 9-2-10 Radiography of RA shows osteoporosis of the bones of the interphalangeal joint, the articular surface becomes narrowed, and subluxation occurs.

5 Ankylosing spondylitis

Ankylosing spondylitis (AS) is a chronic inflammatory disorder affecting the axial skeleton. The disease almost always begins in both sacroiliac joint and lower lumbar spine, and eventually extends to higher levels of the vertebral column. The etiology remains unknown. Etiologic factors may include heredity, immunity, infection, and environmental factors, etc.

[**Pathology and clinical manifestations**]

The incidence of this disease is estimated to be approximately 0.1%. The onset of ankylosing spondylitis occurs between 15~35years. Males are most com-

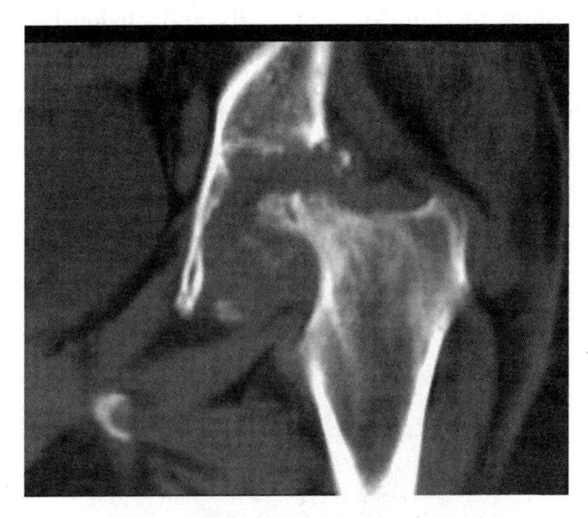

Fig 9-2-11 CT of hip joint RA shows the articular face of left hip has been destroyed.

monly affected. The ratio of the disease in men versus women is about 9 to 1. The main clinical manifestations may be low back pain and stuffiness. The laboratory parameters indicate that rheumatoid factor is negative, elevated erythrocyte sedimentation rates and C-reactive protein levels are elevated, and 90% of the patients with ankylosing spondylitis may be positive for antigen HLA-B_{27}. The pathologic changes of synovial joint alteration in ankylosing spondylitis are similar to that in rheumatoid arthritis, but severe pannus formation is less frequent. Additional pathologic features are related to subchondral bone sclerosis and periosteal elevation. This change is not prominent in rheumatoid arthritis.

[**Imaging appearances**]

1) Radiography

The earliest radiographic signs locate in unilateral sacroiliac joints, especially in the synovium. Several months or years later, the opposite sacroiliac joint will be involved. This symmetric pattern is an important sign in ankylosing spondylitis and may permit its differentiation from other disorders that affect the sarcoiliac joint. The initial radiographic findings include blurring of the articular edges of the joints and osteoporosis. Subsequently superficial erosion and periarticular sclerosis may develop. Because the iliac cartilage is thinner than that of the sacrum, the lesions of ilium develop early and obviously. Ultimately, bone ankylosis ensues, generally within two to five years. Complete disappearance of the joint space eventually occurs (Fig 9-2-12). Erosion of the ischial tuberosity and symphysis pubis is frequent.

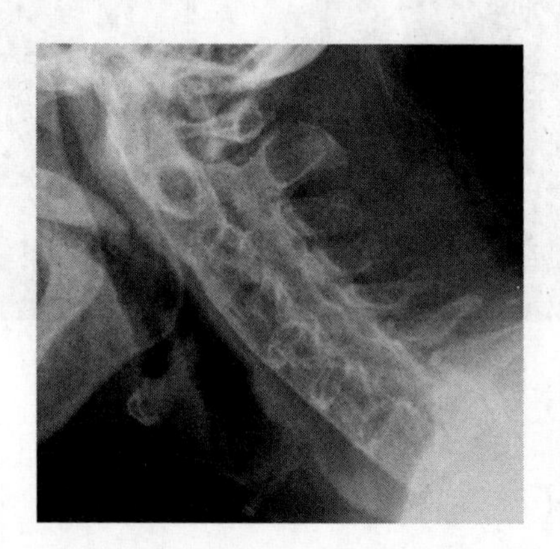

Fig 9-2-12 Radiography of cervical vertebra of AS gives rise to the bamboo spine.

A similar progress takes place in the spine, although this usually is not uniform. There is joint space narrowing and fusion of the apophyseal and costovertebral joints; the vertebral bodies become squared, with sharp corners. Later, there is calcification in the spinal ligament; this, plus the squared vertebral bodies, gives rise to the bamboo spine. General spinal osteoporosis is frequent. Dislocation of the spine is not an uncommon complication.

In long-term cases, involvement of peripheral joints, such as the hips, shoulders, hands, wrists, knees, and temporomandibular joints, may occur. The radiographic changes are similar to those seen in rheumatoid arthritis, but then the osteoporosis and joint space narrowing may be relatively slight, and the bone erosion, sclerosis and bony ankylosis can be relatively severe in ankylosing spondylitis compared with rheumatoid arthritis.

2) CT and MRI

When radiographic findings are normal or inconclusive, CT can demonstrate these destructive and reparative changes better. CT can also detect the lesions of sacroiliac, costovertebral, and apophyseal joints easily and accurately (Fig 9-2-13). MRI can detect inflammatory changes at joints before these destructive-reparative changes take place. MRI signs of early sacroiliitis and subchondral bone marrow edema are increased signal in T2-weighted images and increased contrast-enhancement of the joint cavity, corresponding to synovitis. Bone marrow edematous changes at the ligamentous insertions in the spine are the hallmark of early disease.

[**Diagnosis**]

Ankylosing spondylitis should be considered in young males with chronic low back pain and signs of sacro-iliitis, bilateral symmetrical sacro-iliitis, syndesmophyte formation, ligamentous ossification and articular ankylosis, as well as calcification and ossification of connective tissue.

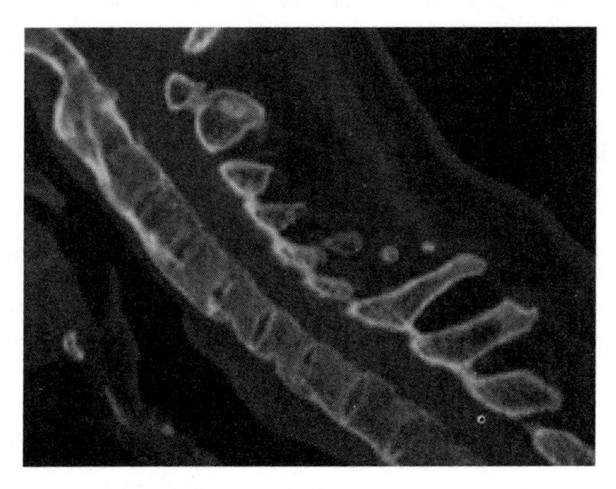

Fig 9-2-13 CT of cervical vertebra of AS: showing the intravertebral bony fusion has occurred.

6 Degenerative joint disease

Degenerative joint disease (osteoarthritis) is the most common form of arthropathy. It is caused by the degeneration of articular cartilage. It is not a real inflammatory disease.

[**Pathology and clinical manifestations**]

Traditionally, degenerative joint disease has been classified into primary and secondary types. The former has been regarded as a process in which articular degeneration occurs in the absence of any obvious underlying abnormality, whereas the latter has been regarded as articular degeneration that is produced by alteration from a preexisting affliction, such as trauma. Many diverse factors appear to be important in the causation of degenerative joint disease. These factors include age, occupation and activity, heredity, inflammation, trauma, minor mechanical disturbance and dysplasia. These factors create a situation in which the intra-articular structures can no longer resist the physical forces. The basic pathologic change of the disease is cartilaginous degeneration. The common manifestations are pain and disability of the ill joint, without swelling and systemic symptom.

[**Imaging appearances**]

Most joints of whole body can have degenerative joint disease. Knee joint is one of the commonest sites of involvement in osteoarthritis. Other common sites include weight-bearing joints (such as hip joints, knee and spine). Degenerations of knee are as follows:

Radiography is the first choice to evaluate the joint degenerations in routine work. The earliest radiographic changes are sharpening and thickening of the articular margins of the bones. Later, subchondral thinning and/or sclerosis of the articular cartilage causes irregular narrowing of the joint space (Fig 9-2-14-A/B, 9-2-15-A/B). The characteristic features of degenerative joint disease reflect the consequences of cartilage loss: a) Joint space narrowing due to loss of cartilage. This is typically worse in the medial tibiofemoral compartment and may result in a varus angulation of the knee joint. b) Marginal osteophytes-reactive new bone formation in response to altered stress on the articular surface. c) Subchondral sclerosis-reactive bone formation in response to stress. d) Subchondral cyst formation-synovial fluid driven into defects of the subchondral bone under pressure. e) Joint subluxation. f) Intra-articular body cartilage fragments are nourished by synovial fluid within the joint; they grow and may calcify or ossify. g) Joint effusion.

[**Diagnosis**]

Degenerative joint disease is a common cause of joint pain, particularly in elderly patients. Joint space narrowing, marginal osteophytes, subchondral sclerosis and cyst formation are characteristic radiological features of osteoarthritis.

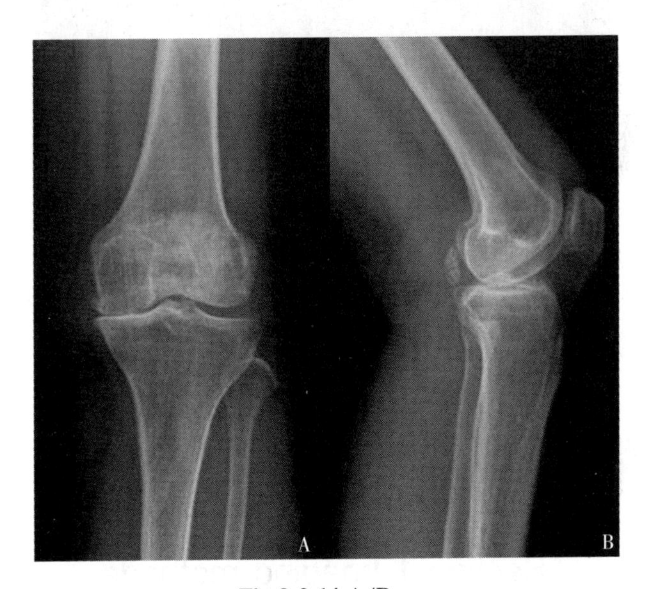

Fig 9-2-14-A/B

Radiography of keen joint osteoarthritis shows the articular face is hardened, the osteophytes and irregular narrowing of the joint space occur.

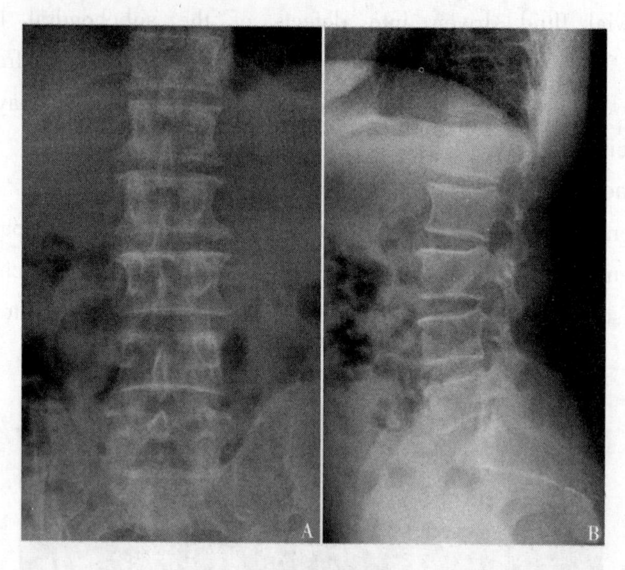

Fig 9-2-15-A/B

Radiography of lumbar osteoarthritis: showing osteophytes occur to lumbar bodies.

Lesson 3 Soft Tissue

Section 1 Imaging methods

1 Radiography

The muscle, blood vessel, nerve, and joint capsule in soft tissue, because of lack of natural contrast, are invisible on radiography, and therefore its use is limited. Sometimes, the angiography is used to evaluate the blood supply of the mass in the soft tissue or to treat disease.

2 CT

The scan method includes plain scanning and enhanced scanning. Plain CT means scanning without intravenous contrast medium. Enhanced CT indicates scanning with intravenous injection of iodinated contrast medium. There are two main purposes of enhanced CT. One is elevating density difference between the lesion and normal tissue in order to discover the lesion. The other is showing the characteristics of enhancement in order to diagnose accurately. CT arthrography implies scanning after arthrography. The transaxial scanning and reformation are used commonly. Usually 2~5mm collimation is adequate after locating on the lateral or coronal scout image. All images should be reviewed at window and center settings appropriate for visualization of both bone and soft tissues.

3 MRI

MRI has the distinct advantage of not using ionizing radiation. Its superior soft tissue contrast resolution and multiplanar capability means that it has superseded CT in the imaging of most soft tissue problems. Soft tissue lesions can be categorized by MRI according to site, morphological changes and signal characteristics. To maximize the potential diagnostic yield, protocols should include sequences in at least two orthogonal planes and with differing weighting to illustrate both the T1-and T2-weighted characteristics of the lesion. Although there are continuing major advances in MRI technology, spin-echo (SE) sequences will suffice in the evaluation of most soft tissue lesions. Reduced data acquisition time with increased image sharpness is an advantage of fast spin-echo (FSE) techniques, also called turbo spin-echo. Both T2-weighted fat-suppressed and STIR sequences are particularly sensitive to small variations in the fluid content of lesions and they are ideally suited for the detection of subtle soft tissue abnormalities.

Section 2 Normal imaging findings of soft tissue

1 Radiography

The soft tissues of musculoskeletal system include muscles, tendons, blood vessels, nerves, fascias, ligaments, and joint capsules. Because of lack of good natural contrast, they can not be differed from each other, appearing moderate density on a plain film.

2 CT

In CT images, fat, muscles and blood vessels can be distinguished from each other. The outermost skin of trunk and limbs appears line-like moderate density; Subcutaneous fats demonstrate low density, with CT value between-100HU~40HU; The muscles, tendons and ligaments between fat and bone appear moderate density; on enhanced CT scans, blood vessels are more clearly shown as high density, and are easily differed from the neural structures.

3 MRI

MRI can display soft tissue structures mentioned above. Fat appears high signal on both T1WI and T2WI, but on fat suppressed sequence show low signal; Muscle show low signal on both T1WI and T2WI; Hyaline cartilage on T1WI shows intermediate signal, while on T2WI shows high signal; Fibrous tissues, tendons, ligaments and fibrous cartilages are all low signal; because of the presence of vascular flow void phenomenon, low signal is shown on T1W1 and T2WI.

Section 3 Imaging signs of soft tissue diseases

Pathological changes in the soft tissue diseases are demonstrated by imaging technology, and can be summarized as the following basic disease manifestations. Understanding and mastering these basic disease manifestations, is very important for diagnosis of the disease.

1 Soft tissue swelling

Soft tissue swelling refers to swelling of soft tissue which is caused by inflammation, hemorrhage, edema or abscess. Its imaging findings are introduced as follows:

1) Radiography

The density of lesions may be different from surrounding soft tissues. Edema can bring reticular changes to the subcutaneous fat layer, while subcutaneous tissues and muscles are ill-defined. If abscess occurs, its edge can be clearer, while surrounding muscular bundles are displaced by its pressure. Tuberculous abscess wall may calcify. The boundaries of hematomas are well-defined or ill-defined.

2) CT

CT is superior to radiography in showing the soft tissue swelling. The edge of abscess is well defined, and in it the liquid density can be visible; the boundaries of early hematoma are ill or well defined, appearing high density.

3) MRI

MRI can distinguish hematoma, and swelling from abscess, which is superior to CT. Swelling and abscess show low signal on T1WI and high signal on T2WI, and the signals are different due to the different stages of hematoma, while the T1WI and T2WI of subacute hematoma show high signal on fat suppression sequence.

2 Soft tissue mass

Soft tissue mass is usually caused by soft tissue tumors or tumor-like lesions. If the bone tumor destroys the cortical bone, soft tissue mass can be formed within the soft tissue; soft tissue mass can be caused by some infections.

1) Radiography

On radiography, usually the edge of benign mass is well defined, adjacent soft tissues may be displaced, and adjacent bones show resorption or bone hardening due to its pressure; malignant tumor generally has ill-define edge, and its adjacent cortical bone is involved. The density varies with different tissues: the density of lipoma is lower than normal soft tissue, and radiography can show the difference; calcification may occur to cartilaginous tumor; myositis ossificans appear matur-bone density in the soft tissue.

2) CT

CT is superior to radiography in showing the size, border, and density of the soft tissue mass, whether it contains fat or not (Fig 9-3-1), and whether calcification or ossification exists; with enhanced scanning, the relationship between the mass and adjacent tissues and blood vessels is shown, tumor and peritumoral edema are distinguished, and liquefying and necrosis, if do occur in the tumor, can be shown.

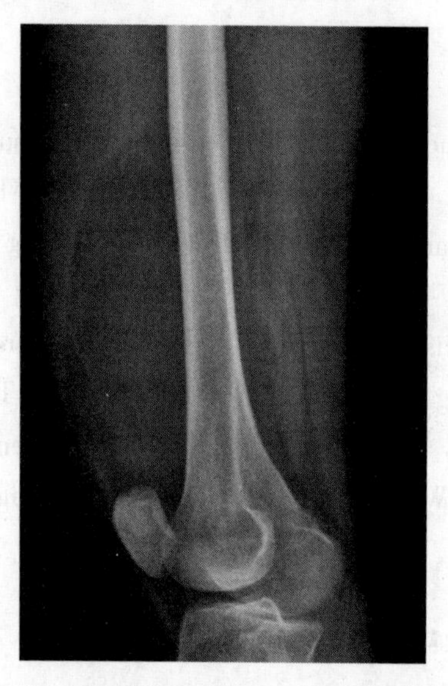

Fig 9-3-1 Radiography of mass around keen joint shows a well-defined low density mass in the leg soft tissue.

3) MRI

MRI is superior to CT in showing the soft tissue mass. The signals of mass are relative to its components and associated imaging sequences. Generally the lumps mostly display homogeneous or heterogeneous long T1, long T2 signal or mixed high signal; liquefied and necrotic areas show long T1, T2 signal, and sometimes the liquid-liquid level can be seen; the lump with fat appears short T1 and long T2 signal, but on fat suppression sequences, its signal can be suppressed. Enhanced MRI and CT scanning can both provide relevant information of blood supply.

3 Calcification and ossification of soft tissue

Calcification and ossification in soft tissue are resulted from bleeding, degeneration, necrosis, tumor, tuberculosis and parasitic infection. They can occur in the muscles, tendons, joint capsules, calcification of blood vessels and lymph nodes, etc.

1) Radiography

On radiography, calcification and ossification display bony density in different shapes (Fig 9-3-2). Different pathological calcifications and ossifications have respective features: the calcification of cartilage lesions is mostly circular, semi-circular or punctate high density; the ossification of myositis ossificans often has flakes, or even visible trabecular bone cortex; most osteoblastic osteosarcomas have cloudy or needle-like calcification or ossification.

2) CT

CT can better display calcification and ossification in soft tissue than radiography. It can also show their shape, size and density.

3) MRI

Calcification and ossification are shown low signal on every MRI sequence, which is less clear than CT.

4 Air in soft tissue

Gas in soft tissue often comes from trauma, surgery or other pathological aerogenes infection. On radiography and CT, it shows very low density in different shapes; on every MRI sequence, it shows no signal. CT can accurately show the amount of gas in the soft tissue.

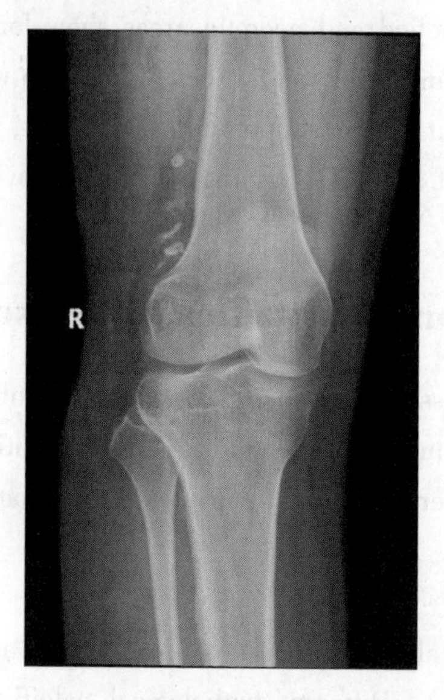

Fig 9-3-2

Radiography of calcifications in leg soft tissue shows multiple bone-like density.

Section 4 Diagnosis of diseases

1 Tendon and ligament injuries

[**Pathology and clinical manifestations**]

Tendon and ligament injuries may be classified as complete tear and incomplete tear. The clinical manifestations of tendon and ligament injuries are pain, tenderness, local swelling, and malfunction.

[**Imaging appearances**]

1) Radiography

Pure tendon and ligament injuries show no positive finding on routine radiography.

2) CT

Plain CT scanning displays that the edge of injury is ill defined and without the normal contour, or even appears fragmented; if accompanied by bleeding, the high density is visible in and around the traumatic ligaments; in addition, the torn fractures and intra-articular effusion can be displayed clearly.

3) MRI

Plain MRI is the best imaging method of revealing ligament and tendon injuries directly: the ligament and tendon can be directly displayed. Under normal conditions, all the ligaments and tendons show low signal ribbon with clear and smooth edge. 1) Incomplete tear: the contour of high signal areas in ruptured tendon and ligament on T2-weighted sequences and fat suppression sequences is enlarged with irregular edges, but some fibers retain low signal; sometimes marrow edema may be accompanied. 2) Complete tear: the low signal of ligaments and tendons is completely interrupted, and is replaced by mixed low signal on T1WI and high signal on T2WI. Its position and direction may also change.

2 Soft tissue inflammation

The causes of soft tissue inflammation are diverse. Imaging is helpful in knowing the location and extent, whether an abscess occurs and whether adjacent bone joints are involved.

[**Pathology and clinical manifestations**]

Soft tissue inflammation can occur in primary or secondary to bony infections. Primary soft tissue infections often have acute onset. Clinical manifestations include redness, swelling, heat, pain, and even fever and elevated white blood cell count.

In acute stage, inflammations mainly display local congestion, edema, inflammatory cell infiltration and tissue necrosis, followed by the formation of abscesses, which can be confined or spread along the muscle space; in chronic stage, calcifications may occur within the inflammation, and sometimes the edge is encapsuled by fibrous tissue.

[**Imaging appearances**]

1) Radiography

Radiography can show partial soft tissue swelling, slightly increased density, blur intramuscular fatty layer, and the reticular opacities in subcutaneous fat.

2) CT

a) On plain scanning, the affected muscles significantly swell, and the intramuscular space and fat layer are obscure; the abscess appears liquid density with uniform wall and smooth inner wall. b) On enhanced scanning, the wall of abscess is enhanced circularly.

3) MRI

MRI is more sensitive in displaying soft tissue inflammation than CT.

a) On plain scanning, the affected muscles swell, the intramuscular space blurs in the early stage, and inflammation shows diffusive long T1 and T2 signals; when abscesses form, pus shows liquid-like low signal on T1WI and high signal on T2WI, and the capsule displays low signal at the edge of it, with uniform thickness and smooth border; on DWI, the cavity of the abscess often shows high signal; b) On enhanced scanning, the wall shows ring-like enhancement, but the cavity of abscess is not enhanced.

3 Soft tissue tumors

Soft tissue tumors, which literally mean masses or swelling, can be classified as neoplastic and non-neoplastic ones or benign and malignant ones.

(1) Lipoma

A lipoma is a benign tumor composed of mature adipocytes, and is the most common soft tissue tumor.

[**Pathology and clinical manifestations**]

Lipomas in soft tissue are superficial and present in adulthood (30~50) as a soft painless mass in the trunk or proximal extremities. They occur more in females than in males, and they are likely to be present for many years.

Simple lipomas are circumscribed encapsulated soft masses entirely made of fat. Occasionally solid components (blood vessels, muscle fibres fibrous septae and fat necrosis) will be present. Histology demonstrates mature adipocytes with no cellular atypia or pleomorphism.

[**Imaging appearances**]

1) Radiography

Lipoma may appear as a well-defined fatty density mass in moderate density soft tissue.

2) CT

Lipoma will appear as radiolucent on radiographs, and low attenuation on CT (−120HU to−65HU) (Fig 9-3-3). A thin capsule and very thin septum (<2 mm) are often seen, and it may change size with muscle contraction. Sometimes, calcification may be present. CT reveals as an unenhanced soft density mass after intravenous administration of iodinated contrast medium.

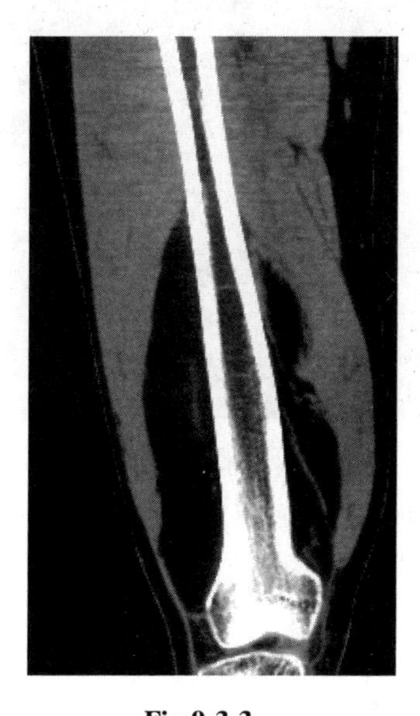

Fig 9-3-3

CT of lipoma in deep soft tissue: showing the well-defined fatty mass grows peri-femur.

3) MRI

Lipoma appears as a well-circumscribed round or ovoid fatty mass with short T1 and T2; on fat-suppressed sequences, it becomes low signal; thin fibrous septa (<2 mm) are often seen, showing low signal on both T1WI and T2WI (Fig 9-3-4-A/B). The mass is not enhanced after intravenous administration of

Gd-DTPA, but the septa are mildly enhanced.

[**Diagnosis**]

Because of its classical image appearance, it can be easily diagnosed correctly.

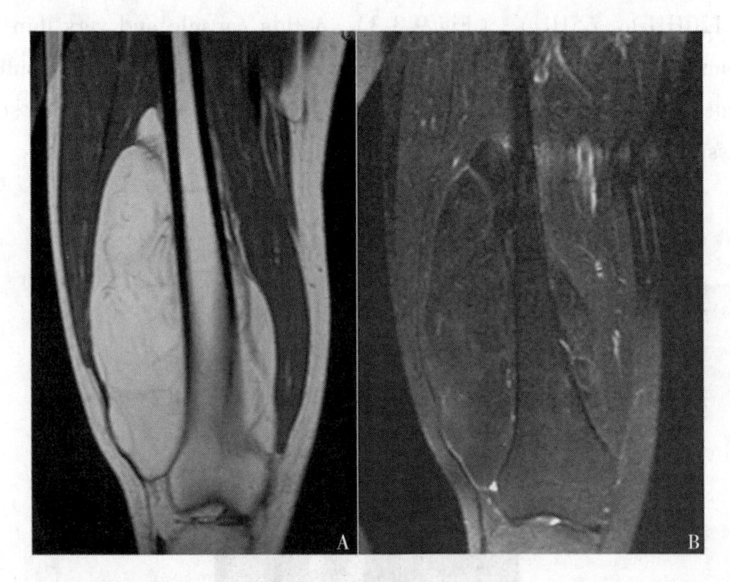

Fig 9-3-4-A/B

MRI T1WI and fat-suppressed T2WI of lipoma in deep soft tissue shows a well-defined high signal on T1WI, and low signal on fat-suppressed T2WI.

(2) Hemangioma

Soft tissue haemangioma is one of the most common benign soft-tissue tumors, which grows slowly.

[**Pathology and clinical manifestations**]

It is dependent on the predominant type of vascular channel identified within them. Soft tissue haemangiomas may be classified in to four histological subtypes: capillary, cavernous, venous and mixed types. Capillary haemangiomas are the most common type, appearing as purple mass with well-defined edge and no capsule, and tend to predominate in the paediatric population (mostly<1year). Usually it occurs in the subcutaneous tissues of the head and face, especially the lips and eyelids. The size of cavernous hemangioma usually is less than 10cm. It is soft and has pseudocapsule. Its section appears cavity-like, which is composed of cyst-dilating lumen and larger vessels with a large quantity of blood in it. It occurs at any age, mostly solitarily; superficial ones appear as rugged blue ridges, while deep ones as diffusive masses with lighter color. Intramuscular hemangioma is the most common hemangioma in deep soft tissue, with possible occurrence of each type, usually in the leg muscles of the youth.

[**Imaging appearances**]

Capillary hemangioma commonly occurs in the skin and subcutaneous tissue. Because of its characteristic appearance, generally it doesn't need imaging examination.

1) Radiography and CT

Calcification is common in cavernous hemangioma, and about 50% of the calcification are phleboliths, which appear as the characteristic "button-like" high density on radiography and CT plain scanning (Fig 9-3-5). On dynamic

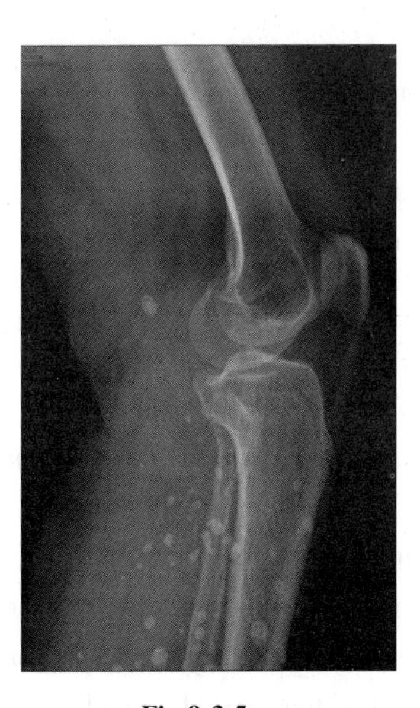

Fig 9-3-5

Radiography of phleboliths of haemangioma shows the button-like high density enhanced CT scanning, the lesion is enhanced gradually characteristically (Fig 9-3-6). At delayed stage, the density of lesion becomes more homogeneous.

2) MRI

①On unenhanced test, the typical cavernous hemangioma appears intermediate to slightly high signal on T1WI and high signal on T2WI as it contains lots of blood vessels filled with blood, and "button like" calcification shows hyposignal on each sequence; in addition, cavernous hemangioma often contains different components, such as fat, fiber, mucus, smooth muscle, bone or calcification, so its signal is usually rather heterogeneous.

②On dynamic enhanced MRI test, its appearance is similar to CT.

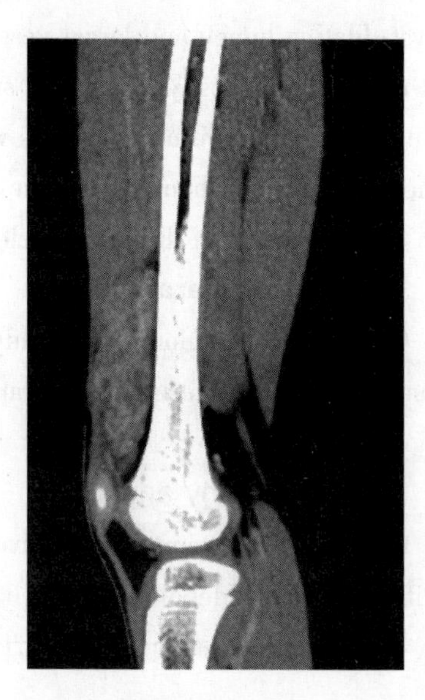

Fig 9-3-6

Enhanced CT of haemangioma in soft tissue shows marked enhancement.

[**Diagnosis**]

The diagnosis of haemangiomas is not generally difficult when finding button-like phleboliths, and gradual enhancement on dynamic enhanced CT and MRI scanning.

(3) Liposarcoma

A liposarcoma thought to be originated from mesenchymal cells is a malignant tumor of fatty tissue. It's one of the most common types of soft tissue sarcomas.

[**Pathology and clinical manifestations**]

Liposarcomas are typically found in adults between the ages of 40 and 60, and are usually seen in the extremities or retroperitoneum. They are histologically classified into 5 types: well differentiated, dedifferentiated, myxoid, pleomorphic, and mixed. Myxoid liposarcoma is the most common subtype. At histological analysis, myxoid liposarcoma consists of well-delineated lobules of myxoid tissue; a characteristic, delicate, arborizing capillary network; and primitive uniform mesenchymal cells with variable numbers of usually monovacuolated and sometimes bivacuolated lipoblasts, Pooling of the myxoid matrix can occur and, if extensive, results in a "pulmonary edema" pattern. Hemorrhage may also be present.

[**Imaging appearances**]

1) Radiography

The larger liposarcoma shows as ill-defined soft tissue mass, and low-density fat can be found in well-differentiated liposarcoma (Fig 9-3-7).

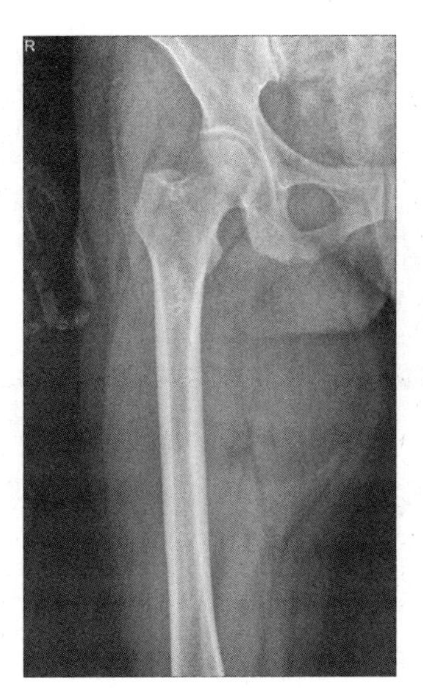

Fig 9-3-7 Radiography of well-differentiated liposarcoma in leg shows fat-containing mass in the leg soft tissue.

2) CT

a) The well-differentiated liposarcoma containing fat may be similar to lipoma, but the former shows slight enhancement. b) The poor-differentiated liposarcoma appears water-like to soft-tissue density, often without adipose component. It has irregular contour and obscure edge, and can be enhanced on enhanced scanning.

3) MRI

a) Since the well-differentiated liposarcoma often contains adipose tissue, fat shows high signal on T1WI and T2WI (Fig 9-3-8-A), but appears low signal on fat-suppression sequence (Fig 9-3-8-B). b) The poor-differentiated liposarcoma rarely containing intratumoral fat content shows as low mixed signal on T1WI and high mixed signal on T2WI, with often more blurred boundaries. On enhanced scan, tumors are often significantly enhanced. Calcification, hemorrhage, and necrosis can occur in some tumors.

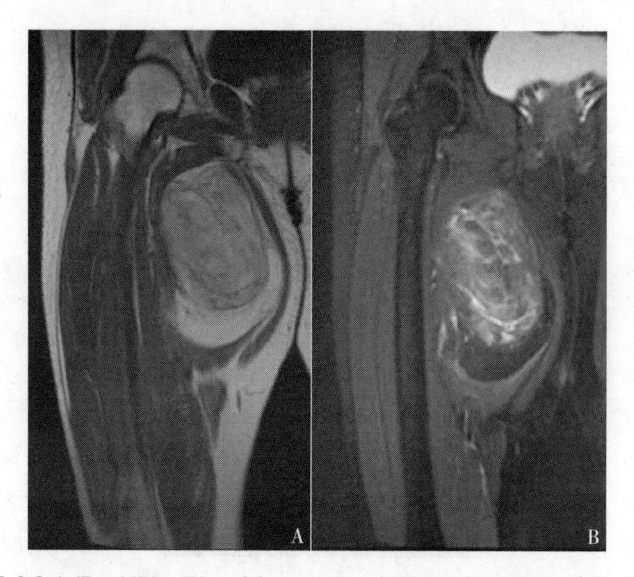

Fig 9-3-8-A/B MRI: T1-and fat-suppressed T2-weighted images of well-differentiated liposarcoma in leg: a fat-containing heterogeneous high signal on T1WI; the fat shows low signal on fat-suppression T2WI.

[**Diagnosis**]

Imaging diagnosis of liposarcoma mainly relies on CT and MRI. Although they are able to find the lesion correctly, qualitative diagnosis is difficult, therefore pathology is a necessity.